D1265880

Color Atlas of

PEDIATRIC NEUROLOGY

Edited by

Richard W Newton

[handwritten inscription]

Ⓜ Mosby-Wolfe

Copyright © 1995 Times Mirror International Publishers Limited
Published in 1995 by Mosby–Wolfe Publishing, an imprint of Times Mirror International Publishers Limited
Printed by Grafos S. A. Arte sobre papel, Barcelona, Spain.
ISBN 0 7234 18799

For full details of all Times Mirror International Publishers Limited titles please write to Times Mirror International Publishers, Lynton House, 7–12 Tavistock Square, London, WC1H 9LB.

A CIP catalogue record for this book is available from the British Library.

Library of Congress Cataloging-in-Publication Data has been applied for.

Contents

Preface

Neurology seemed so daunting as a medical student. The clinical examination itself was so drawn out with its long sequence of points to pursue and interpretation seemingly so difficult. The result is that fear of the subject is still retained by many junior and senior doctors, and that the somewhat indeterminate phrase CNS (tick) is still found with undue frequency in case notes.

Neil Gordon established here in Manchester one of the best staffed departments of paediatric neurology in Britain. The clinical method he taught was one of standing back and looking at patterns of movement so that the diagnosis of mild hemiparesis or limb girdle syndrome of moderate severity was made as the child walked across the room, rather than struggling over whether a particular plantar was deciding to go up or down. With practice, spotting the patterns becomes more easy and the section on clinical examination should help medical practitioners through their sequence of play with children to extract the maximum information possible. Pointers are placed in the text to indicate where short cuts may be taken without losing key data.

The conditions we manage are often long term and carry no fundamental cure. Nevertheless much can be done to help families accommodate and adjust to their new circumstances and the chapter on talking to parents we hope will allow doctors more confidence in the way they deliver information. In order to do this effectively it is essential that doctors examine and overcome their own fear of handicap so that they might talk freely and with confidence, striking a note of optimism with reality rather than negative foreboding. Importance is placed on the choice of words and the differences between impairment, disability and handicap explained.

Each day scientists are bringing us nearer to a fundamental understanding of the conditions we deal with. The mapping of the human genome, the delineation of the gene product, and the understanding of function of biochemicals within cells is a rapidly expanding field. Each year we are able to give parents explanations unavailable in the previous year, and slowly the advances are leading to therapy in many conditions. This has led to major contributions to this text being made by colleagues in inherited and metabolic disease, clinical genetics and, of course, neuroradiology.

We hope this book will be useful as a source of quick and ready reference to help guide general paediatricians and radiologists in their everyday work. It should also be of value as an introduction to our subject for medical students, post-graduates reading for the post-graduate diplomas and for remedial therapists at both undergraduate and post-graduate level.

Above all, we hope the text will convey a clarity that will remove some of the daunting images that have been associated with the subject up to now and induce an appetite for further research and reading.

Richard W. Newton

Acknowledgements

In a book with such a large number of illustrations we have been dependent on a number of people to whom we are indebted. Dr. Anna Kelsey, Consultant Paediatric Pathologist at Royal Manchester and Booth Hall Children's Hospital, and Dr. Tony Barson, Consultant in Perinatal and Paediatric Pathology at St. Mary's Hospital, Manchester, made a major contribution to the book in providing the slides on histology and pathology. Dr. Raafat of Birmingham Children's Hospital must also be thanked.

From the Children's Hospitals, Manchester, Dr. Brennan Wilson, Dr. Ed Ladusans, Dr. Mike Robinson, Mr. Richard Cowie, and Mr. David Gough must all be thanked for their respective help with the radiology, cardiology, neonatalogy, neurosurgery and urology sections. Dr. Tito Testa, Department of Nuclear Medicine, Manchester Royal Infirmary, supplied the SPECT scans. Dr. Jane Fennell provided the chromosome photograph. Professor Sir David Hull, Queen's Medical Centre, Nottingham, and Dr. Andy Spencer, Senior Lecturer in Paediatrics, Keele University, helped us with the picture on Behçet's disease.

Needless to say, there are many others at our Regional Centre who helped by agreeing to be photographed in the course of their work, and we are continually indebted to the children we help to treat and to their families for the inconveniences they allow us to put them through from time to time in the pursuit of postgraduate education.

We are particularly indebted to Mrs. Margaret Cunnah, Mrs. Sandra Fowley and Miss Corrine Fishwick for their painstaking work with the manuscript and illustrations and to Ms Maire Collins, Rachael Miller and Jane Hurd–Cosgrave for their help with its production.

Finally I must express many appreciative thanks to John Bateman and Chris Brown of the Department of Medical Illustration, Royal Manchester Children's Hospital, for their tireless effort in helping us to assemble the illustrations. Without their contribution the book would not have been possible.

List of Contributors

Dr Richard W. Newton, MD, DCH, FRCP
Consultant Paediatric Neurologist
Royal Manchester & Booth Hall Children's Hospital

Dr W. St. Clair Forbes, MA, MB, BCh, DMRD, FRCR
Consultant Neuroradiologist, Salford Royal Hospitals NHS Trust
Lecturer (Part-time) Department of Diagnostic Radiology, University of Manchester

Dr Michael A. Clarke, BSc, DCH, FRCP
Consultant Paediatric Neurologist
Royal Manchester & Booth Hall Children's Hospital

Mr J. R. S. Leggate, BSc (Hons), FRCR
Consultant Paediatric Neurosurgeon
Booth Hall Children's Hospital

Dr Michael J. Noronha, FRCP (London and Edinburgh), MRCPI
Consultant Paediatric Neurologist
Royal Manchester & Booth Hall Children's Hospital

Dr Maurice Super, MD, MSc, FRCP (London and Edinburgh), DCH
Consultant Paediatric Geneticist/Postgraduate Tutor
Royal Manchester Children's Hospital

Dr Pamela I. Tomlin, MA, DCH, FRCP
Consultant Paediatric Neurologist
Royal Preston Hospital

Dr Ed Wraith, FRCP
Director of Willink Biochemical Genetics Unit
Royal Manchester Children's Hospital

Dedication

To Neil Gordon, the father of paediatric neurology in Britain and founder of our Regional Centre, and to our wives and families, for tolerating our continuing contribution to the subject and even more hours at this project.

Judith,
Sarah, Michael and Jennifer

Henry,
Paul and Matthew

Sarah,
Alexander, Jeremy, Georgina and Sophie

Jane,
Gemma, Katie and Anna

Chapter 1: Talking with Families

Richard W. Newton

Attitudes to disability—the effect on clinical practice

There can be no moment more important in the lives of young adults than when they learn that their child has a chronic disabling condition. The news often leaves parents stunned and disbelieving. The words used—epilepsy, mental handicap, cerebral palsy, Down's syndrome—will often be recognised by parents, but they only very rarely have good insight and understanding. It is far more likely that parents will associate these words with negative aspects of life and the overall reaction will be one of disheartenment, despair, disbelief and avoidance.

As the impact of the news is so great, much thought needs to be given to the way information is imparted. Too often it is the lot of relatively junior doctors who, because they know no better, will sidle up to an unaccompanied mother on a children's or lying-in ward, give the news, and then depart, leaving the mother bewildered and unsupported.

Parents will remember those moments for the rest of their lives and, if the situation is not handled well, they may retain resentment for the attending team, creating difficulties later. An impaired relationship of this sort can compromise the help a multidisciplinary team (*see* Chapter 3) has the potential to offer.

There are few doctors who relish the prospect of sitting down with parents to give them news of handicapping or malignant conditions which necessarily affect the quality or length of life. As doctors, we may well think that it would be intolerable to have to face chronic handicap in one's own child. It is only through analysis of one's own fears that such consultations can be approached with ease. This point is reached not only through the process of personal maturity but also through knowledge accumulated with seniority. For these reasons, such consultations are probably best handled by the more senior doctors on the team.

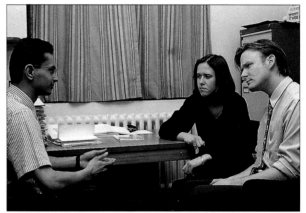

1.1 Undergraduates learning to counsel through role play.

Some medical practitioners may go through their career without ever having addressed this issue; as a consequence initially held prejudices are sustained, and the quality of practice suffers. Research shows that children with Down's syndrome, for example, are less likely than other children to be greeted with the question, "Are you well?" The underlying notion is that health cannot be attributed to a handicapped person. Other studies showed that a child with Down's syndrome and heart disease is less likely to have corrective operative surgery than a child with a urogenital abnormality and the same cardiac lesion. It would seem that preconceived views on handicap do alter management decisions in clinical practice. Greater education of the public (of whom medical practitioners form a small part) on handicapping conditions such as epilepsy and cerebral palsy will serve to alter that prejudgment. Additionally, undergraduate medical curricula should now serve to teach medical students how to conduct consultations where information of a sensitive nature is given to families (**1.1**). Both these influences are likely to help the next generation of doctors in their clinical practice.

Language to use, language to avoid

In their heightened state of anxiety, parents will be influenced by every single word the attendant doctor says. The words will carry great importance and due consideration should be made to the language used at each consultation.

Being too negative

If a doctor with a very glum face and a shake of the head says, "I am very sorry, but I have some very bad news for you. Your child has cerebral palsy", the parents are likely to get a rather different view of cerebral palsy than from that given by a doctor with a relaxed, smiling face saying, "I have some news you were not expecting. Your child has cerebral palsy. This may be something you have heard of but know little about. I shall do the best I can to explain something about it to you." The second approach does not trivialise the serious nature of the task in hand, but it does avoid a negative image of handicap being projected to the parents (*see* **1.2**, below).

Being too positive

There is always pressure on doctors to do something rather than nothing. Traditionally, doctors have always seen themselves in the domain of a healing art where the expectation is to deliver treatment that leads to a cure.

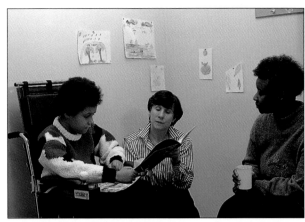

1.3 Family care officer: Neuromuscular Clinic. Families need an advocate.

With neurological conditions, that avenue is rarely open, but paediatricians have a central role in delivering information. This allows children and families a good adjustment to the disability, which in turn allows children to reach their potential and to grow up as confident and as independent as possible.

When a doctor arranges the involvement of physio-, occupational and speech therapy colleagues, it is very easy to present an image to families that this therapy is 'healing' in the traditional way. The reality is that the therapist will suggest to the parents the things that might be incorporated in play which will allow the child the sort of opportunity and encouragement they need to develop to his or her full potential. Advice will be given on positioning and seating and the sort of toys that will encourage the next step in development. Research has shown that outcome is not related so much to the method of therapy used but rather to the extent of the underlying handicap. Therapy may accelerate the acquisition of short-term goals but does not overcome the longer-term compounding effect of the handicap. If the value of therapy is presented in too positive a light, parents may misunderstand and think that 10 hour's physiotherapy a day may be 10 times better than (or at least twice as good as), one hour's physiotherapy a day. Alternatively, they may be led to think that the therapy available in the United States or Hungary is better than the therapy that might be offered by the local preschool support team. Misapprehensions of this sort can lead to emotional and financial strain within a family, and attending paediatricians should strive to establish good understanding very early in this respect.

Advocacy

It should be remembered that whenever a teacher talks to a pupil, the pupil is likely to remember only a third of

---

REMEMBER

• Children are children first, handicapped second.

• AVOID SAYING "epileptic", "Down's syndrome child" or "cerebral palsied child".

• **Do not use phrases which are hurtful to parents.**

• DO SAY "a child with epilepsy/Down's syndrome/cerebral palsy".

1.2 Key points to remember about language to use when discussing children's handicaps with their parents.

what is said, and to misunderstand half of that. So it is when doctors talk to parents. It can be helpful for parents to be accompanied by a representative they know, who preferably has some medical knowledge or previous experience of handicap (**1.3**). A health visitor, social worker, ward nurse, or an advocate from the local preschool support multidisciplinary team could all help in this respect.

Interview technique and timing

Once thoughts on diagnosis are clear, a consultation should be arranged with the parents as soon as possible (**1.4**). The interview should be contrived so that both parents are in attendance. It is usually better to delay this a little so that both parents can be present rather than to be pressurised into seeing one parent alone. For single women, a close relative or friend might be asked to attend where the father cannot.

It is most helpful for the doctor to have the experi-ence and information to hand to answer the questions likely to be asked by the parents. Ideally, the doctor should be familiar to the parents, should greet them cheerfully, and should shake hands with them when they enter the room. The small group should sit in a circle rather than being given the news over a desk top (**1.5**).

If words such as 'cerebral palsy' are used, it is predictable that parents in their stunned state will take in little more after that point. It is most helpful to reconvene the meeting within 24 hours or so, so that further detail can be given. The facts should be given in a simple, truthful and straightforward way (**1.6**). Written advice should complement what is said in the clinic. The parents will often then need a period of a few days to digest what is said and then to return with further, more detailed questions.

It is most helpful if the child is present at the consultation (particularly if a small baby, **1.7**) to show the child is valued as a person regardless of the handicap. The presence of an older child avoids secretive collusion between parents and doctors. If a more open, honest

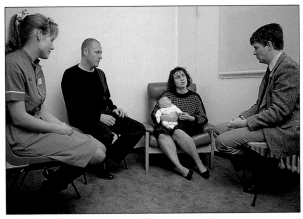

1.4 See both parents together.

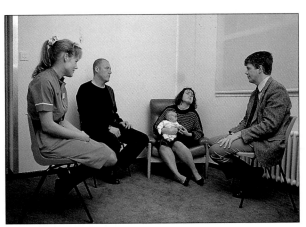

1.5 Make contact informal. Sit in a circle at the same level.

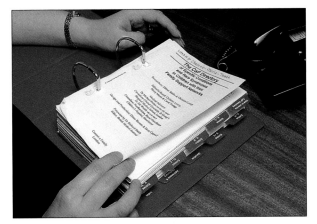

1.6 Contact a Family: information and parents' support groups.

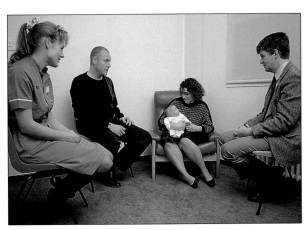

1.7 Have the baby present when the news is given to show that he or she is valued.

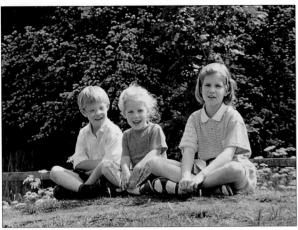

1.8 Involve siblings; address their fears.

After some time their feelings resolve, and 95 % of handicapped babies will go home with their natural parents. Many fathers may harbour thoughts of harming a young handicapped baby which they perceive as being a threat to family happiness; these thoughts are less common amongst women. These thoughts themselves may lead to distress and it is often helpful to talk about that issue at an early stage. Subsequently, parents may find it helpful to be introduced to parent support groups. These act as a useful source of information on the condition involved and are often able to introduce parents to other families who face similar difficulties.

It is most helpful if attending doctors maintain a position of disinterested concern so that if families do take themselves off to see specialists in alternative medicine or visit centres abroad, they know that they will always be welcome back to their local services if their experimentation fails. All too often, professional aloofness is presented as an alternative to the long-term tolerance and understanding that families actually need.

Special circumstances

Two circumstances deserve special consideration: the dying child, and dealing with families following the death of a child. Where a child has a neurodegenerative condition (considered in detail in Chapter 14) parents will find themselves feeling a sense of loss and bereavement not only when death actually occurs but also in the period following the giving of the news. Parents' feelings should be addressed in consultations as an issue separate from the day-to-day management problems of the child. Their wishes should always be respected, particularly when difficult management decisions are addressed: such as, deciding whether to proceed with tube feeding or gastrostomy in a child with metachromatic leukodystrophy in a vegetative state who continues to deteriorate. The needs of the child —as most likely judged by the child—should always be paramount, but due sensitivity should always be paid to the parents' wishes and of course the law.

When a child dies, from any cause, parents often welcome contact with the paediatric team following the death. The contact may be with the paediatrician or attached social worker; the contact may be brief, ensuring that support is adequate and that mourning is following a normal course. Contact is likely to last longer when involvement with the medical team was of long duration or intensive. A follow-up interview provides an opportunity for the doctor to become involved in the bereavement counselling process, to improve on explanation and to dispense with misapprehension. The structure of the interview would do well to encompass aspects outlined in **Table 1.1**, and should be within the scope of all paediatric departments.

relationship follows between child, parents and doctor, adverse psychological consquences can be minimised (**1.8**).

It is known that most parents, on receiving the news that they have a handicapped child, go through a bereavement reaction. In its initial phase, there will be feelings of disbelief and anger, followed by a period of acceptance with slow resolution and adjustment to the problem. It is helpful for the doctor to talk to the parents about the way they will receive the news (**1.9**). Mothers and fathers often react differently and work through their grief at different rates. This may be a source of marital disharmony which may be avoided if parents receive appropriate help at an early stage.

Some professionals talk of parents rejecting the child with handicap but, in reality, in the throes of their grief parents may just feel unable to accept the child and the notion of handicap at that stage (**1.10 and 1.11**).

REMEMBER
Parents want news on diagnosis:

- Together
- As soon as possible
- Sympathetically and in private
- With accuracy.

They also want:
- To be helped to pass on news to family and friends
- To have the baby present.

1.9 Informing families—important points.

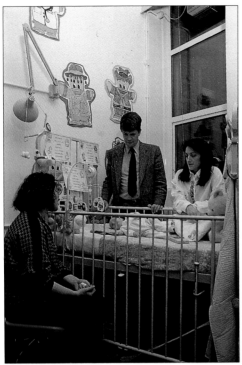

1.10 DO NOT talk across the bed and down to parents.

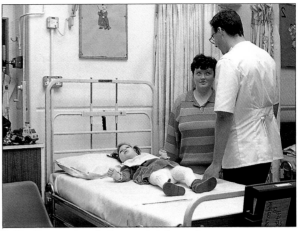

1.11 Ensure the whole team is informed.

TABLE 1.1 Suggested Format for Structured Interviews with Parents Following a Child's Death

(i) Discuss the postmortem examination.

(ii) Re-explain the course of the illness in the light of the postmortem findings.

(iii) Dispense with misconceptions about the illness, death or care.

(iv) Alleviate guilt.

(v) Give counselling on bereavement behaviour of parents and siblings.

(vi) Offer advice on management of existing children.

(vii) Give genetic counselling for family.

(viii) Give an update on transplant recipient, if relevant.

(ix) Accept thanks, donations and offers to help with research.

Chapter 2: Clinical Examination

Pamela I. Tomlin

The clinic visit

A clinic visit should be an enjoyable and relaxing experience for a child. Children should be greeted, made to feel welcome and given an explanation of why they are there and what is to happen. Children will reveal more diagnostic clues if they are not always under observation and if history-taking is done in an atmosphere that encourages confidence. Observation of the young child's play, pattern of movement and behaviour often reveals more than a formal neurological examination (**2.1**). The clinic room should be set out with enough space between the parents and doctor for the child to play, preferably on the floor. A variety of toys should be available. Form boards, paper, pencils and books, coloured bead-threading bricks of different shapes all offer an opportunity for assessment of skill and knowledge. Children usually lose their anxiety as the parents and doctor engage in the dialogue of history-taking, and can then be included. Important history points should be detailed by the child,

and being included in this way prevents even young children feeling confronted when the examination beings.

At the beginning of the examination, it is better to join the young child in play. Then the doctor can encourage the child to adapt to the doctor's activities such as brick-building, showing attention and understanding, giving the correct item from a form board, or threading beads. Manipulation can be observed at this point.

Higher functions

For school children, pencil and paper allow some higher functions to be assessed as the child begins with something well within his ability such as writing his name. Appropriately graded sentences are next offered for writing to dictation. If the child struggles unduly, the effort should be curtailed and the child asked to copy a sentence and then to read it. Some children with language problems can copy but not read back and they find it impossible to write to dictation (**2.2 and 2.3**). Copying

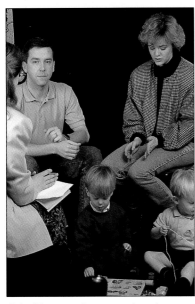

2.1 History-taking—a relaxed atmosphere with the child observed at play.

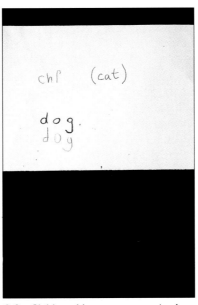

2.2 Child unable to sequence 'cat' to dictation but copies 'dog' easily.

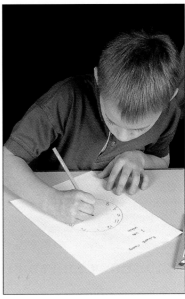

2.3 Writing to dictation, pencil control and spatial organisation.

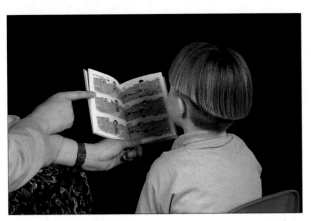

2.4 Clear pictures that show activity encourage the child to talk.

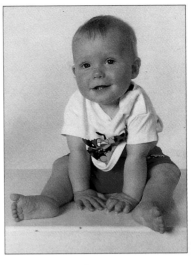

2.5 The bottom shuffler.

simple shapes will test visuo-perceptual function. For children over eight years old putting numbers round a clock face (often difficult for the child with visuo-spatial problems) will reveal how well organised they are. Simple number concept can be tested by saying, "give me ..... (a number) ..... of bricks" (O'Hare *et al.*, 1991). The child can use the bricks to do simple sums and the understanding of arithmetic signs can be checked on paper. Although the doctor will not be an expert in educational problems, obvious difficulties may be observed that have previously been unaddressed. These may have a bearing on the presenting problem, such as behavioural difficulties, headaches or school refusal.

An attempt to assess speech and language should follow. Framing a question which can receive only a "yes/no" reply is not very enlightening, and the direct attention of the examiner may be intimidating to the child. A book of illustrations is more valuable than text (**2.4**). Books with life-like pictures are best; cartoons are to be avoided. Books which illustrate a variety of everyday experience, with sequenced frames that tell a story (such as the Ladybird Talk-About series) are most useful. An eighteen month old may point to specific pictures rather than name them. An older child can begin to talk about the picture. The question, "What is that boy doing in the picture?" or, "What is happening?" will demand more than a one word answer. The doctor can listen for pronunciation, note if the child gets the correct inference and spot faltering telegraphic replies. Expertise in speech pathology is not expected of the doctor, but a child who is obviously struggling and who needs appropriate referral will soon be recognised.

Patterns of movement

Patterns of movement are most informative in neurological examination. In infants or toddlers, observation of movement can often reveal more than an attempt at a more formal examination. The doctor should sit back and watch. Well-motivated movement of any kind is often reassuring regarding higher functions. Bottom shuffling is the commonest pattern of dissociated motor development (Robson, 1970) (**2.5**). When lifted up, the bottom shuffler maintains hip flexion; this pattern of flexion is still detectable with eversion of the feet as the child learns to stand, but it is self-correcting with time. Other patterns of abdominal crawling with symmetrical upper and lower limb movements can be a variant of normal. Commando crawling in the child with spastic diplegia is different. The legs remain extended at the hips and propulsion depends mainly on the upper limbs. The infant who swims erratically on the tummy, revolving in circles without achieving any particular goal and not showing frustration is a source for concern. Such mildly 'dystonic' patterns of movement may be seen in children who gain independent mobility late, at a time when concerns are switching to higher function. They are worthy of further assessment.

A pattern of W-sitting may be seen in children with hypotonia or spasticity (**2.6**). More formal assessment of tone and reflexes will distinguish them. Pronated and flexed posturing of a neglected upper limb may betray a hemiplegia (**2.7**) .

The neonate

Neurological well-being is best reflected by posture and tone in the neonate. Flexor tone predominates in the term infant with an alternating reciprocal pattern of movement (**2.8**). The pre-term infant initially has a predominantly extensor pattern of truncal tone (**2.9**). Axial tone is best assessed by exerting traction on extended arms with the infant in a supine position. A term infant will be capable of aligning the head with the trunk

2.6 (left) W-sitting in a child with hypotonia.

2.7 (right) Flexed and fisted posturing of the right arm in spastic hemiplegia.

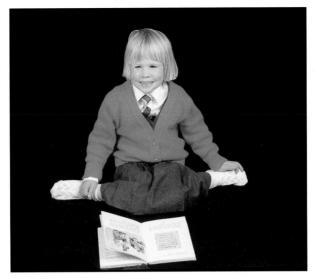

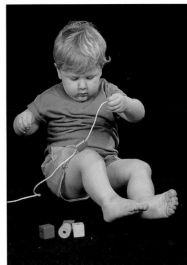

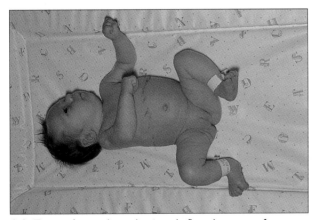

2.8 Term infant with predominantly flexed pattern of tone.

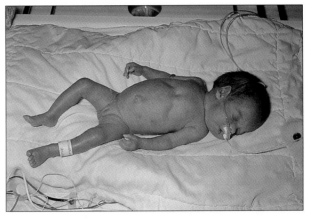

2.9 Pre-term infant predominantly extended.

momentarily (**2.10**). Hypotonia due to a neuromuscular disorder usually affects trunk and limbs; in CNS hypotonia only the axial tone is reduced, leading to head lag on arm traction (**2.11 and 2.12**). In evolving pyramidal disorders, the baby may exhibit an increase in extensor tone when suspended prone (**2.13–2.15**).

Newborn infants will be still and be alert to visual stimuli. Changes in the babies' posture and state (whether they are placid, crying, still or moving) need conscious attention. When lacking, or when random eye movements are seen, attention should be given to the baby's neurological progress by investigation and appropriate follow-up.

Attention should be paid to the persistence or asymmetry of primitive reflexes. This assessment complements the examination of posture, tone and degree of alertness. Eye movements, ophthalmoscopy, and pupillary reaction after 30 weeks' gestation may reveal ocular abnormalities such as choroidoretinitis, cataract, optic nerve hypoplasia, III nerve palsy or Horner's syndrome. Observation will reveal ptosis or facial weakness. A full fontanelle may reflect raised intracranial pressure as may an upward-gaze paresis associated with the setting-sun sign. Conscious level (*see* Chapter 7) and asymmetries in tone or reflexes should be assessed as they would be in an older child.

More formal examination

Depending on the child's maturity, a full cooperative neurological examination can be achieved from the age of three years onwards. The doctor should try in every case, even when the child is initially reluctant, for once the child begins to cooperate, much can be achieved with encouragement. Failure to achieve cooperation may indicate something regarding the child's limitations

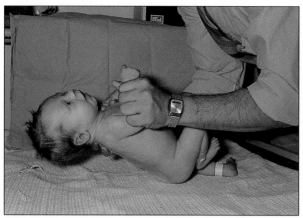

2.10 Normal term infant, arm traction supine.

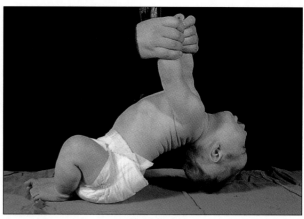

2.11 Arm traction in hypotonia. Central cause. Poor axial but good limb tone.

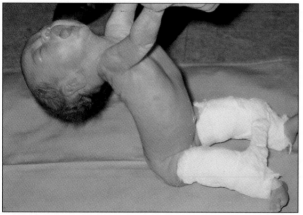

2.12 Arm traction in hypotonia. Neuromuscular. Poor axial and limb tones.

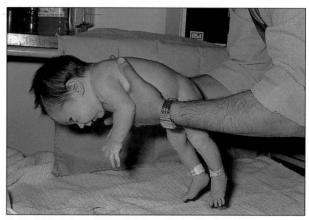

2.13 Normal term infant, prone suspension.

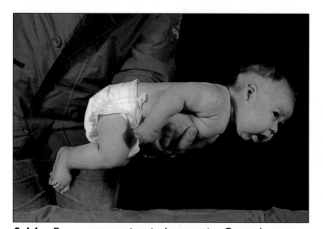

2.14 Prone suspension in hypotonia. Central cause— revealed increased axial tone.

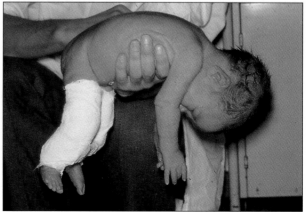

2.15 Prone suspension in hypotonia. Neuromuscular— slumping over hand.

which need further examination in a child-assessment setting.

The examination should include an assessment of the cranial nerves, the balance and coordination of the trunk, upper and lower limbs; additional systems examination such as sensory testing should be included if it is perti-nent to the presenting complaint. Head circumference, growth and blood pressure should be measured in every case. The patient should always be undressed at some stage and examined for neurocutaneous features and muscle wasting. The order of the examination is not important but undressing is best left to the end. The child

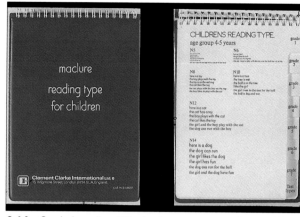

2.16 Graded reading difficulty for assessment of near vision: Maclure Reading Type.

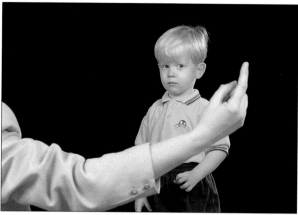

2.17 Binocular assessment of fields in a 3-year-old. The child cannot resist eye-pointing as soon as the finger moves.

will be more cooperative for the earlier examination if he feels dignified, and with that extra confidence will comply with undressing more willingly.

Vision testing—oculomotor muscles

Vision testing can be assessed according to age and reading ability on the Maclure Reading Type (**2.16**). Stycar charts can be used for the pre-reading age group. External ocular movements should be examined for their range and conjugate nature in horizontal and vertical directions. A bright-coloured pin or object should hold the child's attention.

Babies prefer to follow a face. The examiner should allow enough time to detect nystagmus and avoid extremes of gaze for this purpose. Ptosis is usually obvious on upward gaze with the eyelid partially covering the pupil and overactivity of the frontalis muscle. Squints may be revealed on fixation or, if hidden, by intermittent monocular occlusion. The convergence response reassures that both eyes have useful vision. The eye which will not converge may be amblyopic.

Peripheral fields are best assessed by direct confrontation; examiner and child have both eyes open and the child is instructed to look at the examiner's nose (**2.17**). Whilst engaging the child's eye-contact in this

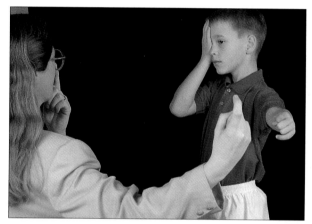

2.18 Monocular assessment of fields in an older child. The child points or calls out as soon as the finger moves.

way, the examiner asks the child to point to whichever finger is moving as they are held at the periphery of the examiner's own visual field. There are very few nasal field defects without a temporal field defect, and screening in this way is quick, effective and objective.

If a defect is revealed, both eyes may then be tested separately (**2.18**). A white pin will assess peripheral fields and a red pin central fields. If the complaint involves vision, then ascertaining that the object is perceived throughout the field from temporal to nasal sides will ensure that no scotoma exists apart from the blind spot. If a field defect is suspected, formal perimetry should follow (*see* **Practice Point 2.1**).

The eye should be examined with a bright pencil torch to look for corneal and iris abnormalities, such as Kayser–Fleischer rings, Brushfield spots and Lisch nodules. These features may sometimes be seen only through slit-lamp examination. The pupil responses are observed for direct and consensual responses. To exam-

PRACTICE POINT 2.1

There are very few nasal visual field constrictions without a temporal field constriction.

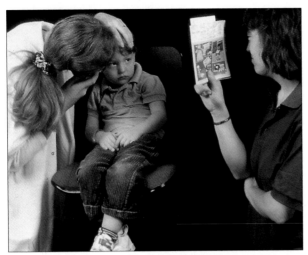

2.19 Cranial nerve sequence: fundoscopy, with nurse distracting the child.

ine the fundi, a nurse or parent should continually attract the child's attention towards a distant object (**2.19**). This is best done before dimming the room, which is not always necessary and sometimes alarms a young child.

In infants, the carer should be discouraged from holding the head, which usually causes the infant to cry. Patience is required to catch the salient features of the retina in infants and allowing them to suckle can be very helpful. If evidence of a retinopathy or retinal scarring is important, then a special attempt at examination with a short-acting mydriatic is essential. An ophthalmologist's opinion, with examination under anaesthetic if necessary, is important whenever visual acuity is questioned (**2.20 and 2.21**).

Further cranial nerve sequence

Facial muscles are assessed by tight voluntary eye closure and asking the child to show the teeth (**2.22 and 2.23**). The child may puff out the cheeks without escape of air from the lips. Some children with dyspraxia find it hard to put on a smile or grimace, and the examiner must be opportune in observing changing facial expressions. If there is a facial weakness of lower motor neurone type, involving the upper and lower face, then the eardrums must be inspected and tests for conductive deafness applied with a tuning fork. The corneal reflex is the most sensitive test of Vth nerve function. A wisp of cotton wool is sufficient, applied lightly to the corneum whilst the face is averted to the opposite side. Light touch and pain perception should be checked in all divisions of the Vth nerve, comparing sensation on both sides of the forehead, cheeks and below the angle of the mouth. An unbent paper clip is to be preferred as it is readily perceived as scratching and is less threatening (needles must never be used) (**2.24 and 2.25**). When

there is Vth nerve involvement a child may be old enough to express an awareness of a difference in sensation as the face is washed and dried. Not infrequently, children describe motor differences as the way the face 'feels' (**Practice Point 2.2**).

PRACTICE POINT 2.2

Sensory V will rarely be abnormal without other signs—the corneal reflex is distressing for children.

Hearing

Hearing cannot be adequately tested in an ordinary outpatient setting, but in school children, tuning-fork tests alongside inspection of the drums is informative. If hearing loss is suspected, formal audiological assessment should be arranged.

Palate and tongue

The anatomy and function of the palate and tongue should be inspected (**2.26 and 2.27**). Palatal movements will always accompany the gag reflex but the child may be alienated by this unpleasant sensation (*see* **Practice Point 2.3**). Some children are shy of saying "ahh" and palatal movements can be seen by asking the child to draw a deep breath and hold it. Nasal escape can be detected by asking the child to say palatal sounds like "cake". If there is a complaint regarding feeding, chewing or swallowing, then a demonstration of the problem with fluids or solids offered in the clinic room will supply a speedy and effective understanding of the problem to the doctor.

The upper limbs

Forward outstretched limbs are inspected for posturing and irregular movements. Erratic small movements may reflect chorea, sub-clinical seizure activity or underlying clumsiness. A tendency to flex at the elbow and wrist on

PRACTICE POINT 2.3

Rather than distress with the gag reflex in a conscious child, ask about chewing and swallowing.

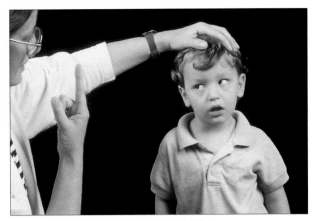

2.20 Cranial nerve sequence: visual following.

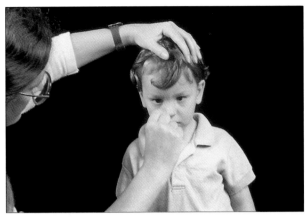

2.21 Cranial nerve sequence: convergence response.

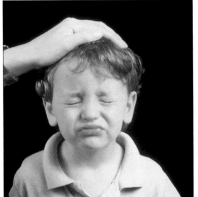

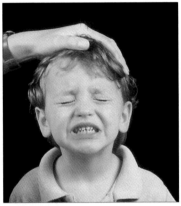

2.22 and 2.23 Cranial nerve sequence: facial expression.

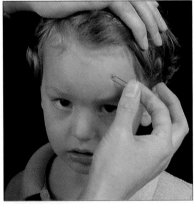

2.24 Cranial nerve sequence: sensory testing.

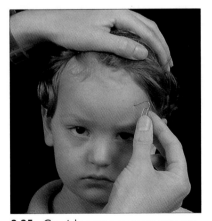

2.25 Cranial nerve sequence: sensory testing.

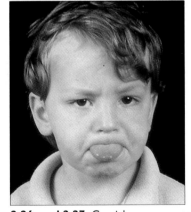

2.26 and 2.27 Cranial nerve sequence: tongue protrusion.

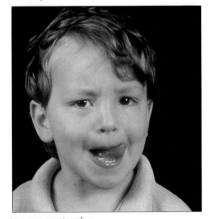

one side points to a hemisyndrome on that side. Turning the palms upwards will reveal limited supination on the spastic side.

Power is best tested symmetrically, particularly to aid the performance and understanding of the young child. Orderly assessment in passing from proximal to distal muscle groups will highlight the need for more thorough testing if weakness is found. Children may be shy of active movement against the examiner but will maintain postures that the examiner tries to overcome, e.g. holding arms laterally outstretched for deltoid power, pushing against the wall for scapula fixation, keeping arms straight or bent to the chest for triceps/biceps function, and maintaining flexion or extension of the wrist and fingers (including spreading and adduction for small muscles of the hand (**2.28–2.31**). These postures hold the

21

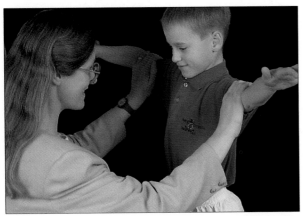

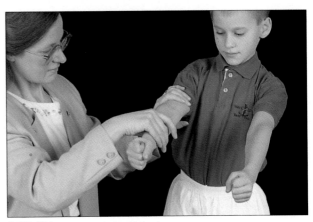

2.28–2.31 Sequence of testing for power proximally to distally. Symmetrical maintenance of posture, or symmetrical effort in the young child gains maximum power.
2.28 Deltoids.

2.29 Triceps.

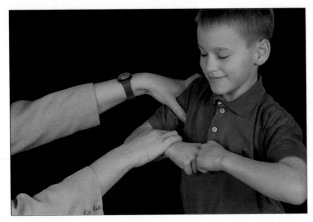

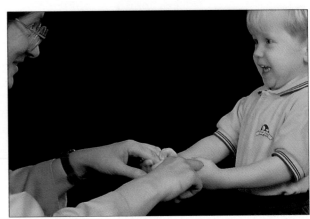

2.30 Biceps.

2.31 Small muscles of the hand.

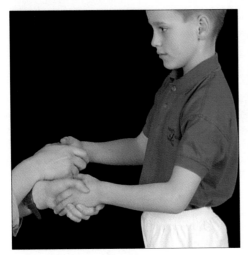

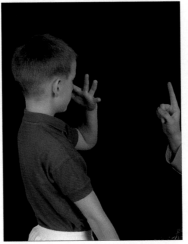

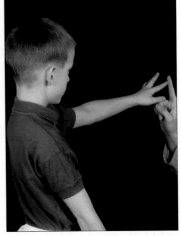

2.32 Testing for tone in the upper limbs, alternating supination and pronation.

2.33 and 2.34 Finger–nose testing, the child fully stretching the upper limb and using the pad of his forefinger involving supination and pronation of the forearm.

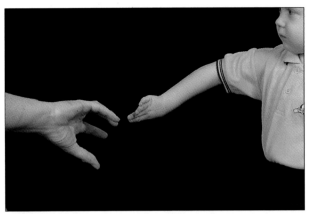 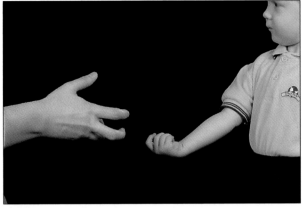

2.35 and 2.36 A 3-year-old's awkward effort at alternating movements.

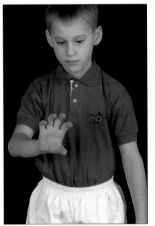 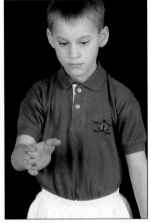 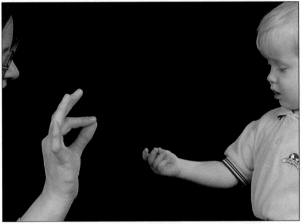

2.37 and 2.38 The 9-year-old's more fluent alternating movement, with no discernible alteration in elbow position with respect to the trunk.

2.39 A 3-year-old achieving finger sequencing which may escape a clumsy older child.

additional advantage of giving the child a mechanical advantage, thus facilitating the discovery of subtle muscle weakness.

The relaxation required for assessment of tone is best achieved directly after testing for power (**2.32**). The movements should be kept simple and always compared immediately with the opposite side. Flexion and extension at the elbow may be confusing as the child tries to join in. Supination and pronation of the forearm make it less easy for the child to superimpose voluntary activity. A pronator catch may be seen and felt as a biphasic movement. In the infant, the upper limbs can also be assessed by holding both hands and gently waggling the limb from the shoulder.

There are a variety of coordination tests, and doctors are well advised to stick to those with which they have become familiar. The dominant hand must be ascertained first, as there will be a natural asymmetry related to that. In the finger–nose test, the child must use the pad of the forefinger to elicit full pronation and extension of the upper limb in reaching out (**2.33 and 2.34**).

If the child is not made to stretch out in this test, an ataxia may be missed as the upper limb is held adducted to the trunk for stability. Pre-school children may not be able to cope with the complexity of instructions for the test, and it is better to break the test down into more simple steps: the child's own nose can be touched several times, followed by the examiner's finger. Alternating movements are demonstrated, beginning with the dominant limb. Active supination/pronation should be attempted with the elbow held as still as possible but away from the trunk (**2.35 and 2.36**). Three- to four-year-old children normally show coarse movement, finding it impossible to keep the elbow still; by seven to nine years of age, they should be rapidly fluent with the elbow held still, but the range of ability is enormous (**2.37 and 2.38**).

Testing finger-and-thumb sequencing movements can be very informative. Most four-year-olds can manage at least the first two fingers in sequence (**2.39**). This test often reveals children who are clumsy due to dyspraxia. They can see what is required but obviously

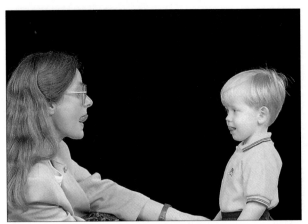

2.40 A 3-year-old pointing to the tongue well to touch the upper lip.

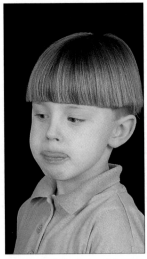

2.41 A 6.5-year-old with dyspraxia unable to achieve the same effect.

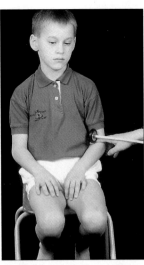

2.42 Upper limb reflexes obtained conventionally in an older child.

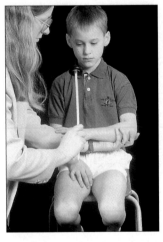

2.43 Supporting the upper limb enhances relaxation in a tense child.

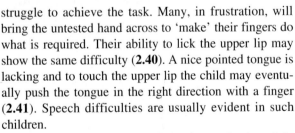

2.44 Gentle but fairly brisk abduction of the hips to assess tone.

struggle to achieve the task. Many, in frustration, will bring the untested hand across to 'make' their fingers do what is required. Their ability to lick the upper lip may show the same difficulty (**2.40**). A nice pointed tongue is lacking and to touch the upper lip the child may eventually push the tongue in the right direction with a finger (**2.41**). Speech difficulties are usually evident in such children.

Reflexes are rarely as informative as in the adult, unless absent or grossly exaggerated (**2.42 and 2.43**). Small children and toddlers may show fear at the sight of a tendon hammer. A flexion reflex at the elbow may be better obtained in them by percussing directly over the brachioradialis at the elbow, and can be achieved in fearful children with percussion by the examiner's fingers.

The lower limbs

Tone is best assessed at the hips and ankles where it is more easy to overcome the child's tendency to join in. Joints should be examined for contractures. Palpation of

the hamstrings on straightening the leg will reveal tight tendons when there is a contracture at the knee. Repeated gentle but fairly brisk abduction of the hips may reveal spasticity if resistance is felt, or hypotonicity if there is obvious looseness (**2.44**). Infants should be observed for active movement at the hip which in neuromuscular weakness is often notably lacking. Alternating patterns of limb movements are the norm from birth up to about five months. Sustained symmetrical extension before this age usually points to underlying spasticity. The range of movement at the ankles should be assessed with the knee flexed and extended, so as not to overlook the contribution of gastrocnemius and hamstrings to any contracture (**2.45 and 2.46**). The foot should dorsiflex beyond 90 degrees. Brisk repeated dorsiflexion of the foot may elicit clonus, which is pathological only if sustained.

To elicit the knee jerk, relaxation is best gauged by supporting the child's foot on the examiner's knee and moving the foot gently up and down (**2.47**). This can be reinforced by asking the child to make a fist, look at it

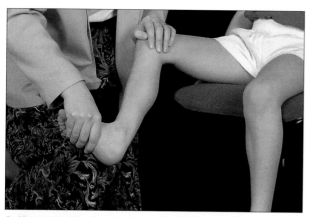

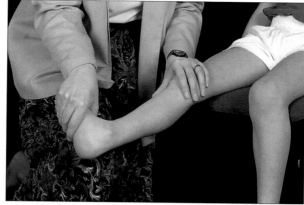

2.45 and 2.46 Assessment of range of movement at the ankle with knee first flexed, then extended.

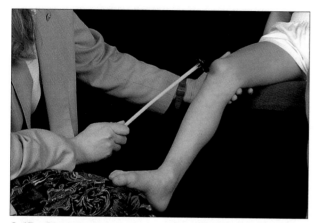

2.47 Obtaining relaxation for the knee jerk by gently supporting the child's foot.

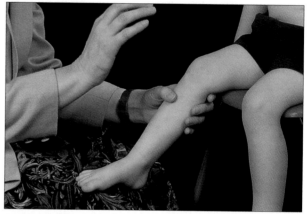

2.48 Finger percussion as an alternative to the tendon hammer in a fearful child.

and squeeze it to command. The examiner's fingers can be as effective in percussion as the tendon hammer with an apprehensive child (**2.48**).

Ankle jerks can be difficult to elicit in infants because handling their feet releases a dynamic increase in tone. Too much emphasis should not be placed on absent ankle jerks in infants. The plantar response should be explained before attempting it. Metal objects are unnecessary and provoke only a withdrawal response. The child should be asked to try to keep the toes still, dampening the tendency to withdraw. The soft pad of the examiner's finger should be used first, progressing to a nail edge if necessary (**2.49**). The stimulus is drawn up from the heel along the outer border of the foot, across and under the toes (**2.50**).

Power is best assessed by observing function. The ambulant child should be observed in getting down to the lying position on the floor and getting up again (**2.51**–**2.53**). In both manoeuvres, an obligatory four-point position after the age of three years suggests hip girdle weakness (Wallace and Newton, 1989). It can be difficult to decide whether the child requires the four-point

position for balance rather than power. If the parents try to entice the child with a toy, the examiner may then assist the child to stand by holding the hands or forearms from behind, without intimidation (**2.54 and 2.55**). It is then often possible to decide whether the child is using the examiner for balance or for pulling power.

Children rarely walk naturally when asked to. It is better to set the child a task of fetching an object, to observe a natural gait. The constancy of the child's base should be observed and the ability to turn round smoothly. Ataxic children have a varying base and often stagger on the turn. They will not manage the 'tight-rope' heel-to-toe walking enjoyed by other children. Standing on one leg and hopping should be achievable between four and five years of age, though ability varies. The child should be given a fair distance for walking in the corridor and should always be asked to run. Running often reveals the awkwardness of the clumsy child, the waddling weakness and lack of spring to the step in the child with a myopathy or the asymmetrical posturing of the child with a hemiparesis.

Fog's test elicits associated movements in the upper

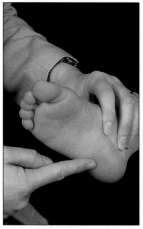

2.49 Gentle stroking of the sole with the pad of forefinger for a plantar response without withdrawal.

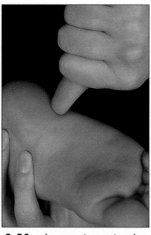

2.50 Increasing stimulus using the thumb nail.

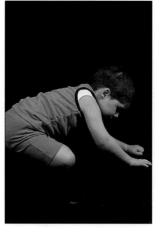

2.51 A child demonstrating an obligatory 4-point position.

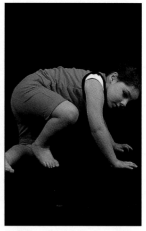

2.52 Getting up from supine —in this case due to ataxia rather than weakness.

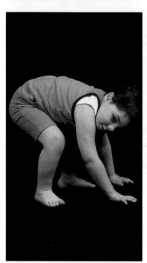

2.53 Getting up from supine due to ataxia.

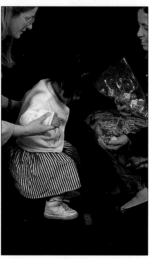

2.54 and 2.55 The mother encourages the child to stand whilst the examiner provides support.

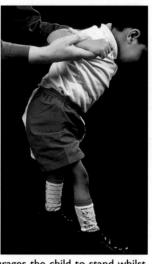

2.56 Normally pronounced and symmetrical associated upper limb postures in a 3-year-old.

limbs, when the child is asked to walk in an unusual pattern such as to heel-walk, toe-walk or walk on inverted or everted feet (**2.56 and 2.57**). In the four-year-old, the upper limbs normally mirror the pattern of movement in the lower limbs. This becomes much less marked or has disappeared entirely by nine to ten years of age (**2.58**). Asymmetries which are marked and reproducible point to a hemisyndrome on the exaggerated side. The signs should not be overread. The more demanding tasks, such as walking on the inner border of the feet, are more likely to reveal a mild, non-significant asymmetry with mildly excessive posturing in the non-dominant arm. Posturing which is bilaterally exaggerated for the child's age points to an underlying developmental dyspraxia or clumsiness which is unlikely to be pathological (*see* **2.66**, example of a quick neurological examination, p. 30).

Examination of the undressed child

This is often more acceptable to the child as one of the last things to be done. The skin can now be examined thoroughly. Depigmented patches typical of tuberous sclerosis often follow the dermatomes and are better seen under ultraviolet light in a darkened room. Achromic naevi are readily distinguished by the cutaneous vessels in their centre. In neurofibromatosis, the number of café-au-lait patches usually increases between birth and five years of age, and the axillae should be carefully examined for freckling. Parents must be examined when skin stigmata are found in the child. The spine should be inspected for mid-line sinuses or lipomas. Scoliosis is best detected with the

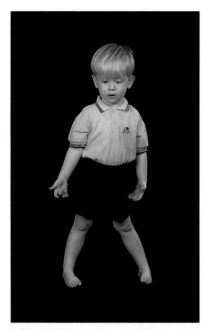

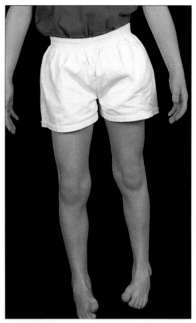

2.57 Walking with inverted feet in a 3-year-old.

2.58 The more mature performance of inverted Fog-walking in a 9-year-old.

child in forward flexion, standing or seated (Black, 1990). A posterior rib hump will be seen on the convex side of the curve as well as unilateral loin fullness. Asymmetry of shoulders or hips may signify a scoliosis.

The limbs can now be inspected for muscle wasting or bulkiness (**2.59–2.65**). More formal testing of power can take place if necessary. Thinking will not be muddled if power is tested in an orderly fashion from proximal to distal muscle groups (*see* above). Similarly for the lower limbs, an approach in terms of joint movements rather than individual muscles may clarify the recording of power and point out a distribution of weakness. The child must be spoken to and encouraged to compete with the examiner throughout. In the juvenile child who is not overweight, full power of hip extension should allow the examiner to lift the buttocks off the couch, holding one leg only. Sustained postures of extension or flexion may be more easily interpreted than requests to pull or push against the examiner. At the ankles, the evertors of the feet should also be examined. These may show weakness in Duchenne dystrophy, peripheral neuropathies or, rarely, low spinal cord lesions.

If muscle wasting is below the knee, particularly when asymmetrical, or if one limb or foot is dwarfed, a careful inspection and subsequent x-ray of the spine should be performed. This is of paramount importance when such asymmetries are evident at birth. Delayed attention to low-cord anomalies may lead to distressing and irreversible incontinence later. The kidneys and

bladder should be palpated and, if felt, the child should pass a measured volume of urine and then be re-examined.

The hips should be examined lying and standing. Lying, the legs must be at right angles to the line joining the anterior iliac spines to assess shortening. Hip movements and the range of abduction can then be compared. In the standing position pelvic tilt can be detected with the examiner's fingers resting on the iliac crests from behind. Trendelenberg's can be tested at the same time. Pelvic tilt may be associated with a scoliosis or with a shortened limb. In Trendelenberg's test the pelvis tilts downwards away from the side of the weight-bearing affected hip.

Additional features of the examination

Sensory testing

When a child presents with acute flaccid paralysis, localised muscle wasting, numbness, pain or altered sensation, then detailed sensory testing is essential (*see* **Practice Point 2.4**). It does not have a regular place in the neurological examination of the child. In spinal lesions, a sweat level can be seen, with reddening and sweating of normally innervated segments and pallor and dryness below the level of the lesion. Frictional changes can be detected by stroking the skin with a metal object. Pin-prick testing will also reveal a spinal level of sensory loss in an infant, so long as testing

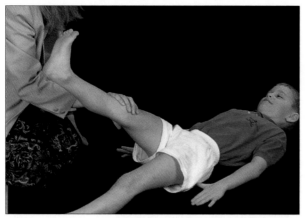

2.59 Lower limb power: sustained hip flexion (psoas).

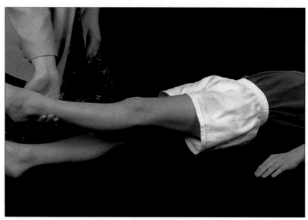

2.60 Hip extension lifting buttocks off floor (gluteal).

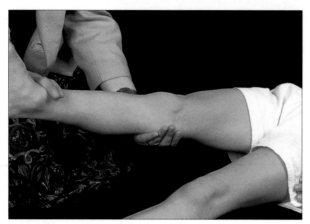

2.61 Knee extension (quadriceps).

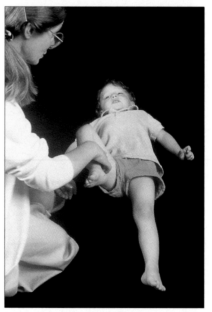

2.62 Knee flexion (hamstrings).

PRACTICE POINT 2.4

If there are no motor signs, there will be no sensory signs without symptoms.

begins from the feet upwards. Once the sensation is perceived, the infant or toddler's objection to the test precludes interpretation of any repeated attempt.

In older children, all modalities should be tested on both sides, following the outer and inner border of the upper limb and the anterior border (including the dorsum of the foot) and posterior border of the leg including the saddle area; always keeping the dermatomes in mind as the examination proceeds. Cotton wool is used for light touch, a neurological pin for pain, and containers of warmed and iced water for temperature sensation.

Anal tone can be assessed by inspection. The neck and trunk should be tested bilaterally, anteriorly and posteriorly. The vibration of the tuning fork is assessed at bony prominences adjacent to joints. To begin with, the child should be given the stimulus where it can be felt normally, and the child needs time to respond as the test proceeds.

Once the area of sensory abnormality is more clearly defined, alternative sensations can be offered with the child's eyes closed. When temperature sensation is affected in spino-thalamic tract lesions, all temperatures may feel warm rather than be lost entirely. For joint posi-

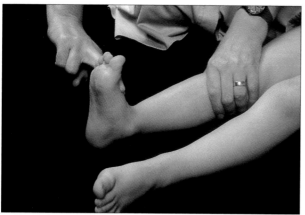

2.63 Ankle dorsiflexion.

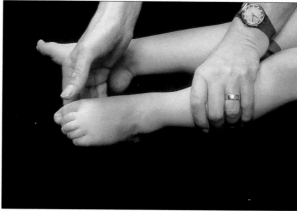

2.64 Ankle plantar flexion.

tion sense, the child must be shown first what each direction of movement is called before he closes his eyes. The child needs encouragement as the test proceeds to sustain concentration. It is best to make one orderly attempt at sensory testing in any one session. Returning persistently to various parts of the sensory examination will probably confuse the examiner as well as the child. Thinking clearly in terms of dermatomes and spinal levels assists the examiner.

Unusual head movements

If an infant or young child cannot keep the head still when following an object, the quality of the head movements should be noted. In oculomotor dyspraxia, the head moves sharply first in the desired direction of gaze, overshooting the fixation point and then coming back to it. The eyes follow the movements of the head but cannot move independently. In nystagmus with visual impairment, the child may make compensatory head-wobbling movements until the null point for the nystagmus is achieved. This is probably to stabilise the image on the retina (Jan, 1991; Jan *et al.*, 1990). The examiner needs to look carefully for the nystagmus as the head is shaking. To achieve fixation with a squint, the child may employ a head tilt. Posterior fossa lesions should be considered in children with head tilt. A mild puppet-like wobbling of the head without ocular abnormalities is usually an extra-pyramidal sign called titubation.

The adolescent

It is a good practice in this age group to direct the history-taking of the presenting complaint towards the adolescent from the beginning of the interview.

In all secondary school children and mature older juniors, it is preferable to examine the patient in a room

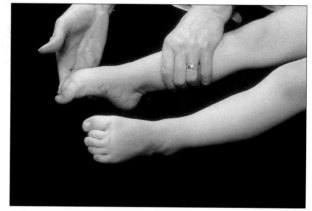

2.65 Foot eversion (peroneals) with assistant discouraging trick movements of hip abduction.

apart from the interview. Though adolescents should never be forced to separate from parents against their will, the majority will welcome the privacy. At such times, the parents will often open up with new and useful information if left in the company of an experienced health visitor or nurse. The doctor will also have a better opportunity to form a relationship with the adolescent. The doctor should always be accompanied for the examination under these circumstances. Whenever possible, adolescents should be given a summary of the doctor's opinion and plan of management, and their views should be sought, before they rejoin the parents. Plans can then be re-outlined to the parents with the adolescent present. It is much better that the adolescent is spoken to, and not spoken about in absentia. The need for a separate interview can usually be readily sensed and should be explained before it takes place.

QUICK NEUROLOGICAL EXAM

Cranials

Pupillary reaction to light and accommodation (II, III)
View optic fundi
Eye movements (III, IV, VI)
Bite and waggle jaw from side to side (V)
Screw up eyes and show teeth (VII)
Say "Agh" (IX)
Shrug shoulders (XI)
Put out tongue (XII)

Temporal visual fields
Visual/hearing acuity when indicated by history

Hold arms outstretched
Finger–nose test
Alternating movement
Touch each finger in turn
Walk—look for toe–heel
(or heel–toe?) gait
—width of base/asymmetry
—waddle of proximal weakness
Fog's test
Gowers' sign

Look for: patterns of movement/
power—pyramidal,
extrapyramidal, cerebellar
or neuromuscular?

Supplementary tasks:

Reflexes/plantar response (if indicated)
Neurocutaneous features
Dysmorphism
Visceromegaly/heart murmur/skeletal signs of storage

2.66 An example of a quick neurological examination.

Chapter 3: The Child with Special Needs

Richard W. Newton

Terms and use

Ten years ago, this section would have been entitled 'mental handicap', but our changing attitudes lead us to use different words which more accurately describe children's strengths and weaknesses. The World Health Organisation (WHO) have been keen to emphasise that some children are born with an impairment which may limit the structure or function of some organs. The functional consequence of this impairment is the disability experienced by the child, but the disability might only actually be a handicap in certain circumstances: for example a child with a flaccid paraparesis due to spina bifida will be handicapped by this disability only when mobility is required but not when watching TV, eating a meal or working at a computer.

The broad term 'mental handicap' does not acknowledge that some children have specific learning difficulties, or that people may have quite severe learning difficulties but in many contexts, be socially quite able. For any given condition, such as Down's syndrome, there is often a spread of abilities, with some children being far more capable than others. Assessments should always be made on an individual basis, and great care taken over the definition of an individual child's strengths and weaknesses.

As discussed in Chapter 1, parents are very appreciative of a positive approach to their child's handicap. Doctors should respond by adopting terms such as 'children with special needs' and by working hard to define those needs on an individual basis and in relation to defined areas of function, such as movement, learning and self-help skills.

Presenting symptoms

Abnormal behaviour in the neonatal period

Apart from obvious dysmorphism, disordered tone, feeding difficulties, irritability and seizures may all signify

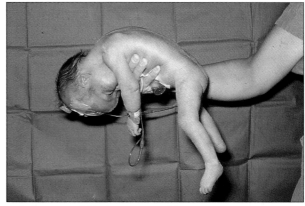

3.1 Learning difficulties: neonatal hypotonia, a common presentation.

continuing neurological abnormality.

Hypotonia in the limbs and axis raises the possibility of a neuromuscular disorder or the Prader–Willi syndrome (**3.1**). Where hypotonia is confined to the axis, there is usually a central nervous system abnormality including the cerebral dysgeneses, or hypoxic–ischaemic encephalopathy when it may be associated with a full fontanelle due to cerebral oedema, irritability, feeding difficulties and seizures (*see* Chapter 15).

Children presenting with abnormal neurological behaviour in the newborn period need full assessment and careful follow-up.

Developmental delay

When children attain developmental skills significantly more slowly than the average child, they may have continuing difficulties with learning in later life. Many standardised tests are available to back up the clinical impression at the neurological consultation. Lack of stimulation due to social disadvantage or prolonged illness in an infant may result in a transient period of relative delay with subsequent catch-up; on the other hand,

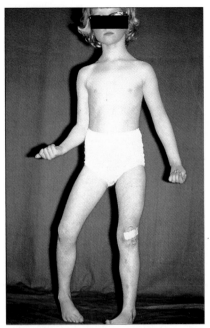

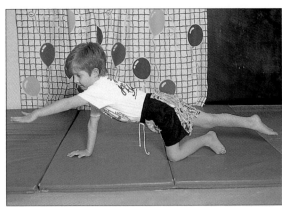

3.3 Physio assessments: testing trunk control and balance.

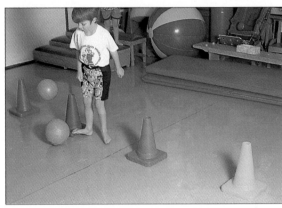

3.4 Physio assessment: testing ball skills and spatial awareness.

3.2 Fog's test: poor dissociated movement in the Clumsy Child syndrome, and here a mild right hemiparesis.

assessment in infancy may serve to over-estimate the ability of children with more severe learning difficulties due to an emphasis in the tests on motor skills.

Funny walks

The emergence of gait disturbance may indicate continuing motor difficulties (*see* Chapter 2) (**3.2**).

Language delay (*see* below).

Trouble at school

Children who present with behaviour problems at school may be having difficulty with balance, coordination or learning. This may act as a source of frustration when for the first time in their lives children are asked, following school entrance, to perform tasks not previously required of them. Assessment of children with balance and coordination difficulties is dealt with in the chapter on clinical examination. The association of poorly set out and untidy work with specific learning difficulties is a common one; full assessment by an educational psychologist is indicated and remedial therapists may be able to offer useful advice to the child and family (**3.3 –3.6**). This will include what tasks might usefully be pursued to encourage good proximal-girdle muscle fixation, to facilitate the distal execution of fine motor skills;

other tasks will improve body image and the sequencing of movement. Tangible success often leads children to feel an improvement in their self esteem which is commonly low in circumstances where they have previously been used to failure.

Speech, language and communication disorders

A disorder of speech and language must be suspected if:
- An 18-month-old male is not obeying commands.
- A two-year-old is saying no words.
- A two-and-a-half-year-old is not using two-word phrases.

Cohort studies show that 15 % of 6–10-year-olds are having some difficulty with speech and language, but spontaneous improvement with age reduces the figure to 5 % of 10–14-year-olds. Boys are twice as commonly affected as girls.

History

The history highlights whether the language problem is isolated or is seen in the context of more global developmental delay. An assessment should be made of language opportunity for the child and whether there is any social disadvantage. Children brought up in a bilingual

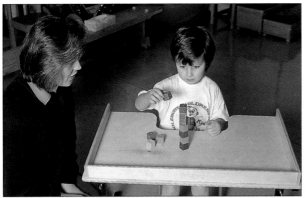

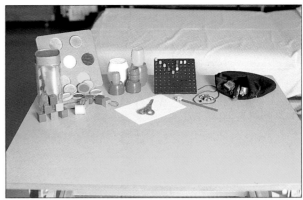

3.5 and 3.6 Occupational therapy. (**3.5, left**) Occupational assessment of hand function. (**3.6, right**) Assessment materials used in occupational therapy.

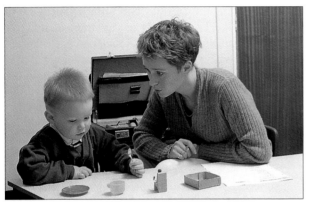

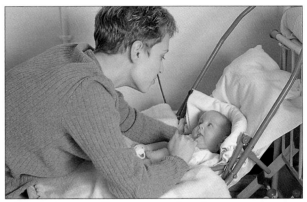

3.7 and 3.8 Speech therapy assessments. (**3.7, left**) Assessment of comprehension of language using formal assessment procedure. (**3.8, right**) Assessment of oro-motor abilities.

environment tend to develop speech later than other children but then catch up. Left handedness or ambidexterity is associated with speech disorder in half the children involved. Elective mutism, commoner in boys, can usually be recognised in the context of unresolved predicament. Children with elective mutism often talk freely in certain situations and continue to communicate with gesture.

Whenever there is indistinct speech and impaired language development, it is important to rule out associated deafness and identify any possibly relevant antecedents in the history.

Physical examination

All children with learning difficulties should be examined for the presence of dysmorphism, signs of a neurocutaneous syndrome or storage disorder. A relatively large head or one showing accelerating growth may reflect an underlying hydrocephalus, the Fragile X syndrome or a leucodystrophy. Particular attention should be paid to the pattern of the speech/language disorder (**3.7 and 3.8**): stammering, dysphonia and dysarthria.

Stammering or stuttering An interruption of the normal

rhythm of speech and may involve involuntary repetition, or prolongation or the arrest of sounds. It is very common and present in up to five per cent of children as they enter school at the age of five. There is male predominance, with a familial tendency. There are many similarities between stammering and simple tics. As children approach certain sounds in a sentence, anxiety about the approaching sequence rises, a stereotyped stutter follows with a release of tension as the sound is passed over.

Dysphonia This is only rarely a cause of speech disorder, accounting for less than one per cent. It may involve the loudness, tone, pitch, inflection or vibrato of sound produced. Most neurological causes are mediated through chest wall weakness or spasticity leading to an abnormal pattern of flow of expired gases over the vocal cords, or to a recurrent laryngeal palsy.

Dysarthria Difficulty with articulation persists in about one in six children beyond the age of five. It results from weakness in bulbar muscles due to a neuromuscular disorder, or poor coordination, or abnormal tone due to pyramidal, extrapyramidal or cerebellar involvement.

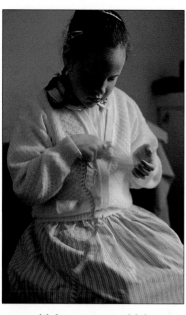

3.9 Manneristic 'flicking' in autism.

pyramidal, extrapyramidal or cerebellar involvement. Dysphagia commonly accompanies the dysarthria. In developmental verbal dyspraxia, some children may find the sequencing and fluency of bulbar muscles difficult to control, as they do any other body musculature. It is rarely an isolated finding and is often seen associated with motor dyspraxia elsewhere, oculo-motor dyspraxia or other forms of learning difficulty.

The definition of language disorder syndrome

Neurological and speech therapy assessment will show whether the child's problem represents a developmental problem, determined perhaps by poor hearing or social disadvantage, which will show eventual catch-up, or whether language development is deviant in some way. Although many combinations are possible, the child's difficulties can be broadly placed within the following groups:

Phonology Many children in the early months and years of language acquisition demonstrate immature articulation or dyslalia: lisping, rhotacism (W for R) and sigmatism (yeth for yes) are common examples of this. Where speech and language is deviant, initial consonant deletion is more common, such as oat for boat.

Lexical syntactic disorders In the early acquisition of language, children commonly make grammatical mistakes such as saying "me want icecream", "I eated my bread". Where language is deviant, there is often a word-finding difficulty, with substitutions or neologisms. Grammatical rules, in particular the complex ones, are often misunderstood.

Semantic disorder This refers to a difficulty in understanding the meaning of language. In simple immaturity, children initially over-extend the meaning of words such as all forms of transport being referred to as car. In deviant semantic language disorder, word-finding difficulties are common and the child may be confused by synonyms.

Pragmatic language disorder This results in the child being confused by the everyday use of language in context. The immature child may demonstrate this by using impolite forms when asking for things, and may have no insight into the use of sarcasm. In deviant forms of pragmatic language disorder, the child may not have the ability to respond to tone of voice; for example, "the door is open", said sternly, may infer that the child should close it. The child may merely acknowledge that the door is open and not respond to the hint to close it.

For each type of language disorder, aetiology should be defined and a treatment plan drawn up.

Developmental language disorders with a poor prognosis
Infantile autism

Autism is one of the pervasive developmental disorders. Its cardinal features are poor social interaction, great difficulty in developing language concept, and play which involves a definite obsessive-compulsive element often associated with poor gross motor ability and more widespread learning difficulties.

Children are often seen to make relatively normal early-developmental progress; a few words of speech may even be acquired, though from the beginning parents have often remarked that the quality of eye contact is poor and children may fail wholly to understand the social meaning of hugging. Developmental progress then slows substantially, with the progress becoming deviant in many areas. Seizures may appear at this stage. Communication may be limited to simple gesture and echolalia is common. Play often assumes an obsessional quality and involves manneristic repetitive flapping, twiddling or flicking (**3.9**). Some children have pockets of ability, particularly with rote learning, memorising lists or form boards. The difficulties with interpersonal communication and communication through speech, however, remain the most dominant features, far more obvious than the child's more general intellectual impairment.

Aspberger's syndrome

As with autism, there are five times more boys affected than girls. This developmental disorder shares with autism the difficulty in communication through speech and language and interaction with other people. Children with Aspberger's syndrome are less intellectually impaired than children with autism, and their difficulties may not be picked up until they are at least three or four years old. Children may have particular difficulty with the pragmatic use of language, being very concrete in their interpretation of speech. Their expressive language may be impolite and their understanding of social context poor, which may lead them be intrusive or quite unaware that they are causing offence. Play is obsessional, and toy cars may be lined or stacked rather than pushed along. Children may spend hours watching or imitating the action of mechanical things such as washing machines. Poor balance or coordination is the rule, and there is an association with epilepsy.

There is a strong case for viewing autism and Aspberger's syndrome as being at different ends of the same developmental spectrum. There are probably many different causes but it is currently suspected that many result from neuronal migration problems (*see* Chapter 11). People with Aspberger's syndrome may be very successful high achievers in adult life whilst others become academic failures and loners. Their difficulties need recognition and support.

The Landau–Kleffner syndrome

The characteristic of this syndrome is that children, either acutely or more slowly over a more prolonged period, develop a profound aphasia, which is most commonly receptive but may be expressive or both, as a specific learning difficulty. This may happen in the context of a well-defined encephalitis/encephalopathic illness or for reasons that are less readily defined. The EEG more usually contains paroxysmal activity—bilateral spikes or spike-waves variable in time and position but most often temporal, and almost continuous during sleep (**3.10**). Seizures may be generalised tonic–clonic or partial. A good third of the children do not have overt seizures, and they are rarely difficult to control. Psychomotor and behavioural disturbances are commonly seen; seizures usually remit before adolescence. Some children show natural remission with spontaneous improvement after a year or so of difficulty; others (and it may be the same group) show remission following steroid therapy. There are anecdotal reports that a sub-pial resection of horizontally orientated fibres from the focus of epileptogenic activity in the temporal lobes improves language performance.

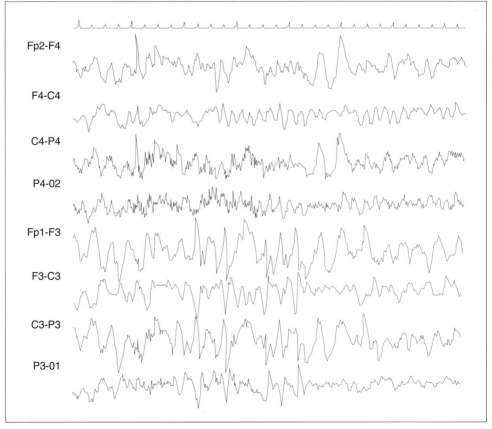

3.10 Landau–Kleffner syndrome: spike-wave discharge poorly localised in left hemisphere.

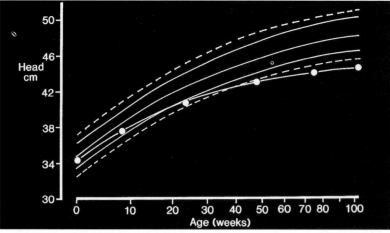

3.11 Rett's syndrome: typical charted head growth.

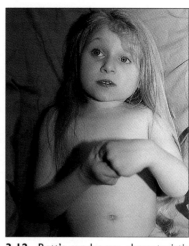

3.12 Rett's syndrome: characteristic facial appearance.

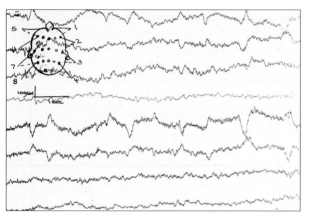

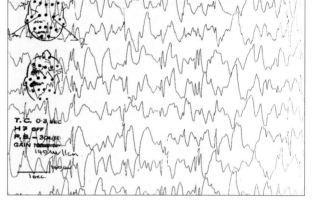

3.13 and 3.14 Rett's syndrome: EEG awake/asleep. Characteristically, seizure discharge appears during sleep.

This condition should not strictly speaking be dealt with in this section, although the pattern of development bears similarities to children with autism. The condition has been described in girls only thus far and is presumed to be an X-linked dominant condition due to spontaneous mutation which is lethal in males. The girls involved show a relatively normal pattern of development into the second half of infancy, although the emergence of the family video has often demonstrated in retrospect that the quality of movement in the girls was probably never quite normal from the start. A period of uncharacteristic irritability may then emerge for several weeks, during which time a degree of loss of developmental skills appears followed by a plateauing of developmental attainment. The rate of head growth slows down so that head size initially within the normal range has fallen below the 3rd centile by the third or fourth year (**3.11**). The girls retain good eye contact and can return a sociable smile, but any single words are lost. Useful hand movement is also lost, precluding the use of gesture to communicate. The hands are often held at the level of the mouth and the girls indulge in repetitive hand movement which may involve flicking of the lower lip or a characteristic wringing of the hands (**3.12**). An extrapyramidal movement disorder with progressive rigidity evolves over the course of many years, and is often associated with the emergence of scoliosis as the teenage years approach. The EEG, although slow for the child's age, shows seizure activity during sleep only (**3.13 and 3.14**). Seizures may be difficult to control. Following the rest of development, the girls retain profound learning difficulties.

Angelman's syndrome

Angelman's syndrome is a cause of severe/profound mental handicap, but there is no specific language disorder. It is mentioned at this stage because girls presenting with the disorder in infancy may show symptoms and signs that are very akin to the presentation of Rett's syndrome (**3.15**). Angelman's syndrome may result from uniparental disomy (*see* Chapter 18). These children, similar to children with Rett's syndrome, have some-

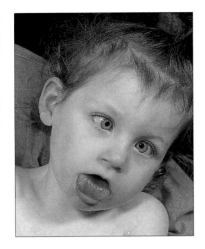

3.15 (left) Angelman's syndrome: characteristic facial appearance.

3.16 (right) Generalised multifocal polyspike- wave activity in Angelman's syndrome.

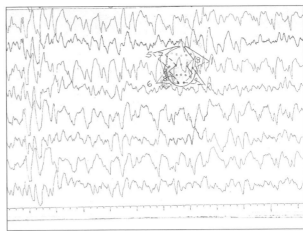

what petite faces with a pointed chin, and may involve themselves in hyperventilation or tongue thrusting. They have generally a pleasant demeanour and a trunkal ataxia. This, linked with jerkiness in limb movement, lead to the initial description of this condition as the Happy Puppet syndrome, a term found by parents to be offensive. Seizures are more common than in Rett's syndrome and the EEG shows seizure activity in the standard waking record (**3.16**).

The diagnostic process

The role of the paediatrician/paediatric neurologist in children with learning difficulties is to help parents to understand the issue of causation, inform the parents of the future outlook, deal with attendant medical problems and arrange genetic counselling.

The history should detail the pregnancy including any drug ingestion or early threatened abortion. The presence of foetal distress should lead to careful scrutiny of the obstetric notes, though it is now generally established that in order to attribute causation to birth asphyxia, the presence of hypoxic ischaemic encephalopathy must be established. A record of cord or early pH measurements and neonatal behaviour is very helpful in this respect. Parents in their own mind often attribute their child's difficulties to the events of labour, and it can be helpful to them to be taken through details of the birth. A detailed family history is clearly of value, especially when supplemented by perusal of family photograph albums. These, together with family video recordings, may give a very good idea about the evolution of a disorder. Many motor disorders such as the spasticity in cerebral palsy or the extrapyramidal involvement in Rett's syndrome may evolve over a period of time, raising the possiblity of a neurodegenerative disorder. Careful scrutiny of the history often reveals that whereas things have changed, skills may not actually have been lost.

Physical examination should pay particular attention to head size, growth, the presence of dysmorphic features, and signs of a neurocutaneous syndrome or storage disorder.

Table 3.1 (overleaf) outlines a rational approach to investigation of children with learning difficulties.

The multidisciplinary team

Once a diagnosis is established it is important to outline a young person's strengths and weaknesses as abilities within a given diagnostic group may vary widely (**3.17 and 3.18**). This picture of ability is best built up by involving remedial therapists used to working together in a team. Physiotherapists give an idea on gross motor skills, balance and coordination; occupational therapists focus mainly on fine motor skills and tasks in everyday living that might be helped with the provision of suitable aids. Speech therapists will offer advice on speech and language development. The clinical psychologists often through formal testing will establish the spread of cognitive ability.

The word 'therapist' may be confusing to parents who may feel that the condition might be 'put right' by therapy or that a child's developmental potential might actually be augmented by intervention (**3.19**). The real aim of therapy is to encourage each child to reach the full developmental potential, rather than fundamentally being able to augment it. Therapists will guide parents in their play with children to encourage the next developmental step. Advice on toys or aids may also be given. Another important role of the physiotherapist is to advise on seating, orthoses and footwear to encourage an optimal posture.

Traditionally, paediatricians have been the coordinators of multidisciplinary teams, though many teams are now moving away from this model. It is important to recognise that some parents are rather bewildered by all

TABLE 3.1   Investigations of Children with Learning Difficulties (LD)

Mild/moderate LD	Thyroid function tests Amino acids (urine) Organic acids (urine)
Special cases:	
Large head	Measure parents' heads CT scan Fragile X (if relatively short, large ear lobes, long mandible)
Dysmorphism	Chromosomes Interrogate computerised data-base for recognisable patterns
Boys	CPK (weakness/motor impairment)
Severe LD	CT scan Chromosomes as above

Note:

• Where more than one child is involved, consider checking amino acids in the mother.

• Where motor impairment (other than dyspraxia appropriate to developmental age) exists concurrently, investigate accordingly (see relevant section).

• With deteriorating school performance, consider unhappiness/depression and neuro-degenerative disorder (see Chapter 14).

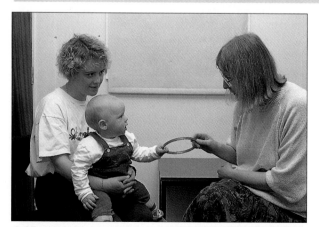 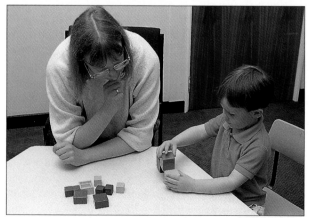

3.17 and 3.18 Psychology assessment: developmental levels can be assessed using various standardised play activities.

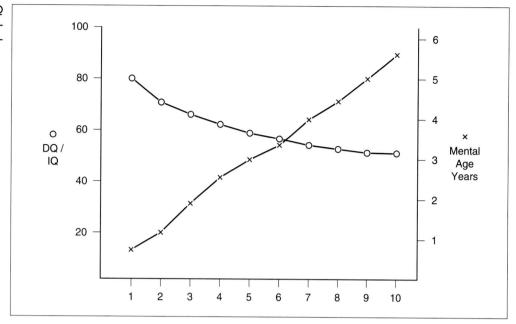

3.19 A fall in DQ/IQ does not mean neurodegeneration, merely slower learning.

the professional involvement, and it is good for one person in the team to be assigned as their advocate, so the parental point of view might be put to other team members. A social worker or health visitor attached to the team might also fulfill this role. Some health authorities employ portage workers who may visit the parents in their homes and advise on useful things to incorporate in play to encourage developmental progress. Developmental check lists may be used to guide the parents in this respect.

Continuing medical care

The care of children with disabilities should be kept as near to their homes as possible. Regular attendance at hospital may be needed for the assessment and surveillance of attendant medical difficulties. The common problems needing medical attention are as follows:

Epilepsy Regardless of causation, where epilepsy is present, due attention should be paid to establishing a diagnosis, categorising seizure type and prescribing anticonvulsant drugs where thought necessary. Medication should be kept to a minimum and given in sugar-free preparations. As in children who are seizure-free for two years, the possibility of slow drug withdrawal should be considered.

Skeletal deformity Prevention is better than cure, with the provision of regular physiotherapy, appropriate aids and orthoses, seating and footwear (**3.20**). In neuromuscular conditions, mobility should be maintained just as long as possible and the spine stabilised when scoliosis emerges.

Gastro-oesophageal reflux This is a common problem in the severely/profoundly handicapped who are immobile. Repeated regurgitation, bouts of wheezing or recurrent pneumonia may all signify its presence. A Gastrograffin swallow, pH monitoring, and oesophagoscopy will define the anatomical abnormality. Where medical treatment with antacids, H_2 receptor antagonists or Gaviscon fails, surgical repair of the hiatus hernia may be indicated. Where the problem is aspiration due to poor coordination of bulbar muscles, the functional problem may be defined with the use of videofluoroscopy (**3.21**).

If the problem is not resolved with attention to positioning and food texture, then a feeding gastrostomy offers a useful alternative. This ensures adequate calorie intake but is best combined with fundoplication to minimise the risk of gastro-oesophageal reflux.

Recurrent chest infections Again, this is mainly a problem in the severely physically handicapped who are immobile. An inefficient cough often accompanied by the swallowing difficulties of bulbar paresis may lead to repeated aspiration and susceptibility to infection. Prophylactic antibiotic therapy may be indicated.

Neurogenic bladder
(*See* Chapter 17.)

Impairment of the special senses
The deaf child

The first priority is always identification of the deafness. If parents suspect their child is deaf, they are probably right. Relevant medical history and notably neonatal jaundice or bacterial meningitis should always lead to

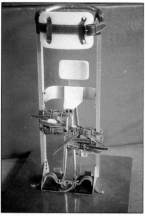

3.20 Standing frame min-imises scoliosis risk and offers children a new per-spective of life.

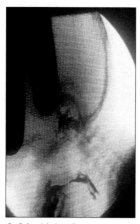

3.21 Videofluoroscopy; defining the functional abnormality in dysphagia.

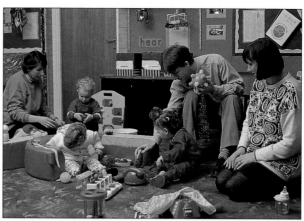

3.22 Activities of the Vision Centre Group: building a pic-ture of the world through tactile and auditory input.

referral for a full hearing assessment. Brain stem audito-ry-evoked potential measurement allows the evaluation of hearing threshold in very young babies and is not dependent on state of alertness.

Early identification allows the early establishment of communication. The provision of hearing aids may ame-liorate the hearing deficit, but sound may still be distort-ed, as evidenced by the very small percentage of children who are profoundly deaf who develop useful speech. The early use of signing helps to develop language concepts, facilitates communication and reduces the risk of behav-iour problems in children with hearing impairment. Advice can be sought from the local social worker for the deaf or the Royal National Institute for the Deaf. The debate continues as to whether the oral/aural approach to communication, which centres on augmented hearing being supplemented by lip reading, or the total approach to communication using signing and lip reading is the best. A satisfactory approach would seem to be to teach signing as a first language with English as a second lan-guage. It must be remembered that a minority of deaf children also have specific learning difficulties. When language concept seems slow to develop further, a full assessment of cognitive ability should be made. Due attention should be paid to the issue of causation and appropriate genetic advice given.

The blind child

Visual impairment is more readily identified than hear-ing impairment. Children from an early stage clearly demonstrate their inability to fix and follow or return their mother's smile at the correct age. Some children with delayed visual maturation 'catch up' with their visual skills within a few months. In others, the impair-ment will remain permanent. Some children with

delayed visual maturation will retain problems with visual or spatial awareness, or have other learning diffi-culties when older. As with deafness, the cause of the blindness must be defined, and appropriate genetic coun-selling given.

Much of early development depends on visual input, as a picture of the world around is built up by the devel-oping infant, and assimilated with information from other sensory modalities (**3.22**). Much of the help par-ents may give their growing children will come naturally to them and is based on common sense. Pity will never replace good encouragement. Input must be made through the other sensory systems, relying on sound, touch and swallow. Body image may be encouraged by attaching bells at first to the hands and later to the feet. In so doing, the growing baby can associate auditory with proprioceptive sounds identified with particular objects. When blind babies are approached, it is helpful to touch them and to call out their name. The baby can be encouraged to feel everyday objects such as the feed-ing spoon, hair-brush and so on. Early mobility may be encouraged by coaxing a child to walk around the cot and later up and down the stairs with the use of handrails. Timidity must be discouraged. Noisy toys will encourage movement but early toys ought to be simple in shape and form and, if possible, associated with a spo-ken word. As the child grows, language will become increasingly important in describing the surrounding world and its meaning.

Children with visual impairment, as any other child, may be integrated into mainstream education. Those chil-dren who are totally blind may well need braille as a medi-um to read, whereas those who are partially sighted may be encouraged to make most use of what vision remains with use of a magnifying lens or electronic magnifier.

Whether a residential school placement or local

3.23 (left) Advisory Centre for Education: parental guidance on the Education Act.

3.24 (right) Most children with moderate learning difficulties capable of being integrated into mainstream education.

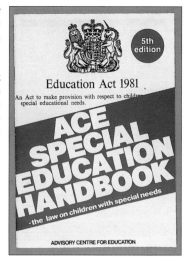

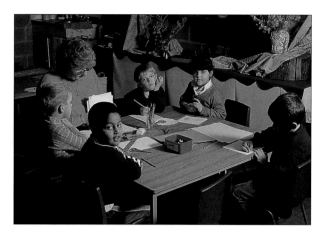

school placement is chosen, one important aim of the educational process must be to make the young person as independent as possible.

Medicine, education and UK law

The Local Education Authority (LEA) and statements of special educational need

The 1981 Education Act ensured the right to integration in mainstream education for children with special needs. Before the age of two years, any doctors involved have a duty to tell the parents and the Education Authority that a child may well have special educational needs (**3.23**). The Education Authority may, with the consent of the parents (and is duty bound to do so at the request of the parents), make an assessment. An officer of the LEA, usually an educational psychologist, starts the process by assessing the child's strengths and weaknesses, and on this basis decides the best educational placement. It is usual for all members of the multidisciplinary team to make a contribution to the statement. When the statement is drawn up, the LEA in theory commits itself to the provision of adequate resources to give integration the best chance of success. Provision of non-teaching aids or for nursery nurses who are able to supervise the activity of children with learning difficulties in the classroom and at breaktime is commonly made. Along with this, provision is made for appropriate teaching support and remedial therapy (**3.24**). Unfortunately, the basic principle of the Act is limited, as integration must be compatible with 'the efficient use of resources'. This resource limitation has at times led children who otherwise would have been more appropriately integrated into mainstream education to be accommodated in special schools.

If it plans to make an assessment, the LEA must give the parents 29 days' notice. Parents must receive notice of any examinations planned, and they have the right to be present and to submit information. Parents refusing assessment of examination of their children without a reasonable excuse are breaking the law and may be fined. If, following assessment, the LEA decides not to make a Statement of Special Educational Need, it must inform the parents of their right to appeal to the Secretary of State. More usually, a statement is drawn up and a draft is sent to the parents. If the parents disagree with any part of it, they must make this known to an officer of the LEA within 15 days. Further evidence may then be submitted within the next 15 days, and final meetings must be made within 15 days of that. The final statement is then drawn up and the parents notified accordingly. If parents still do not agree with the contents of the statement, and appeal to the LEA, there is a further right of appeal to the Secretary of State.

Statements must be reviewed within 12 months, and children who have a statement must be reassessed between the ages of 12 and a half and 14 and a half years. The LEA must see that special educational provision is made and set out in the statement.

The 1988 Education Reform Act allows parents to appeal if the LEA decides to amend a statement (previously appeal rights followed only the initial assessments or reassessments) (*see* **3.25**, a facsimile of page 14 of *ACE Special Education Handbook*, reprinted with permission).

The baseline level of the national curriculum is not attainable by many children with learning difficulties. Discussions are continuing between academic departments of universities and the Department of Education about a suitable curriculum for these children. Further

Summary of procedures

Children under two

Parent can ask for *assessment*;

District Health Authority must tell **parent**, then **education authority**, that child may have *special education needs*;

Education authority may with *consent* of **parent**, and *must at request* of **parent**, make an assessment. It can be of any kind, and may result in a *Statement of Special Educational Needs*.

Children between two and 19

Authorities have a *duty to identify* children *whose special educational needs* call on the **authority** to decide on special educational provision;

Parents can request *assessment* and **authorities** cannot *unreasonably refuse*.

Assessment

Notice to **parents** — *29 days* to comment;

If **authority** decides not to asssess, must notify parent;

Parents must receive *notices* of any *examinations*; have a right to be present and to submit information;

Parents who fail to see that their children turn up for examinations without *reasonable excuse* may be *guilty* of offence and *fined*.

After assessment

Authority may decide *not to make Statement* of Special Education Needs: must inform parent of *right of appeal* to **Secretary of State**;

If **authority** decides to *make Statement*, must serve copy of *draft* statement on **parent**;

If **parent** disagrees with any part:

> *within 15 days* can make *representations*, ask for meeting with **officer**;
>
> *within further 15 days*, ask for other *meetings* with professionals to discuss professional advice provided to authority (which must be given to parent as part of Statement); *within final 15 days* from last meeting, make further *representations* to authority.

Authority, after considering parents' views, can make *Statement* in the same or changed form, or decide not to make it: must *inform* **parent**.

If *Statement* is made, must be sent to **parent** with *notice of right to appeal* in writing to local appeal committee, which can *confirm Statement*, or ask authority to *reconsider* it;

Parent has further *right of appeal* to **Secretary of State**.

After Statement is made

Statements must be reviewed within every 12 months;

Child with *Statement* must be *re-assessed* between age of 12$\frac{1}{2}$ and 14$\frac{1}{2}$.

Parent can *appeal* following any *re-assessment* or any *amendment* of a *Statement*.

Authority must see that special educational provision set out in Statement is made.

3.25 Facsimile of page 14 of ACE Special Education Handbook (reprinted with permission).

anxiety accompanies the fact that mainstream schools may well be less inclined to accommodate children with learning difficulties, as provision for them tends to be expensive, and schools now have their own budgets. School governors are, however, responsible for identifying children with special needs and for satisfying parents that appropriate educational provision will be available in the school. With this in mind, doctors may well encourage parents of children with learning difficulties to become school governers!

The issue of consent

A number of children with learning difficulties are born with life-threatening conditions, some remediable and some irremediable. Medical and nursing staff have a duty to remedy the problem where possible and preserve life. This is an area of potential conflict between parents and health-care professionals. Parents with a sense of fear for what the future holds may see a life-threatening condition in their baby as their 'way out'. At times in the past, doctors have held much sympathy with that point of view and have allowed children to die. Some babies have been sedated and, failing to demand feeds, they have died within a few days of birth. In recent years, a consultant paediatrician was charged with murder (R. v Arthur) in circumstances similar to these. Forensic evidence given in the trial led to the charge being replaced by one of attempted murder, and Dr Arthur was ultimately acquitted, although the trial left many important legal and ethical principles unaddressed. It did make it clear that juries are disinclined to find doctors guilty of murder in these circumstances.

More recently (ReC—a minor) a judge found that it would be 'not unlawful' to let a child die where severe handicap existed and where suffering would be avoided. In recent years, the British Paediatric Association Guidelines have indicated that there are many circumstances in which it would be justifiable to let a child destined to have profound handicap die, so long as the child was facing a life-threatening illness.

The Mental Health Act

Parents of severely handicapped young women are often rightly worried about their daughters' vulnerability to unwanted pregnancy, and a number of sterilisations have been carried out in the past for this reason. At least 36 girls under the age of 18 were sterilised in England between 1973 and 1974 and in 1987. The Department of Health stated that around 90 sterilisations were performed each year on women aged under 19. Under The Mental Health Act (1959), consent could be given on behalf of young people with severe learning difficulties following the notion that guardianship could be held not only by parents but also by Social Services personnel. Medical practitioners involved would share the issues of individual cases, sometimes, if possible, with the girl herself, but certainly with the girl's parents, social workers or other health care professionals, and a decision taken.

The Mental Health Act (1983) replaced this act and significantly restricted the role of guardianship. Consent forms could no longer be signed, and this, together with a case (ReB—a minor) heard before the Court of Appeal in 1987, has given adults with mental disability a new status in law. Those who have enough understanding to give consent to a particular procedure may do so (previously this was not possible: the guardian had to be asked). Proxy consent is no longer valid in law. This must be a welcome development in view of the increasing amount of community care, and a greater awareness of human rights on the part of young people with learning difficulties.

When treatment is not controversial, doctors need to go ahead if possible with the agreement (but not the consent) of parents and usual caretakers of the child. In these circumstances, doctors are deemed to be acting 'in good faith' and showing 'a duty of care'. The principle of necessity is recognised in law to allow doctors to act in an emergency without the consent of the individual.

In ReB—a minor, Lord Justice Dillon said that the court had jurisdiction to authorise the sterilisation on a Ward of Court in wardship proceedings, but this jurisdiction should be exercised only as a last resort, and after all other forms of contraception have been considered. Reaching its decision, the court had considered ReD—a minor, 1976, in which it was made very clear that decisions such as sterilisation should not be within the doctor's sole clinical judgment, where the operation was neither medically indicated nor necessary. Each case would have to be decided by a court on its merits. It is clear from this judgment that when a medical intervention is planned that might be deemed controversial, doctors would be prudent to gain the agreement from a court so that the anticipated controversial intervention "will not be unlawful".

The Children Act

The Children Act (1989) is important recent legislation. It is very comprehensive and replaces previous fragmented legislation as a statement on the law relating to the care and protection of children. One of the most important principles behind the act is that the welfare of the child is paramount, and that children are best looked after within their own families. Where other agencies are required to supervise the care of a child, it is best done in the context of a partnership between those agencies and the family concerned. Much of the act deals with the

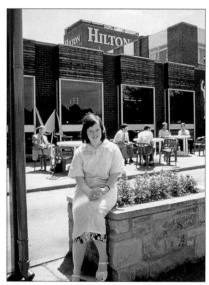
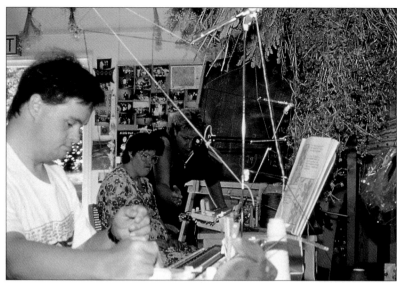

3.26 and 3.27   The aim of intervention: confidence and independence as adults.

issue of child protection, but important consideration is given to children with disability. It is hoped that the creation of a joint register of disabled children between Health, Education and Social Services will greatly facilitate their identification and registration and a coordinated provision of services. This applies not only initially when assessments are being compiled along procedures defined in the 1981 Education Act (*see* above), but also in relation to the provision of respite care and the subsequent placement of adults with severe learning difficulties in residential community houses.

The adult handicapped

Children with special needs will generally have been supervised for up to 19 years by paediatricians and paediatric neurologists before they are transferred to adult services. In many Health Authorities, these adult services have been rather fragmented. The primary aim of medical involvement must be to understand the causation of the problem in so far as is possible, and to offer the family appropriate genetic advice for the benefit of current and future generations. Families must not confuse disability with ill health, and must try to be as independent as possible from medical services. Young peo-

ple and their families must be encouraged to be confident and independent in spite of their handicap (**3.26 and 3.27**). Having said that, it is important for doctors to review young disabled people from time to time to prevent the development of the secondary effects of handicap. It is far better that a preventative approach is taken rather than having to troubleshoot in a crisis. Health Authorities are just beginning to establish posts, often Consultants in Rehabilitation Medicine or Mental Handicap, who will continue the surveyance of the handicapped population through the adult years. This change is to be welcomed.

In addition, Health Authorities in some instances are forming partnerships with local Social Services, and often the private sector, to establish in the community local residences with appropriate support so that young handicapped people can live independently of their parents. Doctors should encourage parents to lobby their local authorities for developments of this sort, to ensure that their children have a future with prospects. The worst time for a young handicapped person to learn to live independently is the day their last remaining parent dies.

Chapter 4: Headache

Richard W. Newton

Epidemiology

Headaches are common in childhood and account for one in four referrals to our general Paediatric Neurology clinics. Waters, in his study of 10–16-year-old schoolchildren, showed that 93 % of girls and 85 % of boys had a headache in a 12-month period, and in 12 % of girls and 9 % of boys, the headache fitted his definition of migraine. Bille showed that the incidence of headaches rises with age, and that migraine is more common in girls as the teenage years are entered (*see* **4.1**).

Differential diagnosis

Most childhood headaches fall into the tension-like headache/migraine spectrum. Only rarely is headache due to disease or illness. Headache is often felt with acute systemic illness, especially when it is accompanied by a fever. Acute sinusitis may lead to severe facial pain with tenderness over the affected bone, but it is doubtful if chronic sinusitis or perennial rhinitis lead to headache, although some children may talk of 'muzzy headedness'. Dental malocclusion can lead to aching and tenderness of the muscles of mastication, especially the masseters: the discomfort is relieved by massage or warmth. Orthodontic treatment can relieve the problem. In other children, problems with accommodation may lead to discomfort around the eyes, and the provision of spectacles alleviates the symptoms.

The possibility of headache representing a cerebral tumour causes irrational fear in many parents and a number of doctors. It is this uncertainty that leads to many hospital referrals. Headache due to an intracranial, space-occupying lesion is only very rarely an isolated symptom. By the time the tumour has caused a rise in intracranial pressure, CSF pathways and neuronal tissues have been compressed. There are almost invariably attendant neurological signs. Ninety per cent of tumours in children lie below the tentorium in the posterior fossa, and truncal ataxia is a prominent feature. Of the 10 % arising above the tentorium, roughly half of these are craniopharyngiomas with associated growth failure. The

Incidence of Headache: Schoolchildren Followed for One Year			
	Age	Any headache (%)	Migraine (%)
Boys (n=4440)	7–10	51	2.9
	11–15	66	3.7
Girls (n=4553)	7–10	50	2.6
	11–15	69	6.2

4.1 Incidence of headache: schoolchildren followed for one year.

headache of raised intracranial pressure is made worse by recumbency, coughing or straining (children with tension headache/migraine usually feel relieved when they lie down). Vomiting, particularly on a recurrent and daily basis, is a common accompanying symptom.

Paroxysmal headaches in children, diagnostic criteria and definitions (after the International Headache Society)

Common migraine (migraine without aura)

This is an idiopathic recurring headache disorder manifesting in attacks lasting 4–72 hours. Typically, the headaches have a unilateral location, pulsating quality, moderate or severe intensity, and are aggravated by physical activity and associated with nausea, photo- and phonophobia.

Classical migraine (migraine with aura)

These bouts affect about 10 % of people who have migraine. They are defined as part of an idiopathic recurring disorder, manifesting with attacks of neurological symptoms unequivocally localisable to the cerebral cortex or brainstem, usually developing gradually over 5–20 minutes and lasting less than 60 minutes. Headache, nausea and/or photophobia usually follow the neurological aura symptoms directly after a free interval of less than an hour. The headache usually lasts 4–72 hours, but may be completely absent.

Some children have migraine with a prolonged aura; this is often referred to as complicated migraine. Neurological symptoms may include an homonymous hemianopia, hemianaesthesia or hemiplegia (**4.2**). The abnormal signs last longer than 60 minutes but less than a week. In some families with familial hemiplegic migraine, the bouts are stereotyped and identical. Basilar migraine refers to migraine with aura, symptoms clearly originating from the brainstem or from both occipital lobes. This predictably gives rise to visual symptoms in both the temporal and nasal fields of both eyes, dysarthria, vertigo, tinnitus, decreased hearing, double vision, ataxia, bilateral paraesthesias, bilateral pareses, or decreased level of consciousness.

Ophthalmoplegic migraine

These bouts involve repeated attacks of headache associated with paresis of one or more oculo-cranial

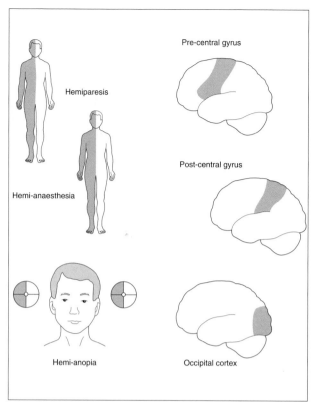

4.2 The wide spectrum of signs in migraine determined by site of involvement.

nerves in the absence of a demonstrable intracranial lesion.

Retinal migraine

This gives repeated attacks of monocular scotomal blindness lasting less than an hour, but associated with headache. An ocular or structural vascular disorder must be ruled out.

Childhood periodic syndromes

These may be precursors to or associated with migraine. It must be remembered that abdominal pain and vomiting is quite a common entity in childhood, and may be due to many factors, including intercurrent infection. This clinical entity, therefore, is poorly defined, and long-term follow-up of children with 'periodic syndrome' shows no significant association with those destined to develop migraine.

It must be noted that children with benign paroxysmal vertigo may present with symptoms similar to those children with basilar migraine. Alternating hemiplegia of childhood involves the onset of bouts of hemiplegia before the age of 18 months. The repeated bouts of hemiplegia involving either or both sides of the body are often associated with developmental delay and at times residual paresis. The relationship of this entity to migraine on the one hand and epilepsy to the other is poorly defined. Frequently, the bouts are resistant to conventional anticonvulsant therapy. Dramatic improvement with flunarizine (not currently available in the UK) or haloperidol therapy is reported in some. Calcium antagonists have been shown to be of benefit and, are probably the drug of choice.

It must be remembered that in that small group of children affected by complicated migraine, and in particular those affected by ophthalmoplegic or hemiplegic migraine, there may be residual neurological signs. Full investigation is warranted (*see* below).

Tension-type headache

This involves recurrent episodes of headache lasting minutes to days. The pain is typically pressing or tightening in quality, of mild or moderate intensity, bilateral in location and does not worsen with routine physical activity. Nausea is absent, but photophobia or phonophobia may be present.

Cluster headache and chronic paroxysmal hemicrania

These headache types which share many features in common are relatively rare in childhood. A number of features distinguish the two. Cluster headache shows a night preponderance with fewer bouts of longer duration in any given cluster (**4.3**). Chronic paroxysmal hemicrania is particularly responsive to indomethacin.

Episodes involve severe strictly unilateral pain orbitally, supraorbitally and/or temporally, lasting 15–180 minutes and occurring from once every other day to eight times a day. Bouts are associated with one or more of the following:

Conjunctival injection	Forehead and facial sweating
Miosis	Lacrimation
Ptosis	Nasal congestion
Eyelid oedema	Rhinorrhoea

Attacks occur in a series lasting for weeks or months, separated by remission periods usually lasting months or years.

The clinical assessment of headaches

Symptom characterisation

It is best to characterise the headache systematically, using the skills learnt as a medical student:
- How many different types of headache are there?

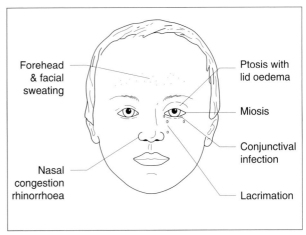

4.3 The features of cluster headache.

- Where is it felt?
- What does it feel like?
- Does is radiate?
- Are there any triggering, exacerbating or relieving factors?

Always ask the children themselves to complement the description given to you by parents. Beware of the language used, many people think the head has five sides: the front, the back, the left, the right and the top! The word throbbing means severe to some, pulsatile to others.

A picture should be painted of the family background. Not only is a familial tendency to have headaches of genetic interest, it may also mean that another family member is acting as a role model for headache behaviour. The predicament at home or at school should be identified. Headache behaviour may represent an attempt by the child to avoid what is perceived to be a difficult situation.

Physical examination

In particular, attention should be made to growth, visual fields, and any dysfluency or asymmetry in the pattern of movement (**4.4–4.6**).

The characteristics of a migraine attack

Parents often notice a prodromal period lasting up to 24 hours or so before symptoms of migraine appear. In this period, the child may be unduly irritable and bad tempered, or lack concentration (**4.7**). An aura may appear, typically lasting about 20 minutes. The location of the cortical dysfunction determines what the child experiences during the aura (*see* **4.2**). The occipital lobe will lead to visual disturbance (**4.8**) and the parietal lobe dysaesthesia or motor dysfunction if the phenomenon

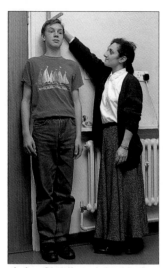

4.4 Childhood headache: measure growth.

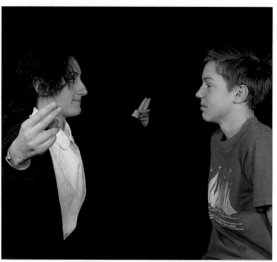

4.5 Childhood headache: assess visual fields.

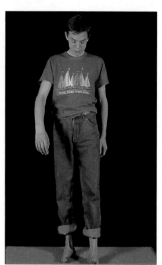

4.6 Childhood headache: assess hemisphere function with Fog's test.

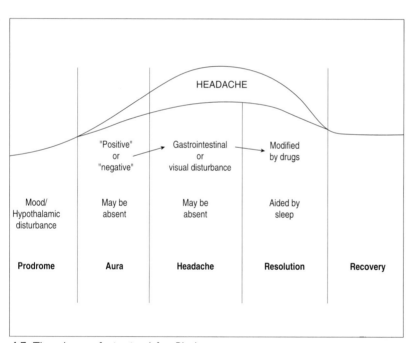

4.7 The phases of migraine (after Blau).

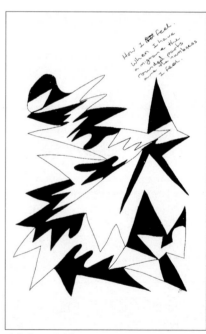

4.8 One child's experience of aura.

spreads forward. The headache itself is at least of moderate intensity, and usually prevents the child continuing with current activity. Some children find that if they concentrate, they are able to delay the onset of this more severe phase. Wretched vomiting is an inconvenience suffered by many at this stage, and a need for sleep is almost universal. Following sleep which may be short, the child often feels relatively refreshed, and in the recovery period often experiences a feeling of great clarity of thought.

The pathophysiology of migraine

A number of theories have been proposed to explain the phenomonology of migraine, laying different emphasis on the relative contributions of vasogenic and neurogenic activity, and Hannington proposed that migraine might actually be a common disorder of blood platelets. Recently, Lance has proposed a unifying hypothesis incorporating each of these components. The theory acknowledges that during the aura phase, there is

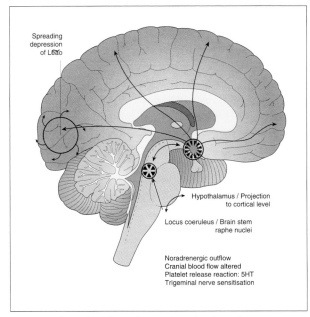

4.9 Lance's unifying hypotheses on pathophysiology.

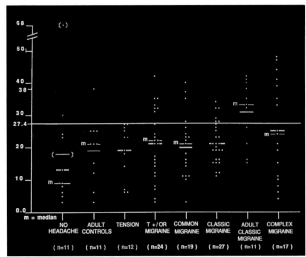

4.10 The association of high platelet adhesiveness with complicated migraine.

increased neurogenic activity in central nervous system structures, with vasoconstriction followed by vasodilatation during the headache phase of a migraine attack. 5-Hydroxytriptamine (5-HT) levels initially rise and then fall during the period of vasodilation.

Lance suggests that the primary event in migraine is in mid-brain structures and particularly the locus coeruleus (**4.9**). Noradrenergic outflow increases and association bundles project activity to a cortical level. A spreading wave of neuronal depression is seen to spread at a rate of about 3 mm/min across the cerebral cortex. If this is confined to the pole of the occipital lobe, a central scotoma is experienced. As the wave of depression spreads more widely, either positive (fortification spectra) or negative (hemianopia) visual phenomena will occur. The wave may spread forward into the parietal lobe giving dysaesthesia, or even further forward into the motor area giving a hemiparesis. It is this spread from posterior cerebral to middle cerebral artery territory that makes a vasogenic cause for this phenomenon unlikely. The increased neurogenic outflow is likely to lead platelets to adhere and undergo a release reaction. At this stage, 5-HT levels will rise, the vasoconstriction becoming more evident, but 5-HT is very quickly cleared from serum and the resulting fall is associated with the vasodilatation phase. The pain of vascular headaches is probably mediated by the trigemino-vascular system. An extracranial vasodilation results from stimulation of the trigeminal nerve. Stimulation of the Gasserian ganglion results in an increase in extracranial blood flow. It has been suggested that the spreading depression depolarises the perivascular sensory nerves of the vessels which make up the trigemino-vascular system. Increased permeability of cerebral arterioles follows, with leakage of plasma and a sterile inflammatory response in some. Pain receptors are activated.

Although Hannington's work showed a significant association between susceptibility to migraine and an increased platelet adhesiveness (**4.10**), we were unable to duplicate this finding in our own study. Whitehouse *et al.* (1989), were to able show that a significantly higher proportion of children with complicated migraine had increased platelets adhesiveness (at least six weeks from the last attack) indicating that if a child is susceptible to migraine and increased platelet adhesiveness, neurological signs are more likely to develop, perhaps through an exaggerated vasoconstriction-ischaemic phase.

The tension-like headache/migraine spectrum

It has been suggested by Waters and others that tension headache and migraine might be part of the same pathophysiological spectrum. A third of the children attending our clinics have headaches that fit the definition of migraine, a third have tension-like headache and a third have both. Individual children may describe one type of headache without associated gastrointestinal features, which may recur with gastrointestinal features; one defined as tension-like headache and the other as migraine. It is possible that brain dysfunction leading to activation of the trigeminal

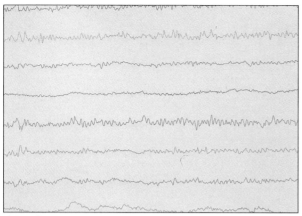

4.11 Dysrhythmic slow-wave discharge in migraine: a non-specific finding.

CT SCANNING FOR:

- Signs of raised intra-cranial pressure
- Under fives
- Short stature
- Complicated migraine

4.12 The indications for CT scanning.

nerve and its branches may give rise to tension-like headache, whereas if a spreading depression at a cortical level is activated, then migraineous phenomena may emerge, and if a platelet-release reaction occurs, complicated migraine may ensue. This, however, remains speculative and the coexistence of two common conditions cannot be discounted.

The investigation of children with headaches

The cornerstone of headache management remains good history-taking and physical examination. A skull x-ray may show signs of raised intracranial pressure, but only extremely rarely in the absence of clinical signs (*see* above). An EEG frequently shows slow-wave abnormality in people who have migraine and there may be a typical visual-evoked potential pattern, but these cannot be regarded as diagnostic tools (**4.11**). Orthodontic assessment is of value if malocclusion is suspected, and psychological assessment either for learning difficulties or family predicament is indicated at times from the history. CT scanning should be reserved for those children with signs of raised intracranial pressure, the under fives, short stature or complicated migraine (**4.12**). A doctor who assures a family that all is well and then sends the child for a skull X-ray is actually giving two messages (**Practice Point 4.1**)!

Practice Point 4.1

REMEMBER:
Investigation undermines reassurance.

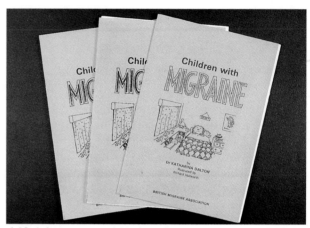

4.13 Information available from British Migraine Association.

The rational approach to treatment

Counselling children and their families

An explanation should be given to children and their families that migraine is a common condition affecting about one in 15 people on earth, and that it does not represent any damaging disease. Families should learn that it is a lifelong periodic disorder with good spells and bad spells, the good spells often lasting many months or years. Useful written advice is available from the British Migraine Association to complement advice given in the consultation (**4.13**).

Avoidance of triggers

Some children or their families notice that ingestion of certain dietary factors more often than not triggers a bout of migraine. Rest after a time of intense concentration may be another susceptible time. However, many children

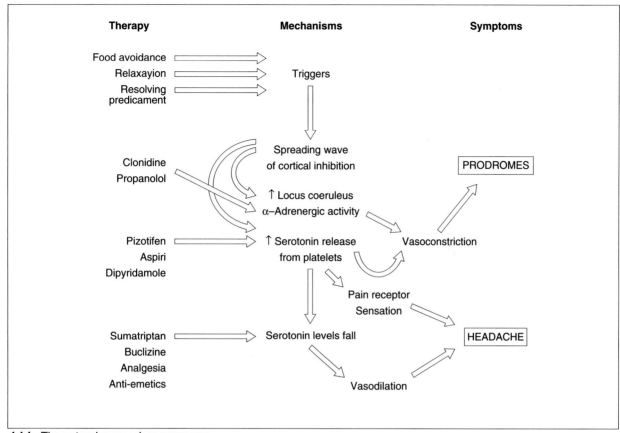

Therapy **Mechanisms** **Symptoms**

Food avoidance
Relaxayion → Triggers
Resolving
predicament

Clonidine
Propanolol
Spreading wave
of cortical inhibition → PRODROMES

↑ Locus coeruleus
α–Adrenergic activity → Vasoconstriction

Pizotifen → ↑ Serotonin release
Aspiri   from platelets
Dipyridamole

Pain receptor
Sensation

Sumatriptan → Serotonin levels fall → HEADACHE
Buclizine
Analgesia
Anti-emetics
Vasodilation

4.14 The rational approach to treatment.

learn they can tolerate these circumstances at other times without headache (**4.14**). One has to postulate that the brain needs to be in a certain susceptible state before a trigger will trigger. The situation needs assessing with some certainty before children are condemned to a life free of chocolate or cheese!

Resolution of predicament

If worry over parental disharmony, illness in a family member or a dead budgerigar is identified, appropriate advice should be given, with due emphasis placed on good communication between family members. Bullying or learning difficulties at school are common stressors for young people. Detailed assessment may need to be made with the help of the child psychiatry or clinical psychology team.

Relaxation therapy

Many young people from the age of eight years onwards find that the pragmatic approach of relaxation exercises helps to alleviate the problem. This often involves biofeedback techniques being learnt over two or three sessions to help them to control their headache rather than the headache controlling their own activity in life.

Medication

For the acute attack The first choice is simple analgesia such as paracetamol (20 mg/kg) taken as early in the headache as possible. This may not abate the bout completely, but is likely to bring useful relief. Children tend to know which of their headaches are likely to be more severe than others.

Anti-emetics are of value, although some children actually find relief in their headache once they have vomited. Metoclopramide can cause dystonic reactions, particularly in younger children. Domperidone is a useful alternative and prochlorperazine is usefully available in suppository form.

Buclizine or other sympathomimetic agents cause vasoconstriction and so lessen the pain associated with vasodilatation. Cafergot and other ergot-related preparations are best avoided in children; they can cause habituation and themselves cause nausea and vomiting quite frequently. Sumatriptan is a newly available drug undergoing trials in children, but seems to be relatively free of side effects and is likely to be of value during the acute attack.

Prophylactic therapy Beta-blockers are thought to

bring benefit by suppressing neuradrenergic activity. In adults, clonidine has not been shown to be any better than a placebo. Propanolol is of benefit, but the dose required is probably at least that to achieve beta-blockade.

Antiserotonin drugs The side effects from methysergide probably preclude its useage in children. Pizotofen is on the whole well tolerated, though causes troublesome drowsiness in some.

The calcium-channel blockers are currently not licensed for use in migraine in the UK and they are probably no more effective than other types of prophylaxis.

Summary of the clinical approach to childhood headaches

The first step is always to characterise the headache and to be confident that the paroxysmal phenomenon does not represent any underlying disease. This confidence should then be transmitted to children and parents by minimising investigations. Written information should complement what is said in clinics. Headache behaviour should be discouraged by identifying and relieving predicament. Therapy should be kept simple, and prophylaxis used only as a last resort.

Chapter 5: Epilepsy

Michael J. Noronha

Definition

An epileptic seizure is the result of a sudden excessive discharge of neurones in the brain resulting in an intermittent symptom complex characterised by repetitive stereotyped disturbances of movement, sensation, behaviour and/or consciousness depending on which part of the brain is involved. Epilepsy is the condition in which the seizures recur, usually spontaneously.

The incidence of epilepsy varies considerably with age: rates are greatest in early childhood, reach a low in early adult life, and rise again in elderly people. Most studies have found incidence rates of 20–70/100,000 per year (range 11–134/100,000 per year) and point prevalence rates of 4–10/1000 in the childhood population (range 1.5–30/1000).

Classification

Epilepsy can be classified in several ways, by clinical events (usually seizure type), electroencephalographic (EEG) changes, aetiology, pathophysiology, anatomy or age. The most generally accepted classification is that of the International League Against Epilepsy (1981) based on seizure type and EEG abnormalities: age and anatomical site are ignored (*see* **Table 5.1**, overleaf), although normal EEG appearances do alter with age (**5.1–5.3**) This classification has been revised to include recognised syndromes which take into account the following:

- Seizure type
- EEG abnormalities
- Age of onset
- Prognostic and aetiological factors.

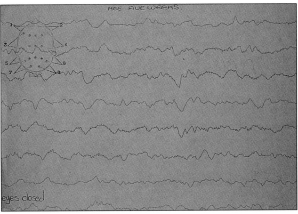

5.1 Normal EEG: 5-week-old infant showing cortical electrical activity predominantly in theta and delta frequency range.

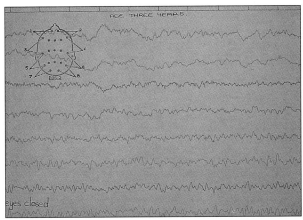

5.2 Normal EEG, 3-year-old: faster activities are now in evidence, with some alpha activity over the occipital regions.

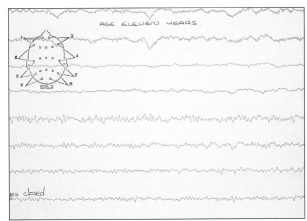

5.3 Normal EEG, 11-year-old. The EEG is well formed, and symmetrical and cortical electrical activity is mainly in the alpha range.

TABLE 5.1 Classification of Seizure Type (ILAE 1981)

1. Partial seizures
   A. Simple partial seizures
      1) With motor signs
      2) With somatosensory or special sensory hallucinations
      3) With autonomic symptoms and signs
      4) With psychic symptoms

   B. Complex partial seizures
      1) Simple partial onset followed by impairment of consciousness
      2) With impaired consciousness at onset

   C. Partial seizures evolving to generalised
      1) Simple partial seizures evolving to generalised
      2) Complex partial seizures evolving to generalised
      3) Simple partial seizures evolving to complex partial seizures, evolving to generalised

2. Generalised seizures
   A. 1) Absence seizures
       2) Atypical absence
   B. Myoclonic seizures
   C. Clonic seizures
   D. Tonic seizures
   E. Tonic–clonic seizures
   F. Atonic

3. Unclassified epileptic seizures

Most childhood epilepsy syndromes (see **Table 5.2**) are age dependent. It should be remembered that similar seizures may occur in different syndromes and that some syndromes are characterised by multiple seizure types. Whilst some epilepsy syndromes are highly specific and a few have been shown to have chromosomal markers, many represent broad concepts only. Furthermore, not all patients fit into the described syndromes.

Aetiology

Genetic factors play an important part in the primary generalised epilepsies. They may also act by increasing the convulsive susceptibility or lowering the convulsive threshold. The genetic predisposition by itself is rarely sufficient to induce clinical epilepsy and the occurrence

of seizures is usually a reflection of the interaction of genetic predisposition to cortical hyperexcitability with the impact of an exogenous insult of some sort. There is no specific pathology for epilepsy and it may occur with almost any pathological process affecting the brain or without any obvious anatomical, physiological or metabolic disorder.

The main epilepsy syndromes of childhood and adolescence are best considered according to age group (see **Table 5.2**).

Benign neonatal convulsions

The following two syndromes can be identified:

Benign familial neonatal seizures   These are rare and usually occur on the second or third day of life. Seizures are of a generalised clonic type, sometimes with apnoeic spells. The outcome is favourable with regard to psychomotor development, but one in seven of these infants develop epilepsy later. The disorder results from autosomal dominant inheritance.

Benign idiopathic neonatal convulsions (fifth day fits) These are uncommon, convulsions are of a clonic type, usually partial and/or apnoeic and occur round the fifth day of life, in an otherwise normal infant. Psychomotor development is normal, and there is no association with later epilepsy.

Pyridoxine dependency

This is rare. Onset may occur *in-utero* or after a few months of life but in over 90 % of cases, seizures start in the first 24 hours of life. The seizures are usually generalised and are refractory to all standard antiepileptic drugs (AEDs). Clinical response to intravenous pyridoxine is usually immediate, and normalisation of EEG may also be immediate but sometimes is delayed for up to four weeks. Most children show intellectual handicap despite early treatment. Doses of up to 100 mg of pyridoxine may be needed to terminate the seizures. A therapeutic trial of pyridoxine should be given whenever the disorder is suspected, and if the seizures are refractory to standard AEDs.

Myoclonic epilepsy in infancy

Severe Rare. The infant is often normal before developing generalised or focal myoclonic seizures, often in the first few months of life. The seizures are resistant to

---

TABLE 5.2 Syndromes of Epilepsy in Childhood and Adolescence

1. Neonatal

: Benign neonatal convulsions
: Myoclonic epilepsy
: Pyridoxine dependency

2. Infancy and early childhood (1 month–5 years)

: Myoclonic epilepsy—severe
: West's syndrome
: Lennox–Gastaut syndrome
: Febrile convulsions

3. Later childhood

: Typical absence epilepsy
: Benign epilepsy with occipital paroxysms
: Epilepsy with continuous spike-wave discharges during sleep
: Landau–Kleffner syndrome

4. Adolescence (11–16 years)

: Juvenile myoclonic epilepsy (Janz syndrome)
: Juvenile absence epilepsy
: Generalised tonic-clonic seizures on awakening

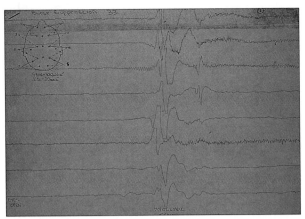

5.4 Generalised sharp- and slow-wave activity in association with a myoclonic jerk.

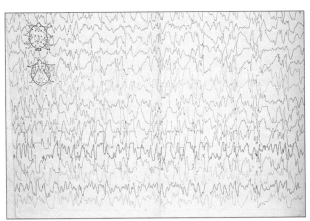

5.5 Hypsarrythmia: generalised high-voltage slow activity associated with spikes or sharp waves recorded in a 10-month-old boy having infantile spasms of recent onset.

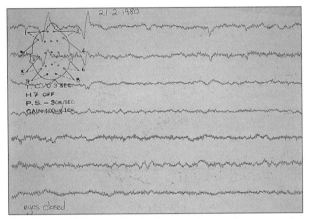

5.6 Repeat EEG recording in the same boy as **5.5** two weeks after treatment with corticotrophin.

treatment and the infants develop severe psychomotor retardation. More than half of them die by one year of age. The EEG manifestations include generalised and localised bursts of spike, or sharp and slow waves with episodic flattening of the background activity. Familial cases are common (**5.4**).

Benign Rare. Characterised by brief bouts of generalised myoclonus occurring in the first or second year of life in normal children who often have a familial history of epilepsy. The seizures are easily controlled with AEDs. Generalised tonic-clonic seizures may occur in adolescence.

West's syndrome (infantile spasms)

The full syndrome with an incidence of between 1:4000 and 1:6000 consists of:

1. Infantile spasms: may be flexor, extensor, head nods or myoclonic. Attacks can occur during waking or during sleep and often in series of up to 30 attacks in quick succession.

2. Mental retardation is almost invariable and usually severe.

3. Hypsarrhythmia on the EEG (**5.5 and 5.6**) a grossly-chaotic mixture of very high-amplitude slow waves with sharp waves and spikes which vary in amplitude, morphology, duration and site.

The incidence is estimated to be between 1:4000 and 1:6000 during infant years. Onset is between 3 to 12 months (peak between three and seven months) and is more common in boys.

Aetiology With the increasing sophistication of investigative techniques, the proportion of symptomatic cases has increased to over 85%. Common causes include hypoxic-ischaemic encephalopathy, metabolic disorders, pre- and post-natal meningoencephalitis, cerebral malformations (dysgenesis) and tuberose sclerosis. The remaining 15% are 'cryptogenic', with no obvious cause and in whom development is normal prior to the onset of the 'spasms'. The prognosis is poorer for the symptomatic group and also if the diagnosis and treatment are delayed. Corticosteroids (ACTH or prednisolone) tend to be the treatment of choice especially in cryptogenic cases. Sodium valproate and benzodiazepines and, more recently, vigabatrin, are alternative therapies. 'Spasms' usually disappear by five years of age whether or not treatment has been given. Complete recovery with cessation of seizures and normal intellectual level is confined to the cryptogenic group.

Lennox–Gastaut syndrome

This syndrome can be considered as an extension of West's syndrome, occurring between the ages of one and eight years with a peak incidence between three and five years. The syndrome consists of:

1. Epileptic seizures: atypical absences, axial tonic

seizures and sudden falls (atonic or myoclonic). Generalised tonic-clonic seizures and partial seizures may also occur.

2. Slowing in mental development, with up to 90 % showing moderate-to-severe mental handicap. Behavioural problems are often associated with it.

3. EEG (**5.7**) shows slow spike-wave abnormalities (1.5 to 2.5 Hz) in the awake state. In sleep, bursts of fast rhythms around 10 Hz are seen.

Aetiological factors are similar to those causing West's syndrome, which may precede the Lennox–Gastaut syndrome in 20 % of cases, with or without a seizure-free period. The seizures are refractory to most anticonvulsant drugs. The ketogenic diet is of use. Anterior corpus callosotomy may reduce or stop the atonic seizures.

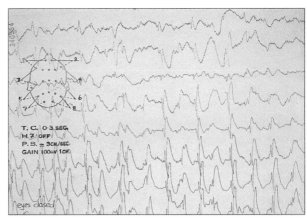

5.7 Generalised slow spike and wave complexes of 2 per second recorded in a child with Lennox-Gastaut syndrome.

Febrile seizures

Seizures associated with fever occur in 3 % of the population between the ages of three months and five years, without evidence of CNS infection (meningitis, encephalitis). The cause of the febrile illness is usually an upper respiratory tract virus infection. A family history of epilepsy or febrile seizures is obtained in 10 % of these children. It must be remembered that up to a third of children with febrile convulsions are actually having reflex-anoxic seizures with different implications for counselling and treatment.

Over 75 % of febrile seizures are 'simple', i.e. brief (lasting less than 15 minutes) and generalised with no neurological sequelae. The remainder are 'complicated', i.e. prolonged (even status epilepticus), may occur in series on the same day (clustering), are often focal or lateralised and may be followed by transient (Todd's paralysis) or permanent neurological features. Recurrence of febrile seizures occurs in one third of these children and a further one third of them will have a third or more seizures.

The risk of subsequent epilepsy is associated with:
• Family history of epilepsy in a parent or sibling.
• 'Complicated' febrile seizures.
• Neurodevelopmental progress abnormal prior to the convulsion.

Children with two of these risk factors have up to a 10 % risk of developing subsequent epilepsy (**Table 5.3,** overleaf).

Prophylactic anticonvulsant therapy is controversial and is usually not indicated as there is no certain evidence that prophylaxis would prevent a prolonged recurrence or the subsequent development of epilepsy. There is also the risk of inducing undesirable cognitive and behavioural side effects. Rectal diazepam may be used to terminate seizures in children who have serial or prolonged attacks.

All parents should be taught the first-aid management of a seizure, given the high risk of recurrence. They should also be taught about the natural history of the condition and its harmless nature (**5.8**).

Typical absence epilepsy ('Petit mal')

Childhood absence epilepsy is a primary generalised epilepsy with the following characteristics:

1. Onset before puberty (peak 4–8 years) and occurring in normal children.

2. The seizure is characterised by impairment of consciousness with abrupt onset and termination usually lasting between five and 15 seconds. Mild clonic movements involving eyelids (blinking at a rhythm of three per sec), lips and of the head may also occur. Attacks are usually very frequent throughout the day.

3. The EEG (**5.9**) shows bilateral, synchronous, symmetrical 3 Hz spike andwave complexes against a normal background activity.

Absence attacks are controlled in 80 % of children with sodium valproate, ethosuximide or clonazepam. In up to 40 % of cases, tonic-clonic seizures develop later. Typical absences rarely persist into adult life. Although children are usually intellectually and neurologically normal, schooling difficulties are not uncommon and may relate either to the child having frequent undetected absence attacks or to the drug therapy.

Benign partial epilepsy with centro-temporal spikes (benign Rolandic epilepsy)

The onset is between three and 13 years (peak 4–10 years) with a genetic predisposition and is commoner in boys. Seizure characteristics include unilateral parathesiae involving the face (lips, tongue and cheek) and/or unilateral tonic, clonic, or tonic-clonic convulsions affecting

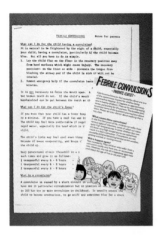

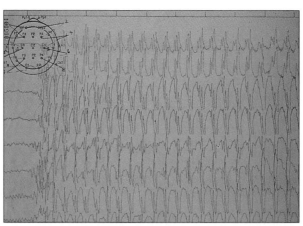

5.8 (left) Literature explaining counselling and treatment for children with febrile seizures.

5.9 (right) Generalised 3 per second spike and wave complexes.

TABLE 5.3 Risk Factors for Epilepsy Following Febrile Seizures

Factors: Partial, Prolonged, Cluster

	Risk of Epilepsy %	
	Nelson & Ellenberg*	Annegers[xy]
NO RISK FACTOR	1.0 (60 %)	2.4
TWO	2.0 (34%)	6–8
≥ TWO	10.0 (6%)	17–22

Note: figures represent percentage developing epilepsy (% in group with that number of risk factors)

* *Paediatrics* 1978

[xy] *NEJM* 1987

Partial epilepsy associated with all three risk factors generalised with >5 febrile seizures and family history.

face, lips, tongue, pharyngeal and laryngeal muscles resulting in speech arrest, dysarthria and drooling. Consciousness is preserved. Attacks last for one to two minutes and often wake the child from sleep. In about half of those with the disorder, generalised tonic-clonic seizures may develop and are usually nocturnal. The EEG (**5.10**) shows centro-temporal spikes in the interictal periods, especially during sleep, and these abnormalities tend to spread and/or shift from one side to the other. The response to carbamazepine is excellent. The seizures and EEG findings cease after puberty, whether or not anticonvulsants have been given. Intellectual status and neurological findings are normal.

Benign epilepsy of childhood with occipital paroxysms

This is an uncommon epilepsy syndrome, with onset usually in the first decade of life, characterised by seizures which include visual symptoms, akin to those in migraine, often followed by hemiclonic seizures or by automatisms. In a third of children, the seizures are followed by headache, often migrainous in character. The EEG features (**5.11**), which occur only during eye closure, consist of paroxysms of high-amplitude spike waves or sharp waves, occurring more or less rhythmically in the occipital and posterior temporal areas of one

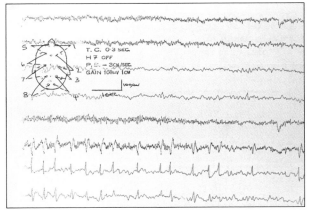

5.10 EEG: spikes and sharp waves localising in the left central region in a child with benign Rolandic seizures.

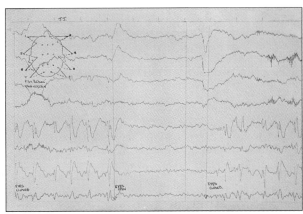

5.11 EEG: asymmetrical occipital spikes that spread anteriorly and present when eyes are closed but are suppressed when eyes are opened.

or both hemispheres. Seizures are usually controlled with anticonvulsant drugs. Prognosis is good with seizures usually remitting by adolescence.

Landau–Kleffner syndrome

Acquired epileptic dysphasia (*see* Chapter 3).

Juvenile-myoclonic epilepsy

The age of onset varies between eight and 26 years with a peak incidence between 12 and 18 years.

It is a primary generalised epilepsy characterised by myoclonic jerks which may be single or repetitive, affecting mainly the upper limbs with preserved consciousness. The myoclonic jerks predominantly occur shortly after waking or following sleep deprivation.

Generalised tonic-clonic seizures are also common, but partial seizures are experienced by some. Absence seizures (of adolescence) may also occur.

The EEG shows polyspike wave discharges accompanying clinical attacks of myoclonus and a photosensitive response is also common. The prognosis is excellent with a good response to sodium valproate, but relapses are common if the drug is withdrawn and the AED will have to continue into adult life. The gene for this disorder has been located on chromosome 6.

Juvenile absence epilepsy and generalised tonic-clonic seizures on awakening

Absences are infrequent and are associated with generalised tonic-clonic seizures on awakening in 80 % of cases. These epilepsies belong to the group of primary generalised epilepsies. There is a strong genetic predis-

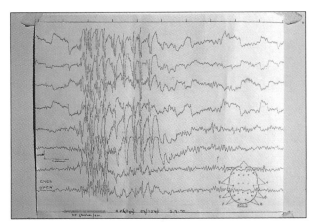

5.12 Marked photosensitive response with generalised polyspike and slow wave complexes observed at 25 flashes per second.

position and photosensitivity (**5.12**) is common. The EEG shows fast generalised spike and wave activity. Seizures are usually controlled with anticonvulsant therapy. Prognosis is favourable and intellectual deterioration does not occur.

Partial epilepsy

Partial seizures are common at any age. Their onset is limited to one part of the cerebral hemisphere (**5.13**). The site of neuronal hyperexcitability determines the symptoms experienced by the child (see **Table 5.4**), and the spread of the activity determines whether consciousness is lost or whether there is secondary generalisation.

Where partial seizures are resistant to anti-epileptic drugs, accurate siting of the focus may allow a surgical cure.

TABLE 5.4 The Spectrum of Partial Seizures

Simple partial seizures (awareness retained)

With motor signs— .	e.g. Focal motor (Jacksonian) Versive movement of head and eyes
Somatosensory or special sensory symptoms—	e.g. Visual Auditory
With autonomic symptoms With psychic symptoms—	e.g. Dysphasic Dysmnesic (deja vu, jamais vu)
Experiential—	e.g. Complex hallucinations

Complex partial seizures

Simple onset with impairment of awareness—with automation

Partial seizures with secondary generalisation

Differential diagnosis

The diagnosis of epilepsy is clinical and is based on a detailed description of events experienced by the child before, during and after the attack and, more importantly, on an eye witness account. If there is any doubt about the nature of the attacks, the clinician should resist the temptation to attach a label and commence anticonvulsant therapy and should rely on the passage of time and further description of symptomatic events to reach a firmer conclusion. Modern neurophysiological techniques allow definite evidence of a seizure disorder to be identified in the vast majority of cases (*see* **Practice Point 5.1**).

Conditions that are often confused with epilepsy

1. *Syncope.* The loss of consciousness is usually preceded by an aura of unsteadiness and nausea. The child usually slumps to the floor toneless, but on rare occasions convulsive movement may follow. Extreme pallor is the rule with cold and clammy peripheries. Recovery is usually quite rapid, although nausea or light-headedness may persist for a while. Teenagers are most predisposed to syncope, which often follows rising from a sitting position (orthostatic hypotension), standing in school assembly (particularly when it is hot), or pain. Exercise-induced syncope should be met with a full cardiological assessment for paroxysmal cardiac arrythmias. Some cases are familial.

2. *Cyanotic breath-holding attacks.* This is a toddler age-group phenomenon. Anger or frustration will lead many toddlers to hold their breath in inspiration. The resulting valsalva manoeuvre leads to falling venous return and blue breath-holding syncope.

3. *Reflexic anoxic (pallid syncopal) attacks.* Some children, usually again in the toddler age-group, have an inherently high vagaltone. They often have a first degree relative with a tendency to syncope. In response to a variety of stimuli, such as a fever, minor head trauma or

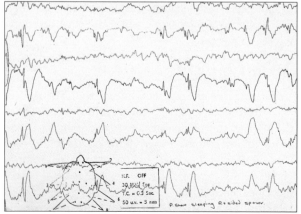

5.13 EEG—persistent slow-wave abnormality associated with spikes or sharp waves localising in the right mid- to anterior temporal region.

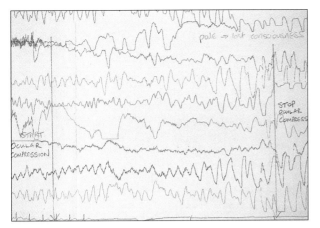 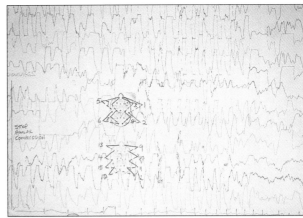

5.14 and 5.15 Ocular compression: shortly after commencement of ocular compression, there is absence of QRS complexes on the ECG channel. This is accompanied by facial pallor and loss of consciousness. ECG returns to normal shortly after stopping ocular compression, with reversal of clinical features.

cold ice-cream, vagal out-flow increases and syncope ensues. Convulsive movement may follow but the children are initially very pale. Ocular compression leads to significant bradycardia or asystole with reflex slowing of the EEG (**5.14 and 5.15**). Under strictly controlled conditions in the EEG laboratory this can be a useful diagnostic test if preceded by a good explanation for the parents. The natural history is for slow resolution of the problem as the children grow older.

4. *Sleep disorders/benign sleep myoclonus.* Night terrors, sleepwalking, hypnagogic hallucinations.

5. *Migraine*—especially 'basilar' migraine.

6. *Episodic vestibular disturbance*—'vestibular neuronitis'.

7. *Cardiac dysrhythmias*—supraventricular tachycardia, heartblock (*see* above).

8. *Masturbation.*

9. *Daydreaming.*

10. *Benign myoclonus of infancy.* Many young babies are seen to have jerky-like movements, particularly as they go off to sleep. This benign sleep-related disorder can be diagnosed from the history.

11. *Psychogenic attacks.* Non-epileptic seizures, pseudo-seizures, hyperventilation, panic attacks. Non-epileptic seizures are common, and are often mistaken for epilepsy, particularly because many of them bear a superficial resemblance to it. It has been estimated that up to 40 % of children referred with the label of epilepsy do not in fact have epilepsy.

There are many children with epilepsy who at some stage in their lives feign seizures, presumably in some way to try to understand a disorder and its effects for which they might otherwise have no cognisance, or to manipulate their environment. Their predicament should be identified and a solution sought.

PRACTICE POINT 5.1
Management of seizures

- Establish diagnosis;
- Define seizure type—partial or generalised;
- Define which epilepsy.

This allows parent information and a rational approach to drug therapy and investigation.

Investigations

1. Routine biochemical tests are not indicated except if the clinical features suggest a biochemical disorder such as hypoglycaemia or hypocalcaemia. Routine skull x-rays usually provide no useful information.

2. EEGs (**5.16 and 5.17**) provide valuable information that may:

   a. help to confirm the clinical diagnosis;

   b. help to obtain the classification of epilepsy, i.e. generalised or partial;.

   c. show changes that increase the suspicion of an underlying structural lesion: the presence of a focal slow-wave abnormality may suggest the necessity of some form of neuro-imaging.

3. Neuroradiological imaging: although CT brain scanning of unselected children with epilepsy shows a high incidence of abnormalities, the great majority of these abnormalities are non-specific and have no therapeutic implications. CT scan abnormalities are commonly found in children with focal rather than generalised seizures, focal neurological signs, and focal EEG abnormalities.

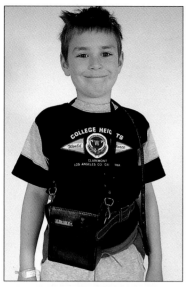

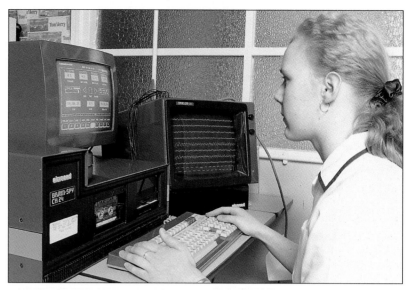

5.16 24-hour ambulatory cassette EEG recording: scalp electrodes applied and the cassette recorder supported by a harness.

5.17 Monitor and computer for the read-out of the 24-hour EEG tapes.

PRACTICE POINT 5.2
Drugs and Epilepsy

* Single drug;
* Sugar-free preparations;
* Work towards target dose in 3–4 weeks (to minimise side effects);
* Serum levels only when necessary (assessing compliance, possible side effects, poor response and target dose exceeded).

MRI scanning is capable of detecting subtle structural lesions not evident on a CT scan and is particularly useful in those children in whom surgery for epilepsy is being considered.

Treatment

The risk of recurrence after a single febrile seizure in children varies widely, but is probably about 50 %. It is usual practice not to treat a single seizure in Britain. Most children with epilepsy will achieve long-term freedom from seizures with anticonvulsant therapy, but the adverse effects of these drugs should not be discounted. In previously untreated children followed up prospec-

tively, the longer the seizures continue, the less likely it is for children to go into remission, and the intervals between untreated tonic-clonic seizures often decrease. Factors that may weigh in favour of withholding therapy include seizures that are infrequent and more than perhaps 12 months apart; occasional nocturnal seizures; and some types of seizure disorders, such as the benign partial epilepsies of childhood.

Once it has been decided to start treatment, the lowest dose of a single effective drug should be used (*see* **Practice Point 5.2**). First choice drugs and other useful agents are listed in **Table 5.5**. The dose of a drug should be increased until there is satisfactory control of seizures or until the maximum tolerated level has been achieved before abandoning the drug and resorting to another AED. Polypharmacy should be avoided, as the risk of undesirable side effects is greatly increased, and the therapeutic benefits minimal.

Toxicity of anticonvulsant drugs

These may be:
1. Acute and dose-related. This is usually a non-specific encephalopathy characterised by nystagmus, ataxia, dysarthria, confusion and drowsiness related to toxic drug levels. Impairment of behaviour and cognitive function in children may be caused by any AED but commonly with phenobarbitone, phenytoin and benzodiazepines. These side effects usually resolve with reduction of the dose.
2. Idiosyncratic reactions. Mild maculo-papular rashes are not uncommon with carbamazepine, phenytoin and

TABLE 5.5 AEDs for Different Seizure Types

Seizure type	First line	Second line
Partial seizures		
Simple partial Complex partial Secondarily generalised	Carbamazepine Valproate	Vigabatrin Gabapentin Lamotrigine Phenytoin Phenobarbitone Clobazam
Generalised seizures		
Tonic-clonic Tonic, clonic	Valproate Carbamazepine Clobazam	Lamotrigine Vigabatrin Phenobarbitone Phenytoin
Absence	Valproate Ethosuximide	Lamotrigine Clonazepam Acetazolamide
Atypical absences	Valproate Clonazepam Clobazam	Lamotrigine Carbamazepine Phenobarbitone Phenytoin Acetazolamide
Myoclonic	Valproate Clonazepam	Lamotrigine Phenobarbitone

barbiturates. More severe exfoliative eruptions or the Stevens–Johnson syndrome are rare. Involvement of the haemopoietic system with neutropaenia, agranulocytosis, aplastic anaemia and lymphadenopathy has been reported in association with AEDs. Acute fatal liver failure has been associated with sodium valproate, more commonly in children under three who also have a neurological handicap.

3. Chronic toxicity. This can affect any system, and complications are numerous. Important ones in childhood relate to impairment of memory and cognitive function, hyperactivity and behavioural disturbances, hepatocellular enzyme induction, rickets, particularly in severely retarded children on deficient diets, gum hyper-trophy and coarse facial features (particularly with phenytoin), and teratogeneticity.

Stopping anticonvulsant therapy

As AEDs have been associated with various acute and chronic side effects, and in particular their subtle effect on behaviour and cognitive function, there is a strong argument for withdrawing AEDs in children who have had a significant period of remission (free of seizures for two years or longer). The AEDs should be withdrawn gradually, preferably over a period of months. The overall risk of relapse is about 20 % in children. The factors that have an adverse effect on the prognosis for cessation of epileptic seizures include partial rather than pri-

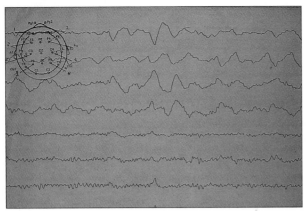

5.18 Persistent slow-wave abnormality over the right hemisphere suggesting an underlying abnormality.

mary generalised seizures, symptomatic rather than idiopathic epilepsies, an episode of status epilepticus, increasing frequency and duration of seizures before treatment or remission, and some specific epilepsy syndromes.

The role of surgery in the management of epilepsy

Criteria for surgical treatment of epilepsy include:
1. Undoubted epilepsy.
2. Resistance to appropriate drugs in adequate dose given over a reasonable period of time.
3. Psycholoigcal dysfunction consequent on the seizure disorder. Surgical approaches include:
1. Resection of a discrete zone of epileptogenic tissue, as in anterior temporal lobectomy. This is applicable only to patients with partial seizures arising from a single localised area of brain which is both structurally and functionally abnormal (**5.18**) and which can be removed without causing a serious deficit.
2. Removal of a large mass of grossly dysfunctional brain, as in hemispherectomy. This is very effective in patients in whom one hemisphere has been virtually destroyed and, provided the insult occurred early in life, no increase in neurological deficit results.
3. Interruption of the pathways of seizure propagation, as in callosotomy. This is a palliative measure to prevent secondarily generalised tonic-clonic or atonic seizures leading to repeated injuries.

Surgery for epilepsy can follow only careful electrophysiological, neuroradiological and psychological assessment. This necessarily entails the involvement of an experienced team in a regional centre.

Status epilepticus

This may be convulsive or non-convulsive. Status epilepticus is defined as recurring seizures, without recovery of consciousness, for 30 minutes or more.

Convulsive status is a medical emergency with a significant morbidity and mortality. It may develop in the course of established epilepsy or as the initial manifestation of epilepsy. Prognosis is related to the aetiology and the time interval between the onset of seizures and the start of effective therapy. Cerebral damage may be due to hypoxic-ischaemic insult secondary to the inability of the cerebral circulation to provide adequate nutrients for the increased demands of the continuous neuronal activity.

The mainstay of therapy is to maintain cerebral perfusion pressure, oxygenation, and to control continuing seizure discharge with AEDs. Cardio-respiratory protection is important, as hypoxia is common and sudden respiratory collapse may occur. Admission to an intensive care unit is desirable as intubation and artificial respiration may be necessary if the seizures persist. The systolic blood pressure should be monitored and supported. Where the period of coma is prolonged or seizures continue, the intracranial pressure should be monitored and controlled (*see* **Table 5.6** and Chapter 7).

Anticonvulsant therapy should be given with two aims: firstly toobtain immediate suppression of seizures, and secondly to provide long-term anticonvulsant protection. An immediate intravenous bolus of diazepam or clonazepam should be given to control the seizure and this is often all that is needed. If intravenous diazepam fails to control the seizures, or if they recur after initial suppression, then an infusion of intravenous phenobarbitone should be given over a period of 5 to 10 minutes. If the seizure continues relentlessly, which is rare, it may be necessary to use intravenous thiopentone anaesthesia. EEG monitoring is advisable in refractory status epilepticus, especially as, in an anaethetised, paralysed and ventilated patient, this may be the only way of detecting epileptic activity.

TABLE 5.6 Management of Status Epilepticus

A. Immediate management
1. Assessment of vital functions—establish i.v. line: blood sampling (glucose, urea & electrolytes, anticonvulsant drug levels).
2. I.V. diazepam (0.25–0.5 mg/kg not faster than 2 mg/min). Rectal diazepam 0.5 mg/kg may be used if i.v. line is not established; or i.v. lorazepam (0.05 mg/kg over 2.5 mins).

B. Second stage
3. Monitoring of vital functions and correction of metabolic disturbances if present. Tracheal intubation if necessary.
4. Investigation of possible cause of S.E., especially metabolic and infections.
5. I.V. administration of pyridoxine 100 mg (under 2 years of age).
6. Treatment of cause, if possible (meningitis, metabolic).

C. Third stage
7. If seizures are not controlled by i.v. or rectal diazepam in 5–10 mins, can repeat dose of diazepam or proceed to:
8. I.V. phenobarbitone (loading dose 15–20 mg/kg). (N.B.—this is preferably done under close supervision in an intensive care unit.)

D. Fourth stage
9. If the above measures fail, then administer general anaesthesia with i.v. thiopentone. Neuromuscular blockade may be necessary for maintaining ventilation. EEG monitoring will be necessary.

Chapter 6: Central Nervous System Infection

Michael A. Clarke, Richard W. Newton, W. St. Clair Forbes

Central nervous system sepsis and neurological disorders

Central nervous system (CNS) sepsis is to be considered in most acute neurological disorders, particularly when children present with coma and/or seizures. At the time of presentation, CNS bacterial infection frequently cannot be excluded with confidence, and should always be treated if suspected without waiting for laboratory confirmation. Failure to treat infection whilst laboratory results are awaited can result in chronic disability or mortality.

Bacterial meningitis

Bacterial meningitis occurs most frequently in the neonate, in infants and younger children, but sporadic cases particularly of meningococcal and less frequently pneumococcal meningitis are seen through all age groups (*see* **Table 6.1**). In the neonatal period, coliforms and Group B streptococcus are the commonest pathogens. Listeria monocytogenes is becoming increasingly common but there is no quick sensitive method for laboratory diagnosis and gram staining may be unreliable. In the neonatal period in particular the signs of meningitis are not specific but meningitis must always be considered in a neonate with seizures.

When normal-term infants become ill on the postnatal ward or in the first few days at home, septicaemia and less frequently meningitis due to Lancefield Group B beta-haemolytic streptococcus may be the cause. If diagnosis is delayed, death may rapidly ensue.

Outside the neonatal period, *Haemophilus influenzae* and *Neisseria meningitidis* are the commonest causative organisms. In the infant and child, seizures and impaired consciousness may be presenting features. Neck stiffness may be absent in deep coma. Careful inspection for the petechial rash of meningococcaemia (**6.1 and 6.2**) must be made in any child with fever and headache. One hundred and ten children died from meningococcal disease in 1991 in the UK (Begg, 1992); the case fatality rate was 5–10 %. This has not fallen for 30 years, in spite of the availability of effective antibiotic treatment. Mortality from meningococcal disease is reduced (particularly in the most severely ill) if parenteral pencillin or chloramphenicol is given before admission to hospital. This does not alter the rate of microbiological diagnosis that can still be made; the rate of positive nasopharyngeal swabs for meningococci is not affected by administration of antibiotics before admission.

Organisms can be identified by Gram staining and

TABLE 6.1 Meningitis: Commonest Infecting Organism and Age (in order of frequency)

Neonate	One month – 4 years	4 years – 14 years
Coliforms	Haemophilus influenzae	Nesseria meningitidis
Group B streptococcus	Nesseria meningitidis	Streptococcus pneumoniae
Streptococcus pneumoniae	Streptococcus pneumoniae	Haemophilus influenzae
Listeria		

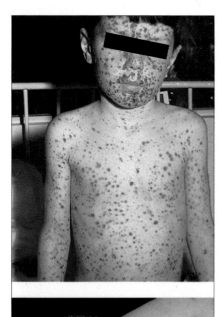

6.1 and 6.2 Petechial rash of meningococcaemia (**6.1, top, and 6.2, bottom**) (Figure 12.21 A & B from Zitelli, *Atlas of Paediatric Physical Diagnosis*, 2nd edition, Wolfe, 1992 (reprinted with permission).

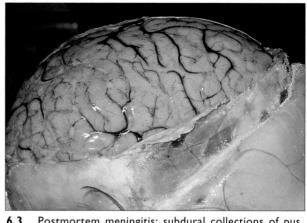

6.3 Postmortem meningitis: subdural collections of pus. Note striking brain swelling.

culture of CSF (**Table 6.2**) in at least 80 % of children with bacterial meningitis. Administration of antibiotics before admission to hospital makes this less likely to be successful but does not alter the degree of pleocytosis, or the protein or glucose level in the cerebrospinal fluid. In the neonatal period, meningitis may not be accompanied by a CSF pleocytosis. It is wise, where meningitis is suspected but not proven, to await CSF culture results before discontinuing antibiotics. Where cultures are negative, antibiotics should continue for 72 hours. This decision will be influenced by the possibility of sepsis outside the CNS.

Increasingly sophisticated methods of CSF bacterial antigen detection are available when a lumbar puncture has not been performed as an initial investigation. Techniques such as counter-current immunoelectrophoresis and latex particle agglutination are of value but should not override clinical judgment. Outside the neonatal period, only 5 % of the normal population have a single polymorph per ml of CSF, and a white-cell count of greater than six per mm^3 or above is abnormal. In the case of a traumatic tap, it is said that the CSF white-cell count increases by one white cell for every 700–800 red cells, although it is not wise to interpret

such guidelines without reference to the clinical situation.

Pyogenic meningitis is almost invariably associated with raised intracranial pressure (**6.3**) and this has important implications for the timing of lumbar puncture and for management. The clinical contraindications to lumbar puncture are detailed in Chapter 7. If there is any doubt about the safety of lumbar puncture being carried out at presentation, it should not be done.

In children who are severely ill with meningitis, many of the signs at presentation may be the result of raised intracranial pressure: abnormal posture, seizures, impaired consciousness, focal signs, and cranial nerve abnormalities. Papilloedema is rarely present in the acute situation and fontanelle tension is variable.

Raised pressure in the early stages of meningitis results from cerebral oedema or obstructive hydrocephalus. Cranial CT scans are usually but not invariably abnormal when intracranial pressure is elevated. The dangers of coning in meningitis are real. In a recent study of infantile meningitis in England and Wales (Louvois *et al.*, 1991), 18 children (including four neonates) were reported to have coned after lumbar puncture. Lumbar puncture should not be done until the matter of raised intracranial pressure has been considered and managed.

The management of meningitis entails the sterilisation of the CNS, the reduction of the effects of vasculitis and the control of raised intracranial pressure. Recommendations for antibiotic treatment depend on the organisms present, and their sensitivities. The appropriate initial antibiotic therapy of bacterial meningitis for children at different ages where a definite bacteriological diagnosis has not been made is outlined in **Table 6.3** (overleaf). Household members who have intimate contact with the index case should have prophylactic treatment with Rifampicin (*see* **Table 6.4**, overleaf).

TABLE 6.2 Meningitis: Diagnosis by CSF Findings

	Appearance	Cells	Glucose mmol/l	Protein mg/100 mls
Normal	Clear	0–5 (lymphs)	2.2–4.4	15–40
Bacterial	Turbid	100–>20,000	<0.5–1.5	100–200 Higher in neonates or with 'block'
Tuberculous meningitis	Clear or opalescent	30–500 (early PMN—later lymphs)	0–2.0	Up to 300 or more
Viral	Clear	25–500	>2.2	50–100
Guillain–Barré syndrome	Clear	Normal	Normal	Slight to marked increase
Botulism	Clear	Normal	Normal	Normal
Fungal	Clear	0–500 (lymphs)	1.0–2.0	100–500
'Bloody tap'	Pink or red Clears in successive tubes	As in peripheral blood	Normal	Normal to slightly elevated
Subarachnoid haemorrahge	Grossly bloody supernatant xanthochromic	As in peripheral blood	Normal to slightly elevated	Normal to slightly elevated
Subdural haematoma	Clear or xanthochromic	Normal to 20 (PMN)	Normal	Normal to moderate increase
Cerebral abscess	Clear	10–60 (lymphs)	Normal	20–80
CNS tumour	Clear	Occasionally up to 500 (PMN or lymphs)	Normal	Normal to slight increase: markedly high if 'block'

The effectiveness of antibiotic treatment in reducing mortality and morbidity from bacterial meningitis has led to the consideration of other factors leading to CNS damage and their treatment. The need to monitor and control raised intracranial pressure has been mentioned. The destructive nature of the inflammatory response and the way it damages nervous tissue has been the subject of some study. The initial event in bacterial meningitis is disruption of the blood-brain barrier (which can be measured by determining the ratios of the concentration of CSF to serum albumin). Impairment of the blood-brain barrier results in increased brain water-cerebral oedema. Following this, there is an influx of polymorphs with a reduction in glucose, elevation of lactate, indicating

TABLE 6.3 Treatment of Bacterial Meningitis: Organisms Not Yet Known

Neonate	Ampicillin 100 mg/kg/day for first week, then 200 mg/kg/day) PLUS Cefotaxime (100 mg/kg/day for first week, then 200 mg/kg/day)

Infants (0–3 months)	Ampicillin
	<1 week 150 mg/kg/day in 2 divided doses; >1 week, 200 mg/kg/day in 3–4 divided doses
	    PLUS
	Cefotaxime
	<1 week, 100 mg/kg/day in 2 divided doses; >1 week, 200 mg/kg/day in 3–4 divided doses
	    OR
	Ceftriaxone
	<4 weeks, 50 mg/kg/day as single dose; 1–3 months, 100 mg/kg/day as loading dose, then 80 mg/kg/day thereafter

>3 months	Cefotaxime 200 mg/kg/day (maximum 12 g/day) in 3–4 divided doses OR Ceftriaxone 100 mg/kg/day (maximum 2–4 g/day) as a loading dose, then 80 mg/kg/day thereafter

TABLE 6.4 Rifampicin Prophylaxis of Meningitis

Meningococcal disease	**Rifampicin**
Infants less than 1 month old	5 mg/kg/dose bd for 2 days
Infants and children	10 mg/kg/dose bd for 2 days
Adults	600 mg bd for 2 days
Hip disease	
Infants less than 1 month	10 mg/kg/dose od for 4 days
Infants and children	20 mg/kg/dose od for 4 days
Adults	600 mg od for 4 days

anaerobic metabolism, and probable mitochondrial dysfunction (maintenance of blood-brain barrier is an active process) and the appearance in the CSF of tissue enzymes, such as keratin, phophokinase, and lactate dehydrogenase indicating cellular damage. Animal studies of meningitis have shown that rapid bacteriolysis resulting from antibiotic administration increases the intensity of the inflammatory response. The complement cascade is induced by bacterial products such asendotoxin and is initiated by cytokines, including prostaglandins, tumour necrosis factor and interleukin I. This work has led to the study of the possible therapeutic benefits of steroid therapy; calcium channel blockers have yet to be assessed.

The Meningitis Working Party report (1992) indicates that children with haemophilus meningitis may benefit from the use of early adjunct therapy with dexamethasone, particularly in the reduction of deafness. The case for its use in pneumococcal meningitis is minimal and there is very limited information available for meningococcal disease. Animal studies (and some evidence from human studies) show that steroids reduce brain oedema, the inflammatory response and degree of blood-brain barrier dysfunction. Further study is needed but it seems reasonable to administer dexamethasone (0.15 mg/kg) before the first dose of antibiotics in suspected meningitis.

Monoclonal IgM antibodies (centoxin) produced by meningococci, though expensive, showed promise as a treatment for the disseminated intravascular coagulation found in overwhelming infection, but have now been withdrawn.

Complications and prognosis of meningitis

Though nearly 40 % of children have neurological abnormalities one month after bacterial meningitis (**Table 6.5**), most have resolved by a year later. The commonest long-term neurological sequel of bacterial meningitis is sensori-neural hearing loss affecting 10 % of children. However, 4 % of children are left with multiple neurological deficits and 7 % have at least one or more late seizures not associated with fever. Morbidity and mortality are much higher in neonatal meningitis. Key factors in reducing morbidity and mortality are the early use of appropriate antibiotics, the availability of paediatric intensive care, management of raised intracranial pressure and the management of the inflammatory response. It has become standard practice to restrict fluid intake in the early stages of treatment to attempt to prevent cerebral oedema and to prevent complications from anticipated inappropriate antidiuretic hormone production (shown by fluid overload and hyponatraemia). Fluid

TABLE 6.5 Complications of Meningitis

Acute
— Raised intracranial pressure
— Inappropriate ADH secretion
— Seizures

Subacute
— Subdural empyema
— Cerebral abscess
— Subdural collections
— Seizures

Long-term
— Deafness
— Hydrocephalus
— Epilepsy
— Cognitive impairment
— Physical handicap

restriction may not be appropriate. Serum osmolality is raised on admission in children with bacterial meningitis but it becomes significantly lower 24 hours later in children given maintennance **plus** replacement fluid when compared to children who have fluid restriction. These findings suggest serum osmolality levels are appropriate for the degree of the hypovolaemia.

Complications requiring treatment may occur in the days or weeks following presentation of bacterial meningitis. The CT finding of an increase in extracerebral fluid, with or without ventricular enlargement, may occur for a number of reasons. It can be difficult to distinguish communicating hydrocephalus from rapidly progressing atrophy due to neuronal necrosis. Periventricular lucencies (usually thought to indicate raised intracranial pressure with transependymal egress of CSF) may be present in both situations. Clearly, it is not appropriate to shunt if the cause of ventricular enlargement is brain atrophy. Intracranial pressure monitoring may be necessary. Severe necrosis of neural tissue is most likely to occur in the neonate and young infant, and serial measurement of the head circumference and the development of overriding cranial sutures may provide a guide as to the appropriate course of action.

Extracerebral fluid collections and raised intracranial

pressure may also result from the development of subdural collections. An expectant approach is usually best, but care mustbe taken that subdural empyema is not present, in which case the subdural fluid is infected. This is found in 10 % of fluid collections.

Ventriculitis (infection of ventricular system) and ependyma are particularly likely to occur in neonatal meningitis. Cerebrospinal fluid taken via the lumbar route may be sterile, though ventriculitis is in fact present. Treatment is contentious, but intraventricular antibiotics may not be necessary with the third generation cephalosporins which have good CSF penetration.

Aseptic meningitis

The child with subacute or chronic meningitis who fails to respond to adequate antibiotic therapy presents the paediatrician with a worrying and perplexing problem. Most of these children will present with fever, nuchal rigidity and headache, probably after an insidious prodromal illness of general malaise and anorexia. The CSF initially may show pleocytosis changing to lymphocytosis within a few hours or a day or two. Antibiotic therapy for at least 48 hours is appropriate until cultures are shown to be negative, along with supportive therapy with fluids, analgesia and antipyretics.

The enteroviruses account for 80 % of all cases of aseptic meningitis in American studies. The UK picture is similar in infancy, but the mumps virus is a more common pathogen in the one to nine year old age group. This may change with the advent of mumps, measles, and rubella vaccination, which itself has been implicated in producing aseptic meningitis. Other common causes include herpes simplex, adenovirus, measles, cytomegalovirus, rubella, varicella, Epstein–Barr, influenza, parainfluenza and rotavirus. The Epstein–Barr and Coxsackie virus in particular may run a subacute or chronic course. The illness may be accompanied by a rash which can be specific. Convulsions are rare in the absence of a pre-existing seizure disorder. Generally, younger children are irritable and resent handling, whilst older children complain of myalgia, photophobia and retrobulbar pain with evidence of nuchal rigidity in only about 50 %.

It is generally accepted that after 12 hours of illness, almost all (97 %) of the cellular response in CSF will be lymphocytic and that antibiotics can be withheld if the patient seems othewise well. CSF sugar may be low in up to 20 % of patients and CSF protein may be increased in up to 50 %. Laboratory tests for bacteria (*see* above) should be negative but be complemented by specific viral culture of CSF and other sites, including throat, faeces and urine, as well as the measurement of serum viral-antibody titres. Raised

alpha-interferon levels usually indicate a viral meningoencephalitic illness, but slightly raised levels may also occur in bacterial infection. Viral identification can shorten antibiotic courses and reduce time spent in hospital.

After 48 hours of treatment the main alternative diagnoses toconsider with a sterile polymorphic or pleocytic CSF are partially treated bacterial or tuberculous meningitis (TBM). Partially treated meningitis is particularly likely if there is a history of a course of oral antibiotics given for an intercurrent infection. This treatment may render microbacterial techniques unreliable, and it is reasonable at this stage to stop all antibiotics in order to clarify the situation. If deterioration ensues, antibiotic therapy may be reinstituted.

Tuberculous meningitis

Tuberculosis (TB) of the CNS occurs in all ethnic groups; diagnosis and treatment are difficult. Late diagnosis carries an associated high morbidity and mortality. The incidence of TB of the CNS is increasing in part as a result of the Acquired Immuno-deficiency Syndrome becoming more common. In children, TB of the CNS is often a complication of primary infection with or without miliary spread. TB of the CNS should be considered in any child with a subacute history of fever, headache, seizures, vomiting, behavioural change or impairment of consciousness. Respiratory symptoms may or may not be present. It is important to note that tuberculous meningitis (TBM) results from Rich's focus produced in an intensive inflammatory response, particularly at the base of the brain. There is an associated vasculitis which may result in convulsions, cranial nerve palsies, dyskinesia, hemiparesis, or signs of a mild radiculopathy.

The CSF sugar is typically low, but may be normal in up to 10% of patients. When the ratio of blood to CSF sugar is greater than 2:1 in the presence of a lymphocytic meningitis, TBM must be given very serious consideration. The Mantoux test may remain negative for some weeks due to anergy following primary exposure; the combination of lobar consolidation on a chest x-ray (**6.4**) and aseptic meningitis is a particularly strong indication for anti-tuberculous therapy. The decision to treat is rather easier when the x-ray shows classical miliary mottling, or examination of the fundi reveals choroidal tubercles.

Cranial CT scan with contrast is essential for diagnosis; tuberculoma may not be evident on an unenhanced scan. Lumbar puncture may be negative for culture of acid-fast bacilli, this diagnosis being made only on ventricular drainage. Acid-fast bacilli have to be searched for assiduously in CSF specimens. The use of the polymerised chain reaction to detect antigen or metabolic products of tubercle bacilli shows promise.

6.4 (left) An abnormal chest x-ray and meningitis suggests tuberculosis or mycoplasma.

6.5 (right) Severe TB meningitis— ventricular drain in situ to aid control of intracranial pressure.

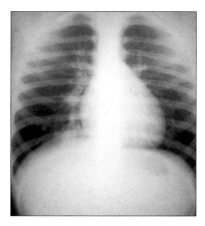

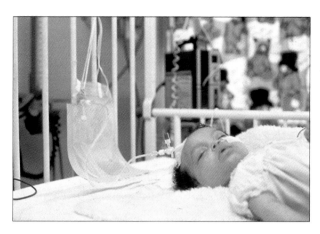

Treatment of tuberculous meningitis involves administration for at least a year of two anti-tuberculous therapeutic agents that penetrate the blood-brain barrier and tuberculomas. Isoniazid and Pyrazinamide are the mainstay of continued treatment during this period. Steroids are of value when there is progressive neurological disorder or deteriorating consciousness, once appropriate anti-tuberculous chemotherapy is begun (**6.5**).

Other causes When a child with lymphocytic CSF does not improve as expected, a full reappraisal of the history and findings is appropriate, and thoughts on differential diagnosis should be broadened. Possibilities are rarer bacteria (*see* below) an immune paresis with opportunistic infection, a fistula, autoimmune disease or toxins.

Five per cent of all children with acute lymphoblastic leukaemia have CNS disease at presentation. The CNS is the most common site for relapse. Usually-associated signs of bone marrow failure (anaemia, thrombocytopenia, recurrent infection) will aid diagnosis. Rarely, primary CNS lymphoma may present in this way. Itis essential that bone-marrow investigation is performed before any use of steroids.

In an immunocompromised or severely debilitated child, fungal infection may spread to the CNS from specific skin or oral lesions.Stains for fungi, swabs, cultures, antibody titres and urine microscopy should identify the cause. When the degree of debility is severe, and particularly when there is marked and rapid wasting of muscles, it may justified to administer a course of amphotericin.

Neurological manifestations of nervous system infection with *Borrelia burgdorferi* (a spirochaete) are protean. It is a multisystem disorder affecting the skin, joints, nervous system and cardiovascular system. Borrelia inhabits the gut of the *Ixodes* tic. The tic is widespread throughout the UK but found in greater numbers in woodland.

Man is infected by the bite of a tic producing (in most cases) a slowly enlarging patch of erythema (ery-

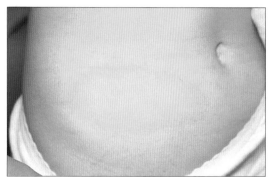

6.6 Lyme disease: Erythema chronicum migrans . (Reprinted with permission from Cohen, *Atlas of Paediatric Dermatology*, Wolfe, 1993.)

thema chronicum migrans) (**6.6**). A non-specific flu-like illness may occur at this stage. These symptoms may be followed by cranial poly- or mononeuropathies, aseptic meningitis, transverse myelitis, post-infectious polyneuritis and encephalitis. A history of skin lesion or a tic bite is not always obtained. Diagnosis is difficult, and serological studies may not be positive at the time of neurological presentation. Specific IgM is the most valuable serological test and intrathecal synthesis of specific antibodies which immunoblot the spirochaetal antigen may also (in due course) be helpful diagnostically. Treatment in childhood is usually with penicillin or erythromycin. Nervous system disease must be treated aggressively as chronic encephalopathy may ensue. There is increasing evidence in neuroborreliosis that intravenous cephalosporins are superior to penicillin, because of the latter's relatively poor penetration.

The protozoon *Toxoplasma gondii* may cause meningitis in immuno-suppressed children. It is usually accompanied by lymphadenopathy. The histology of an affected node may give the diagnosis, as may the presence in the serum of specific IgM. Treatment with sulphonamides, pyramethamine or spiramycin is effective.

Leptospirosis results from contact with infected animal urine (mainly rats), usually in contaminated water or

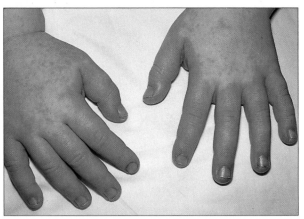

6.7 Kawasaki disease: swollen erythematous hands, often with desquamation. (Reprinted with permission from Zitelli, *Atlas of Paediatric Physical Diagnosis, 2nd edition*, Wolfe, 1992.)

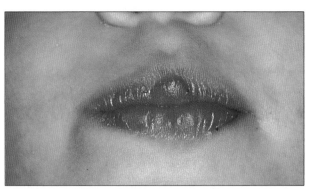

6.8 Kawasaki disease: characteristic clinical findings include erythema and fissuring of the lips. (Reprinted with permission from Cohen, *Atlas of Paediatric Dermatology*, Wolfe, 1993.)

from farm machinery. After an incubation period of 10 days, the illness typically produces a high fever, sweating, headaches, conjunctival suffusion, muscle tenderness and pain with meningitis. Cardiac or renal failure may occur, with spontaneous improvement after three weeks. Diagnosis is based on cultured blood and urine and rising antibody titres after the first week. Penicillin and tetracycline may be ineffective clinically, though they remain the treatment of choice along with supportive therapy.

Mycoplasma pneumoniae is reported to cause CNS disease in 7 % of those admitted to hospital with associated upper or lower respiratory tract illness. A meningoencephalitis which may be severe is the commonest result, but polyneuropathy or transverse myelitis may also occur.

Neurobrucellosis may also cause meningoencephalitis. It is usually contracted from animals known to harbour the organism, or from the ingestion of unpasteurised milk products. Sweating, abdominal pain, fever, hepatosplenomegaly and arthritis commonly accompany the illness. Axonal polyneuropathy has been reported. Brucella melitensis may be isolated from CSF and there may be rising antibody titres. Tetracycline, streptomycin, and rifampicin have all been used in combination for children, usually with a full recovery.

Kawasaki disease or mucocutaneous lymph node syndrome is a relatively uncommon disorder. It predominates in the under-fives and, though uncertain, infective agents have been implicated in its aetiology. Presentation is with persistent fever, characteristic skin rashes with desquamation of the extremities (**6.7 and 6.8**), mucosal and buccal involvement and lymphadenopathy. It may be associated with aseptic meningitis though rarely is an isolated feature. The association of aseptic meningitis with an auto-immune vasculitis is dealt with in Chapter 9.

Aseptic meningitis may follow the administration of certaindrugs. These include, OKT3 (in renal transplantation), immunoglobulin (in idiopathic thrombocytopenic purpura and Kawasaki disease), isoniazid, sulfamethiazole, co-trimoxasole andazathioprine. A cellular response has also been reported in lead poisoning, though meningism is rare and reduced conscious level common.

It must also be remembered that migraine at times leads to a cellular response in the CSF, particularly in complicated migraine. If the hemiplegia is fleeting, the child's presentation at hospital may be with headache and the picture of an aseptic meningitis. Migraine may also present with fever, neck stiffness and aseptic meningitis. Although uncommon, recognition of this syndrome should help to avoid unnecessary invasive investigations.

The clinician needs to be aware that aseptic meningitis may well be the presenting feature of a number of less common, but important conditions specified here. While the diagnosis is being investigated, due attention should be paid to the child's parents, who will also be feeling worried and perplexed. Adequate time needs to be allocated to inform them of investigation and treatment strategy at each stage, in order to maintain their confidence at a time when the medical team themselves may be feeling unsure.

Recurrent or chronic meningitis

Recurrent bacterial meningitis can result from anatomic alabnormalities of the inner ear or cranio-vertebral axis. The causes are acquired (following trauma) or

6.9 Mid-line fistula —predisposing to recurrent meningitis.

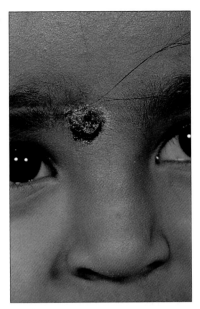

6.10 Excision of the fistula shown in **6.9**.

congenital, immunedeficiency or distant untreated foci of infection.

In any child with recurrent meningitis, a communication between the CNS and the exterior must be assiduously sought. Congenital abnormalities of the inner ear leading to fistulae may present with recurrent meningitis. Otoscopy is usually normal, and diagnosis requires expert neuroradiological and possibily radioisotope investigation. CSF fistulae may also result from trauma or infection.

Recurrent meningitis (often with unusual organisms for age), may result from infection via a midline dermal fistula (**6.9 and 6.10**) (often referred to as a sinus), usually associated with spina bifida occulta. The fistula can occur at any point in the midline, though the natal cleft is the commonest site. There may be associated cord tethering, intraspinal dermoid, lipoma or cyst or diastematomyelia.

The second commonest site for a fistula is the occiput, and there may be associated cerebellar or brainstem signs of hydrocephalus. Infection of a dermoid cyst and proximal end of a neurodermal sinus may result in intranspinal abscess rather than meningitis.

Any neurodermal sinus that ends above the sacrum should be dealt with neurosurgically. Surgical results are poorer when definitive treatment is delayed until after the occurrence of meningitis.

Cerebral abscess

Intracerebral abscess results from suppuration in adjacent anatomical structures such as otogenic abscess or sinusitis. Such parameningeal abscesses are usually single. Abscesses maybe associated with meningitis. When the source of infection is distant, as in cyanotic congenital heart disease, or pulmonary suppuration, abscesses may be multiple. Children with cyanotic heart disease are particularly at risk, and account for 10 percent of cases. About 25 % of intracranial suppurations are empyemas. Delayed development of an empyema months or years after surgical and accidental trauma is well recognised. They occur anywhere in the subdural space, but especially posteriorly.

Compound skull fractures, and penetrating wounds (including neurosurgical procedures) of the cranium, may also result in abscess formation. The commonest presenting features are headache, seizures, fever and impaired consciousness. Focal neurological signs are absent in at least 30 % of cases. Papilloedema is rarely present in a young child.

Lumbar puncture is dangerous and never diagnostic. Meningitis and cerebral abscess may coexist. If abscess is suspected, cranial CT scan with contrast must be undertaken before lumbar puncture. Appropriate neurosurgical treatment of cerebral abscess is controversial, but cerebellar and temporal-lobe abscesses, which usually arise from ear or mastoid infections, should be treated neurosurgically.

More than one organism is often isolated, anaerobes being particularly common. Appropriate antibiotic treatment is cefotaxime and metronidazole, but close collaboration with microbiology colleagues is essential. Organisms are isolated from only 80 % of cases.

Poliomyelitis

There are three strains of poliovirus; they cause disease by invasion of the anterior-horn cell. Polio usually presents with a non-specific flu-like illness associated with viraemia, followed within five to seven days by features of an aseptic meningitis. Resolution of the temperature may occur after 48 hours or so, followed by a relapse (the dromedary-hump temperature chart). Only 2 % of infection with poliovirus leads to paralytic disease. Pain is a prominent symptom at the time of onset of paralysis.

Asymmetric flaccid paralysis of lower limbs is the commonest presentation, with areflexia, neurophysiological evidence of a radiculopathy and no sensory loss. This may be followed by paralysis of upper limbs and lower motor neurone facial weakness. Bulbar involvement is rarely an isolated finding. Ventilation may be required if there is involvement of bulbar and respiratory musculature.

It is rare to isolate poliovirus from the CSF. Diagnosis is by positive culture of wild, or vaccine-like, virus from the stool and serological evidence of a rise in antibody titres. Definitive virological diagnosis remains difficult in vaccine-associated cases.

Recovery of some function is the rule rather than the exception in paralytic poliomyelitis. The relationship of poliovirus infection to motor neurone disease in later life remains a matter of considerable debate.

Control of poliomyelitis is by vaccination either with live (Sabin) or inactivated (Salk) virus. Polio vaccine is the main cause of poliomyelitis in the developed world in either recipients of vaccination or contacts with recipients—both are very rare. Bulbar involvement is rare in vaccine-associated cases. Polio vaccination can cause a severe and atypical poliomyelitis in immune-deficient children or adults. A polio-like illness can be caused by a number of other enteroviruses, particularly Coxsackie.

Varicella–zoster virus

Primary infection leads to chicken pox which may be followed by a post-infectious cerebellopathy, characteristically two to three weeks after the rash appears. Resolution may take some weeks and posterior-fossa tumours need considering. Reactivation of a latent infection leads to shingles, with a characteristic eruption appearing over the affected dermatome. Invasion of the associated posterior-root ganglion makes the disease very painful. It is rare to see this before the teenage years unless the virus was acquired *in utero*. Intra-uterine infection may also lead to foetal loss, a serious neonatal multisystem illness or cicatricial skin lesions and bone hypoplasia.

Central nervous system disease due to toxins

Tetanus

Central nervous system involvement follows infection of a wound with the spore-forming anaerobic gram-positive

bacterium *Clostridium tetani*. The incubation period may be up to three weeks, during which time the bacilli multiply, producing tetanospasmin: a protein absorbed through motor nerve endings. The toxin interferes with neuromuscular transmission, selectively blocking inhibitory neurotransmission, leading to the characteristic tetanic spasms of muscle.

Early manifestations may be pain with neck and back stiffness; trismus and dysphagia are common. The condition may deteriorate leading to a generalised increase in extensor tone and opisthotonus; death may ensue from respiratory obstruction.

In neonatal tetanus the organism most commonly gains entry to the body through the umbilical stump. Onset of disease is a tabout 14 days of age, with feeding or swallowing difficulty. Convulsions or cyanotic spells are common.

Management involves treatment of the bacillus with penicillin, administering the anti-toxin and sedating, paralysing and ventilating where necessary. Active immunisation prevents the disease.

Diphtheria

This gram-positive rod produces an exotoxin which may cause tissue necrosis. Asymmetrical polyneuropathy occurs in 10 % of infected people after the first week of the illness. A palatal paralysis is most commonly seen, but extra-ocular muscles may also be involved. Limb paralysis is rare.

Treatment is with the use of anti-toxin and supporting ventilation where necessary.

Botulism

Clostridium botulinum is an anaerobic spore-forming bacillus widely distributed in soil and marine sediments. The heat-resistant spores can survive in improperly-processed foods. The toxin is absorbed from the intestine and then irreversibly blocks acetyl choline release to give a flaccid paralysis. A bulbar paresis is the most common presenting feature. Paralysis ofextra-ocular muscles may follow, leading to a symmetrical descending paresis (**6.11**). Constitutional disturbance, including fatiguability and drowsiness, is common. Constipation, vomiting and abdominal pain are seen in up to a third. A remarkably dry mouth and fever are less common. Examination of the cerebrospinal fluid is normal, helping differentiation from the Miller–Fisher syndrome. Treatment with the anti-toxin may help to shorten the period of constitutional disturbance, but probably doesnot reduce the length of paralysis. The mainstay of therapy is supportive care with ventilation as necessary. Early involvement of the public health services to identify the source of the toxin is very important.

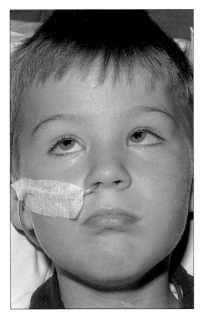

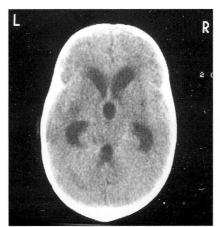

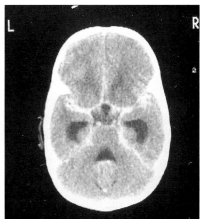

6.12 and 6.13 CT scan: meningitis—(**6.12, left**) plain study(**6.12, right**) showing striking meningeal enhancement following contrast injection.

6.11 Right VI nerve palsy and bulbar paresis in botulism.

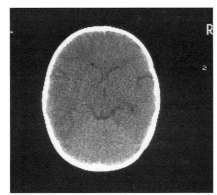

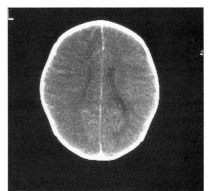

6.14 and 6.15 CT scan showing infection following meningitis—(**6.14, left**) early swelling in illness; (**6.15, right**) later atrophy.

Neuroradiology in infections of the CNS

Acute bacterial meningitis

Computed tomography, magnetic-resonance imaging and ultrasound in infants may all aid the investigation of childrenwith suspected infection.

Role of imaging

1. In cases of diagnostic difficulty at presentation.

2. Prior to performing a lumbar puncture, especially wherethere is a suspicion of raised intracranial pressure.

3. Development of focal signs during treatment.

4. Failure to respond to treatment.

5. To detect the complications of meningitis.

6. To monitor post-meningitic hydrocephalus.

7. To investigate the possible causes, especially in cases of recurrent meningitis, e.g. cerebrospinal fluid fistulae due to dural defects, congenital or post-traumatic, and congenital abnormalities such as dermal sinuses, encephalocoeles and meninglomyelocoeles.

The CT-scan appearances are usually normal in uncomplicated meningitis. However, pronounced contrast enhancement of the meninges of the basal cisterns may be seen (**6.12 and 6.13**). In some cases, the attenuation of the CSF may be increased due to the presence of pus, and may resemble a subarachnoid haemorrhage in severe cases. Pus contained within the ventricles will cause an increase in the attenuation values of the CSF and will layer in the supine position.

Low attenuation changes in the grey and white matter are common; they are seen in over 50 % of children. In over 70 % of children with *Haemophilus influenzae* meningitis, these changes are located near the frontal poles bilaterally. The low attenuation changes progress to atrophy and/or encephalomalacia in 70 % of cases, with resolution in the remainder (**6.14 and 6.15**). MR scanning will show the abnormalities shown by CT. Increased signal in the periventricular white matter may be due to ventriculitis or result from interstitial oedema of hydrocephalus or widespread vasculitis. MRI may show signs of recent haemorrhage.

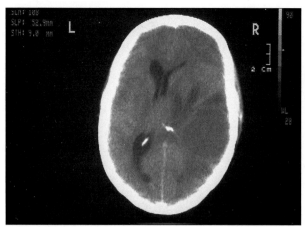 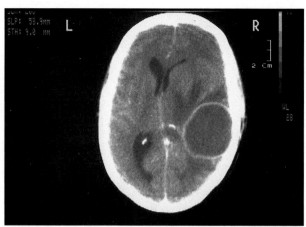

6.16 and 6.17 CT scan showing intracranial abscess. **6.16 (left)** Thin isodense rim seen on plain scan. **6.17 (right)** Enhancement seen with contrast.

Complications such as intracerebral infarctions, venous sinus thrombosis, ventriculitis or intracranial abscess, hydrocephalus or intracerebral haemorrhage secondary to a ruptured mycotic aneurism may all be visualised on either CT or MR scanning. In the very young, subdural effusions may be seen in cases of *Haemophilus influenzae* meningitis. These are demonstrated on MR or CT as a fluid collection or low-density area over the surface of the cerebral hemisphere, and may be unilateral or bilateral.

Ventriculitis is more severe in neonates than in older infants and children. The CT appearances may include focal contrast enhancement within the ventricular system and along the ventricular wall, or subsequent development of polycystic loculation within the ventricles.

TB meningitis

Role of imaging
1. To establish the diagnosis.
2. To demonstrate the extent of the disease.
3. To detect the complications (ischaemic infarcts, hydrocephalus due to cisternal and intraventricular obstruction, and calcification).

Only about 5 % of scans will be normal. Establishing a diagnosis may be difficult and delayed in some cases.

The CT findings in tuberculous meningitis are the presenceof basal exudates, recognised following intravenous contrast as diffuse enchancement of the basal cisterns, particularly around the mesencephalon. The feature, however, is not pathognomonic of TB and may be found in other types of granulomatous basalarachnoiditis. Hydrocephalus is readily recognised and the presence of the ischaemic changes are noted on CT scanning as areas of low attenuation in the deep white or grey matter. The ischaemic lesions may be detected at an earlier state on MR scanning.

Tuberculomas (granulomas) are the frequent parenchymal abnormality. On CT, they are round or oval in shape, usually isodense or slightly hyperdense and show marked enhancement of nodular or annular type. There is usually surrounding oedema. The frontal region and cerebellum are the most frequent sites. Lesions close to critical sites within the ventricular system may produce hydrocephalus due to obstruction, e.g. at the foramen of Monro or aqueduct. Healing of these lesions may result in a calcified focus.

Areas of ischaemia or infarction are usually associated withthe presence of basal exudates. Cerebral atrophy and hydrocephalus may result from CNS tuberculosis.

Intracranial abscess

Role of imaging
1. The diagnosis (size, shape, site, multiplicity).
2. Management following treatment.
3. Assessment of complications.
4. Detection of recurrence.

Intracerebral abscess

Most abscesses are unilocular and the wall is thinner on the medial aspect. Abscesses may be multiple, resulting from haematogenous spread.

The CT features of an intracranial abscess are:
1. Early stage of cerebritis: area of hypodensity with irregular area of enhancement with mass effect.
2. Late cerebritis: ill-defined area of ring enhancement representing inflammatory reaction.
3. Early capsule stage: ring enhancement.
4. Late capsule stage: thin, isodense rim clearly visible on plain CT (**6.16 and 6.17**). This represents the collagenous capsule.

Contrast enchancement in the wall is valueless as an

indicator of persisting activity. Routine scanning of patients is unnecessary, unless haemorrhage has occurred or drainage is unsatisfactory.

Pitfalls in diagnosis include:

1. Areas of cerebritis may not be considered on CT alone, due to their non-specific nature.

2. Posterior fossa abscesses may be overlooked due to the presence of artefact.

3. Cerebral oedema and areas of ring enhancement may occur normally following surgery.

MRI shows the abscess on T2W images. The collection shows increased signal even when the adjacent brain appears oedematous. Changes in the adjacent cortex and underlying white matter are shown with great sensitivity, as well as the paranasal sinus disease or intradiploeic infections.

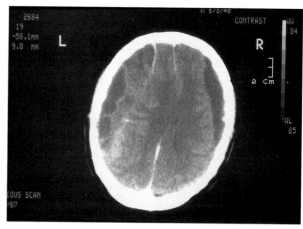

6.18 CT scan showing subdural empyema.

Intracranial empyemas

Empyemas are collections of pus in the subdural or extradural spaces. Contrast-enhanced CT must be performed to show the collection. They are usually crescentic in shape (**6.18**); however, most parafalcine collections are flat. The attenuation of the collection is similar to or slightly greater than CSF and bubbles of gas may be seen within it. There is usually enhancement of the medial membrane, which has a density greater than the adjacent brain. Abnormalities may be visible in the brain before the collection is recognised. Mass effect may be greater than expected from the size of the collection. An area of low density may be seen in the adjacent brain in 25 %, and there may be enhancement of the gyri. Areas of cerebritis or intracerebral abscess may be seen in 10 %.

On MRI the subdural collections are hypointense on T1-weighted and hyperintense on T2-weighted images compared with the underlying brain tissue. However, the changes are less marked than those seen in CSF, due to the cellular debris in abscess cavities affecting the signal intensity. This difference allows empyemas to be distinguished from CSF collections in most cases. The brain and underlying empyema may lose corticomedullary

definition. This is thought to be due to oedema of brain parenchyma underlying the subdural empyema with resultant diminution in the T1 difference between grey and white matter.

Role of sonography in the diagnosis of CNS infections

Sonography is the modality of choice in the evaluation of ventriculitis and other continuing intracranial infections. The sonographic features of ventriculitis include the development of low-level echogenicity of debris within the ventricle. Inventriculitis, there is typically some degree of periventricular echogenicity. Sonography is an excellent method to follow the effectiveness of treatment in children with ventriculitis, by monitoring the appearance and clearing of ventricular debris. Complications of intracranial infections such as ventricular oculation, cerebritis, abscess and cystic encephalomalacia may be detected. Abscess formation is usually well visualised sonographically, and appears as a cystic space.

Chapter 7: Encephalitis and Encephalopathy

Michael A. Clarke, W. St. Clair Forbes

Introduction

'Encephalopathy' is a non-specific term which is now accepted to imply a dysfunction of the brain in which either arousal and/or the content of consciousness are abnormal. The term 'coma' is used when both the level of arousal and content of consciousness are grossly impaired. This is not the case in persistent vegetative state, where the level of arousal may not be greatly disturbed, though the content of consciousness is clearly abnormal (see **Practice Point 7.1**). Plum and Posner (1980) described coma as a state of unrousable psychologic unresponsiveness in which the subject lies with eyes closed. A person in coma shows no understandable response to external stimulus or inner need.

The commonest cause of non-traumatic coma in childhood is infection. In 82 children presenting to the Hospital for Sick Children, Great Ormond Street with coma (Cole, 1991), infective encephalitis or meningitis were identified in 51 children, with encephalitis the commonest cause. The next largest group were children who had suffered hypoxic-ischaemic insults following cardiac arrest or drowning or near-miss Sudden Infant Death syndrome. Reye's syndrome and metabolic causes were identified in nine. Other important causes of non-traumatic coma in childhood are status epilepticus, non-accidental injury, blocked shunts in children with hydrocephalus, vascular disease, complex migraine, diabetes mellitus, liver failure and inherited metabolic disorders. In a neonate and young infant, biochemical causes in particular must be considered, including non-ketotic hyper-glycinaemia, hyperammonaemia, mitochondrial cytopathies, beta-oxidation defects and peroxisomal disorders.

Clinical assessment

Level of coma

There have been a number of attempts to produce satisfactory coma scales for children but none has been entirely satisfactory. Figure **7.1** (overleaf) shows the paediatric coma scale and normal values which vary with age. The key clinical feature in assessing coma in children is the localisation of pain. There is frequently confusion about what this means. This does not mean that if a painful stimulus is applied to a child's limb that the limb is merely withdrawn. Localising pain means a purposive response to painful stimulation applied to the area supplied by a branch of the trigeminal nerve or the upper cervical dermatones. When such a stimulus is given, asymmetry of facial movement may indicate either upper or lower motor neurone facial paresis.

Observation of posture is important. Abnormal posturing may be persistent, intermittent, occur spontaneously or only with stimulation. In decerebrate posturing the child is in coma, with the neck extended, arms extended and hyperpronated, legs extended and feet plantar-flexed. In decorticate posturing, the arms are adducted, shoulders externally rotated, elbows and wrists flexed, and legs extended (**7.2**). The two abnormal postures do not have anatomical localising value but may be, and indeed fre-

---

Practice Point 7.1 Levels of Consciousness

When discussing the level of consciousness, two factors must be considered:

1. Level of arousal

2. Content of consciousness.

Comparison of Adelaide Paediatric Scale and Glasgow Coma Scale (after Reilly *et al.* 1988)

Paediatric Scale

Eyes open			Best verbal response		
Spontaneously	4		Orientated	5	
To speech	3		Words	4	
To pain	2		Vocal sounds	3	
None	1		Cries	2	
			None	1	

	Best motor response	
	Obeys commands	5
	Localises pain	4
	Flexion to pain	3
	None	1

7.1 Glasgow coma scale for children.

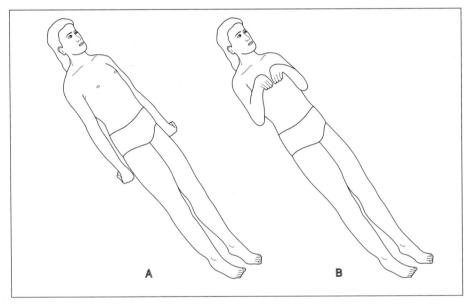

7.2 Abnormal posture in coma. a) Decerebrate. b) Decorticate.

A

B

quently are, associated with raised intracranial pressure. This may be caused by any condition in which there is severe disturbance of function of the cortex or brainstem. Abnormal posturing may be lateralised and may indicate imminent brain shifts due to raised pressure.

The examination of ocular motility is crucial in assessing the severity of coma. Paresis of conjugate upgaze when the neck is flexed is one of the earliest signs of raised intracranial pressure. The oculo-cephalic reflexes are demonstrated in (**7.3**). A child with abnor-mal oculocephalic reflexes is unlikely to localise pain. In deep coma, these findings indicate brain stem dysfunc-tion. The presence of the corneal reflex should be assessed. Fundoscopic examination may reveal retinopa-thy in some inherited metabolic disorders, or haemor-rhage following central nervous system bleeding (trau-matic or not). Raised intracranial pressure is only rarely accompanied by papilloedema in children.

The light of an ophthalmosope is not an adequate stimulus for the examination of the pupillary responses;

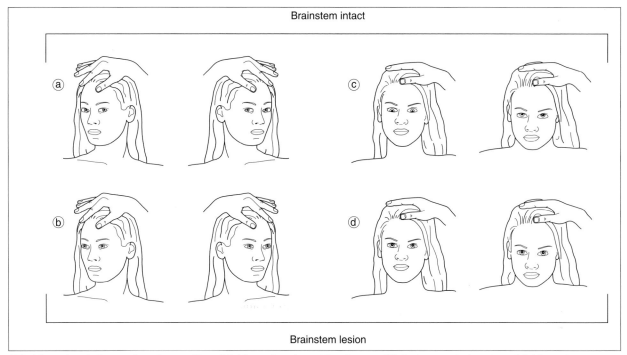

Brainstem intact

Brainstem lesion

7.3 Normal and abnormal ocular motility. **(a)** Normal on lateral head turn. **(b)** Brainstem dysfunction. **(c)** Normal upgaze on neck flexion. **(d)** Absent upgaze on neck flexion. NB. Cervical spine instability must be excluded prior to testing.

a bright torch should be used. A unilateral Horner's syndrome in which the pupil is constricted with anhidrosis over half the body is one of the earlier signs of transtentorial herniation. In a mid-brain lesion, the pupils are fixed in the mid-position; hippus may be present. A unilateral sixth or third nerve palsy may indicate imminent shifts within cranial compartments due to raised intracranial pressure.

Abnormalities of respiration both of rate and of depth are frequent in coma and have localising value. Central neurogenic hyperventilation is rare and, if present, implies dysfunction of the mid brain and pons but other causes, particularly abnormalities of acid-base status are much more likely in childhood. Cheyne–Stokes respiration suggests an abnormality of the thalamus and hypothalamus. Apnoea with end-inspiratory pauses has good localising value and suggests dysfunction inthe mid or lower pons. In medullary dysfunction, breathing is ataxic, completely irregular, deep and shallow breaths occurring randomly.

Raised intracranial pressure may accompany coma. In simple terms, raised intracranial pressure is due to too much water in the intracranial compartment. In cytotoxic cerebral oedema, there is predominant swelling of neural cellular elements and an abnormality of intracellular–extracellular osmolar gradient. In vasogenic cerebral oedema, which commonly accompanies mass lesions, there is an excess plasma filtrate and in the extracellular space, and in interstitial oedema there is transependymal

movement of cerebrospinal fluid, usually due to raised pressure within the ventricles.

In each of the above, there is a disruption of either the blood-brain or blood-CSF barrier (**7.4**). The site of the blood-brain barrier is the capillary endothelial cell. Water moves easily through the blood-brain barrier. The capillary endothelium is characterised by tight junctions between the cells. There are no intercellular channels for the passage of water-soluble compounds. Brain capillaries therefore act as a continuous phospholipid membrane, and the ease with which substances pass through this barrier is related to their lipid solubility, molecular weight and hydrodynamic radius. Hydrophilic, large, polar, protein-bound molecules do not easily pass through the blood-brain barrier, and for many such substrates there are brain-specific carrier mechanisms. The blood-brain barrier is almost certainly the site of initial dysfunction in many disorders in childhood leading to coma.

Brain compliance, the relationship between intracranial pressure and the volume of intracranial contents, is not linear. **7.5** shows that, after a certain point, small changes in thevolume of intracranial contents are associated with very large rises in intracranial pressure. Pressure–volume relationships are not constant. This can be demonstrated by using the analogy of a party balloon. When a balloon is initially inflated, considerable pressure is needed to produce a small change in volume; after a certain point, a much smaller change in pressure

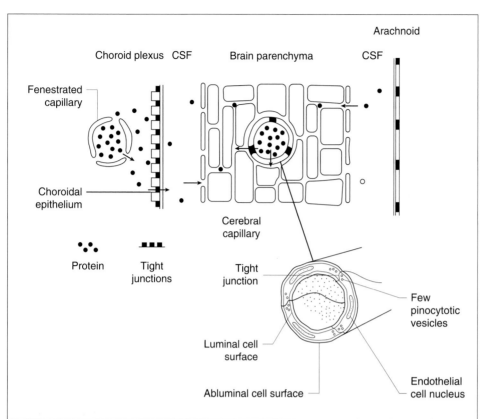

7.4 Diagrammatic representation of blood-brain barrier.

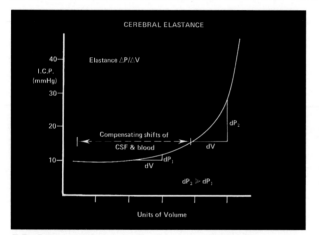

7.5 Brain compliance: pressure/volume relationship.

When not to do a Lumbar Puncture:
>   Consciousness impaired
>   Abnormal Oculocephalic reflexes/Pupils
>   Lateralized Signs/Abnormal Posture
>   After recent seizures
>   Papilloedema

7.6 Contraindications to lumbar puncture.

produces a much larger change in volume. The significance of pressure-volume relationships and their non-linear relationship is important when using neuroradiological techniques to make an assessment of intracranial pressure. Though generally there is a good relationship between abnormalities on cranial CT scan such as ventricular size, or the loss of sulcal pattern and perimesencephalic cisterns, this is not always so. The pressure can be elevated, occasionally markedly, when there is no evidence of this on the cranial CT scan.

Intracranial pressure may be raised in a child in coma. Failure to localise pain, paddling or cycling movements, ataxia, a return of primitive reflexes or abnormal postures may all indicate raised intracranial pressure. At least half the children with raised intracranial pressure show no evidence of papilloedema, and its absence therefore does not indicate that a lumbar puncture is safe in a child in coma. The natural history of papilloedema, if intracranial pressure is not relieved, is optic atrophy. This is of particular importance in children who have shunt-dependent hydrocephalus in which there may have been previous episodes of raised

Acute Childhood Encephalopathy
Sequence of immunological findings:

Breakdown of blood-brain barrier ⟶ Raised IgG index ⟶ Appearance of oligoclonal bands in CSF

Shown by abnormal: Reflects intrathecal IgG synthesis   A 'focused' immune response

Albumin CSF Ratio $\dfrac{\text{IgG CSF}}{\text{IgG serum}} \div \dfrac{\text{Albumin CSF}}{\text{Albumin serum}}$

Albumin serum

Normal $< 4.3 \times 10^{3}$ Normal < 0.6

7.7 Blood-brain barrier and intrathecal antibody synthesis in viral encephalitis.

intracranial pressure. Once opticatrophy has occurred, papilloedema will not recur even in the presence of raised intracranial pressure. As there are difficulties in being able to determine on clinical examination whether intracranial pressure is raised or not, lumbar puncture is ill-advised in circumstances shown in **7.6** (with failure to localise pain, abnormal oculo-cephalic reflexes, lateralised signs: abnormal posture after recent seizures, papilloedema).

The pathogenesis of encephalopathy

The commonest cause of coma in childhood is infection. In children seen in this department in coma where primary metabolic disturbance or bacterial infection have been excluded, there was a clinical or viral infection in over 80 % of cases but a specific virological diagnosis made in less than a quarter. Seventy-five percent had seizures close to or at the onset of coma and a CSF leucocytosis was by no means invariable.

Although the commonest identifiable cause of sporadic encephalitis in children is herpes simplex Type 1 virus, most cases are due to enteroviruses. Failure to make a specific virological diagnosis in most children with encephalitis is due to specific problems of virological diagnosis, particularly related to the large number of different types of enterovirus, and the fact that it is rare for the laboratory to receive adequate samples. To maximise the chance of making a virological diagnosis, throat, stool and urine samples need to be sent for viral culture on three occasions and blood and CSF should be sent on two occasions, 10 days apart. Brain biopsy has little role in the diagnosis of viral encephalitis.

Though specific diagnosis can be made in a small number of children only, there are indications that viruses are aetiologically involved, not only because of the frequent clinical history of viral infection, but also because Interferon-Alpha can often be detected in blood or cerebrospinal fluid in these children.

There is a characteristic sequence of abnormal neuroimmunological events seen in children with viral encephalitis (**7.7**). An initial disruption of the blood-brain barrier is evidenced by an abnormal albumin ratio. Subsequently, the blood-brain barrier frequently returns to normal, but there is evidence of intrathecal antibody synthesis as shown by an elevated IgG index or by detection of oligoclonal banding in the cerebrospinal fluid. Detection of oligoclonal bands in encephalitis shows there are immunoreactive cells present within the central nervous system that are of restricted response, hence the term oligoclonal. In most children with encephalitis, the antibody specificities of this oligoclonal response are not known, though it is likely that there is oligoclonal intrathecal antibody production to both neural and viral elements.

The outcome of viral encephalitis is often poor, with less than 50 % of previously normal children recovering completely, and with mortality approaching 10 %. **7.8 and 7.9** show the cranial CT scans of a child presenting with simple partial seizures involving the left arm with progression to coma. This child was shown to have herpes simplex encephalitis; a scan taken at onset shows vascular stasis in the temporo-parietal region. The scan taken after recovery from the acute episode shows a gross loss of neural tissue in the region of the Sylvian fissure.

It is highly likely that in many children diagnosed as having viral encephalitis, there is no viral invasion of the brain. This is particularly likely to be so if there has

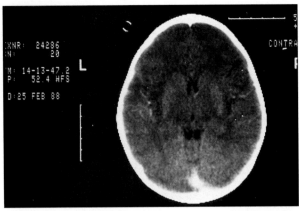 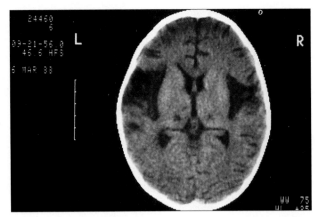

7.8 and 7.9 Herpes simplex encephalitis. **7.8 (above left)** acute stage—vascular stasis and low attenuation. **7.9 (above right)** Atrophic changes six weeks later.

been a period of recovery between the viral infection and the onset of neurological disorder. Some of these children's magnetic resonance scans show abnormal signals from myelin, and neuropathologically, demyelination can be found.

Investigations in encephalopathy

A wide number of investigations need to be considered in the child presenting in coma without obvious cause. Clearly, infection of the central nervous system needs to be considered as discussed above.

The following investigations should be considered:

blood urea and electrolytes	urinary organic acids
blood glucose	urinary ketones
blood gases	urinary porphyrins
blood urate	urinary toxicology
blood lactate	urinary aminoacids
liver function tests	blood cultures
ammonia	
blood for virology and immunology	

swabs, urine and faeces for bacteriological and virological study.

Muscle biopsy may be helpful in the diagnosis of lipid-storage myopathies associated with central nervous system features, as in the fatty-acid oxidation defects and other mitochondrial cytopathies. When safe, CSF should be examined and lactate estimated along with the albumin ratio to give an indication of blood-barrier function, and the IgG index to indicate whether intrathecal antibody synthesis is present. This can be complemented by isoelectric-focusing electrophoresis of cerebrospinal fluids searching for oligoclonal bands, viral culture and specific viral antibodies.

The electroencephalogram is an aid to diagnosis but more particularly to management and prognosis. High-voltage diffuse slow-wave activity occurs in encephalopathy from any cause. Continuous EEG monitoring using a cerebral function monitor may be helpful in detecting frequent epileptic activity.

Management

The management of children in coma requires admission to a paediatric intensive-care unit. If sepsis is suspected, it is wise to treat with penicillin and chloramphenicol, or a cephalosporin and acyclovir. Management then centres on the maintenance of normal metabolism, fluid balance, the control of seizures and intracranial pressure.

Normal intracranial pressure varies with age: 2 mm Hg in neonates, 5 mm Hg at 12 months, 6–13 mm Hg at 7 years of age and 15 mm Hg at 13 years of age. At any time, an intracranial pressure greater than 20 mm Hg requires treatment.

The absolute level of intracranial pressure is not as important as the cerebral perfusion pressure (the difference between the mean arterial pressure and the intracranial pressure). The cerebral perfusion pressure needs to be maintained above at least 40 mm Hg for there to be an adequate blood supply to the central nervous system. The cerebral perfusion pressure in neonates is 20–25 mm Hg.

In a normal brain, autoregulation adjusts the diameter of the cerebral arterioles and hence links cerebral blood flow to metabolic requirement; cerebral blood flow is constant with a cerebral perfusion pressure of 60–100 mm Hg. Autoregulation is frequently lost in coma and this has a number of factors. If cerebral perfusion pressure falls below 60 mm Hg, autoregulation ceases and cerebral blood flow becomes directly related in a linear way to cerebral perfusion pressure. If arterial oxygen saturation falls, cerebral blood flow can increase as long as cerebral arterioles can dilate, but again if arterial oxygen saturation falls below 50 or 60 mm Hg in this aspect, autoregulation also ceases. If arterial CO_2

7.10 (left) Cerebral autoregulation.

7.11 (right) Intracranial pressure monitoring—access sites.

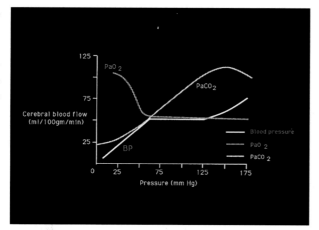

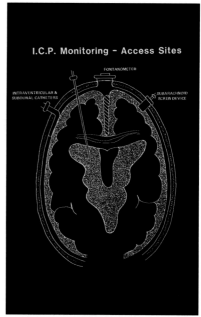

concentration increases, cerebral blood flow can increase, but again autoregulation may be lost. If arterial CO_2 saturation falls, cerebral blood flow decreases and this is the rationale for hyperventilation. The relationships of these parameters to changes in cerebral blood flow are shown in **7.10**.

Intracranial pressure is most ideally measured by an intraventricular catheter, but this presents difficulties in swollen brains. The most common method of measurement is by the placement of a subdural catheter attached to a pressure transducer. Other methods are to use a subdural screw which is screwed into the skull with a pressure device against the dura (**7.11**). Devices for measuring anterior fontanelle pressure in infants with an open fontanelle have not received wide acceptance and are often unreliable.

Doppler blood-flow studies are non-invasive but do not give a direct measure of cerebral perfusion pressure. They do allow judgments to be made about flow in cerebral arteries and may indicate ischaemia and that autoregulation has ceased. Intraparenchymal devices have been used without side effects for measuring intracranial pressure. The major difficulty with devices measuring intracranial pressure is drift in the measurement and the constant need to readjust to baseline. Infection is a rare complication.

In addition to measurements of absolute numbers, the wave form resulting from intracranial pressure monitoring is important in clinical management. The value of a continuous printout of pressure wave form, the detection of plateau waves, poor brain compliance and other pathological states is invaluable (**7.12**), and is necessary when interpreting the significance of absolute levels of intracranial pressure.

In neurointensive care, arterial oxygen concentration shouldbe kept greater than 60 mm Hg and CO_2 25-28 mm Hg. The headof the bed can raised up to 45 degrees, adequate sedation is essential, as is fluid restriction to 50 % of requirements. A central venous pressure line is invaluable in managing fluids. Adequate sedation with barbiturate, anaesthetic agents or benzodiazepines is essential. It is important to note that suction, physiotherapy, and painful procedures will raise intracranial pressure in the inadequately sedated patient and fever increases the cerebral metabolic demand for oxygen. Acute rises of pressure can be treated with hyperventilation or Mannitol 1.5 g/kg. It is important when giving Mannitol to monitor the serum osmolarity, and there is no point in Mannitol being given to a person who is maximally dehydrated. There is a danger of rebound cerebral oedema with Mannitol which diffuses into neuronal tissue and fluid follows. Mannitol should be givenwith diuretics, particularly frusimide, as the two act synergistically.

Steroids should not be routinely given. They do have an undoubted role in perifocal vasogenic oedema and do decrease the inflammatory response. The role in acute pyogenic meningitis is discussed elsewhere. There is evidence that they activate the sodium pump and prevent the release of lytic enzymes which serves to minimise the disruption of the blood-brain barrier.

Status epilepticus requires vigorous management and is discussed in Chapter 5. Seizures may not be evident if a child is paralysed for ventilation (**7.13**). It is in this situation that cerebral function monitor can be invaluable.

The value of intracranial pressure monitoring has not

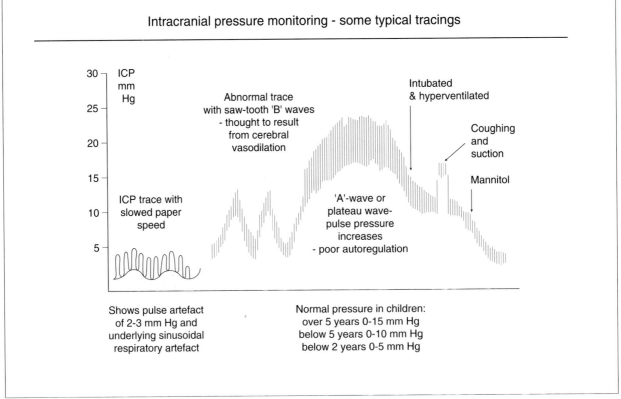

Intracranial pressure monitoring - some typical tracings

ICP mm Hg (y-axis: 30, 25, 20, 15, 10, 5)

ICP trace with slowed paper speed

Abnormal trace with saw-tooth 'B' waves - thought to result from cerebral vasodilation

'A'-wave or plateau wave- pulse pressure increases - poor autoregulation

Intubated & hyperventilated

Coughing and suction

Mannitol

Shows pulse artefact of 2-3 mm Hg and underlying sinusoidal respiratory artefact

Normal pressure in children:
over 5 years 0-15 mm Hg
below 5 years 0-10 mm Hg
below 2 years 0-5 mm Hg

7.12 Intracranial pressure monitor in:some typical tracings. a) Normal. b) Diminished brain compliance. c) Plateau waves.

EEGs have important prognostic implications in the assessment of non-traumatic coma. Evidence of multi-organ failure rather than absolute levels of intracranial pressure reached is more important prognostically.

Future developments may include the measurement of arterio-venous oxygen and lactate differences combined with measures of intracranial pressure and cerebral perfusion pressure. This may allow the prevention of ischaemia and acknowledges the fact that there are great local differences in the central nervous system in a person in coma with loss of cerebral autoregulation. These differences are related to cerebral metabolic demand for oxygen and the likelihood of ischaemia in any given area.

Calcium channel blockers may hold promise for the prevention of neuronal damage and there are further possibilities for the modification of inhibitory neuro-transmitters.

Non-traumatic coma is a common and serious paediatric neurological emergency. Appropriate management requires skilled neurointensive care and is not an appropriate activity for those seeing such children only occasionally.

Neuroradiology in herpes simplex encephalitis

Computed tomography reveals abnormalities in 95 % of cases but only in 78 % in the first five days. The earliest abnormality is the poorly defined non-specific low-density abnormality in one temporal lobe. This subsequently becomes more definite, with additional involvement of the inferior frontal lobe and insula. In 90 %, the insula has a distinctive sharp medial margin indicating sparing of the striatum. In over 80 %, the changes will eventually be bilateral, whereas the earlier scans show bilateral changes in only 10 %. Local mass effect develops with time, but becomes prominent in only 75 %. Contrast enhancement ispresent in 70 % of cases, though is rarely present in early scans and is seldom marked. Haemorrhage is recognisable at some stage in about 15 %. It is most common in the most medial part of the temporal lobe, bordering on the crural cistern and can be mistaken for subarachnoid haemorrhage. Severe cases may show generalised cerebral oedema. In the intermediate stage of the illness, CT scanning will show a decrease of mass effect, and in the late stage will show focal or generalised cerebral atrophy. These features may be of use in assessing the prognosis.

MRI provides clear evidence of the disease and bilateral involvement at an earlier stage than CT. Extensive signal changes are often also present in the periventricular white matter. T1-weighted images often fail to reveal any abnormality unless haemorrhage or extensive necrosis has occurred. The T2-weighted images show multiple areas of increased signal which may resemble those of multiple sclerosis.

Relation Between Discharges in Initial EEG and Outcome in Non-Traumatic Coma

(Tasker *et al.*, 1988)

Discharges	Outcome		
	Good	Moderate	Poor
None	17	2	16
Continuous	1	0	0
Isolated	2	2	3
Electrical storms	0	1	4

Worst EEG and Outcome in 20 Children with Non-Traumatic Coma with Adequate Cerebral Perfusion Pressure

(Tasker *et al.*, 1988)

Worst EEG	Outcome		
	Good	Moderate	Poor
1. Diffusely slow (0.5 – 3 cycles/second) or periods of low amplitude (< 50 μU) or both lasting < 5 seconds	13	1	1
2. Generalised low voltage	0	0	2
3. Isoelectric	0	0	3

7.13 EEG and outcome in non-traumatic coma.

Chapter 8: Neuromuscular Disorders

Michael J. Noronha

Neuromuscular disorders include the myopathies, neuropathies and neurogenic atrophies. In myopathies, the pathology is confined to the muscle itself, with no associated structural abnormality in the peripheral nerve. In the neuropathies or neurogenic atrophies, there is an abnormality along the course of the peripheral nerve from anterior horn cell to the neuromuscular junction. Both the myopathies and the neuropathies can be further subdivided into hereditary and acquired ones, and into acute and chronic syndromes, and further categorisation is based on the characteristic pattern of the particular disorder.

The term muscular dystrophy is used for the genetically determined, progressive, degenerative myopathies and the spinal muscular atrophies, and motor neuropathies are neurogenic disorders in which the lesion is in the anterior horn cell or the peripheral nerve. These syndromes can be subdivided further on the basis of their clinical features and their mode of inheritance. The congenital myopathies are a group of genetically determined muscle disorders in which specific structural abnormalities can be recognised in the muscle but tend not to run a progressive course like the muscular dystrophies. The metabolic myopathies are akin to the congenital myopathies but represent those syndromes in which a specific abnormality has been identified, usually related to carbohydrate or lipid metabolism. The cardinal feature of the myotonic disorders is continued active contraction of a muscle which persists after the termination of voluntary effort. The various acquired neuromuscular disorders include inflammatory, endocrine and toxic conditions affecting either the peripheral nerve or the muscle itself.

The cardinal symptom in neuromuscular disorders is weakness and the history often reveals failure to achieve motor skills or loss of specific motor skill or ability (**8.1–8.3**). Hypotonia generally accompanies any significant degree of weakness, but it may also occur in the absence of weakness. The course and distribution of weakness should be elicited as well as variability in the

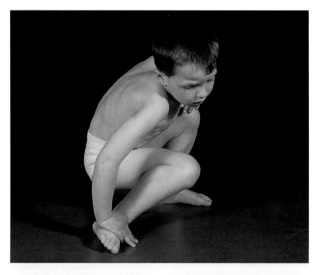

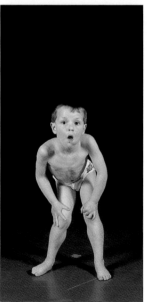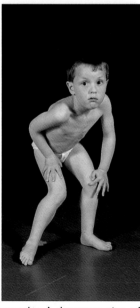

8.1–8.3 Duchenne muscular dystrophy. A demonstration of the 'Gower's manouevre'. Notice that the child, when requested to stand from a lying position, after rolling over because of truncal weakness, finally climbs up on his knees before standing (see **Practice Point 8.1**).

muscle weakness from day to day. A detailed family history is essential to establish a possible genetic mechanism. It is noteworthy that in a young child, a lot more information on the degree and localisation of muscle weakness can be acquired by observing spontaneous activity before trying to do a formal neurological examination (*see* Chapter 2).

Special investigations

Investigations of value in the differential diagnosis of neuromuscular disorders include serum enzymes, electrophysiological procedures, biopsy of muscle and peripheral nerve, and recombinant DNA studies. Biopsy usually gives a more exact and definitive diagnosis, whilst DNA studies may define the genetic nature of the disorder. The results should always be analysed in conjunction with the clinical picture.

Serum enzymes   Serum creatine kinase is elevated in conditions with degeneration of muscle. In Duchenne and Becker dystrophies the elevation is marked, but in many of the other neuromuscular disorders, the serum creatine kinase is likely to be normal or only slightly elevated.

Electrophysiological investigations   Nerve conduction velocity is a relatively simple technique and can be performed without much discomfort to the patient. The conduction velocity is dependent on the diameter and degree of myelination of the nerve fibre. In diseases affecting the peripheral nerve, the pathology may be primarily in the axon itself (axonal or neuronal neuropathy) or in the supporting Schwann cells, giving a segmental demyelination (demyelinating neuropathy). In the demyelinating neuropathies, the nerve conduction velocity is markedly slowed to half the normal rate or less. In the axonal neuropathies, the conduction velocity may be normal or only slightly depressed. In myasthenia gravis, the fatiguability of the muscle can be demonstrated by the reduction in size of the evoked muscle action potential following repetitive stimulation of the nerve.

Electromyography is unpleasant, as it entails sampling of muscles with a needle electrode. The amount of information obtained depends on the degree of cooperation of the child. The particular electrical patterns recorded may give some help in differentiating between myopathic or neuropathic disorders (**Table 8.1**).

Muscle and nerve biopsy   A muscle biopsy is essential for any patient with a neuromuscular disorder in order to establish a definitive disorder as accurately as possible. The biopsy may be obtained by means of a special biopsy needle with little discomfort to the patient (**8.4 and 8.5**). The size of the sample is small but usually adequate for light microscopy and electron microscopy. Open muscle biopsy is indicated if needle muscle biopsy fails, and also if a larger amount of muscle is required for biochemical analysis.

Several histological and histochemical stains are done routinely on every biopsy and usually provide adequate diagnostic information (**8.6–8.13**). Firstly, these techniques may identify if the muscle is normal or abnormal. Secondly, in abnormal muscles, a broad distinction into neurogenic and myopathic disorders can be made. Thirdly, certain specific histological or histochem-

TABLE 8.1 E.M.G.

'Neurogenic' disorders	— Fibrillation potential—positive sharp waves at rest. — Motor units increased ('giant motor units'). — Decreased interference pattern on maximal contraction.
'Myopathic' disorders	— No spontaneous activity at rest. — Motor units polyphasic and reduced in amplitude. — Interference pattern complete on maximal contraction.

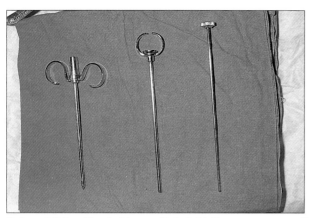

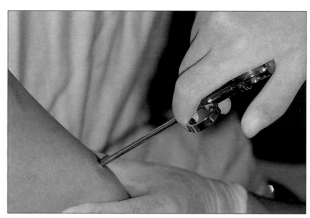

8.4 and 8.5   Muscle biopsy: (**8.4, left**) Percutaneous needle muscle biopsy with trochar and cannular. (**8.5, right**) Needle inserted in quadriceps femoris muscle and is about to be removed.

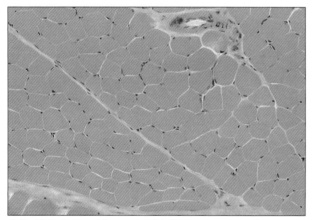

8.6   H & E: provides general information on architecture, fibre size, splitting, nuclei and morphometry.

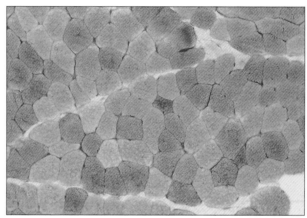

8.7   Periodic acid Schiff (P.A.S.): demonstrates glycogen granules and cell membranes and other myofibrillar membranous structures.

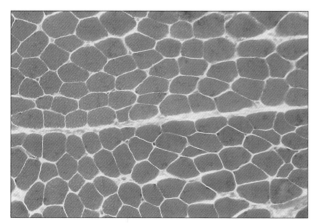

8.8   Modified Gomori trichrome: enables delineation of nuclei, fibrous tissue, myofibrillar material and intermyofibrillar substance.

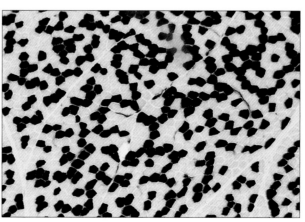

8.9   Adenosine triphosphatase ATPase: uses pre-incubation buffer at differing pH, usually pH 9.4, 4.5 and 4.3 to identify fibre type. Seen here at pH 4.3 (Type I dark).

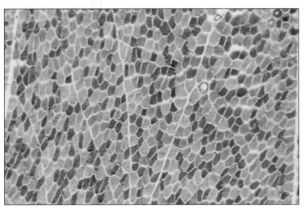

8.10 Nicotine adenine dinucleotide tetrazolium reductase (N.A.D.H.). Allows fibre-type differentiation with the reaction localised in mitochondria.

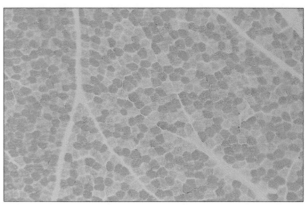

8.11 Cytochrome oxidase: reaction localised in mitochondria.

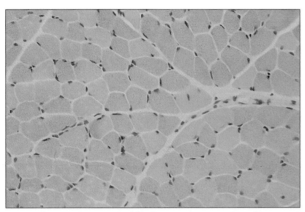

8.12 Oil-red O method (ORO): enables basophilic fibres and sarcolemnal nuclei to be recognised.

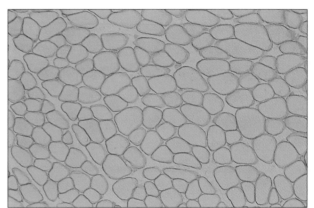

8.13 Dystrophin: immunohistochemistry shows a golden-brown membrane staining in normal muscle.

ical features may enable a more definitive diagnosis to be made, e.g. excess glycogen in storage disorders, or ragged red fibres in the mitochondrial disorders. Finally, the distribution, nature and severity of the changes in the neuromuscular disorder can be assessed. Dystrophin staining techniques may be helpful in the differentiation of Duchenne and Becker dystrophies. Electron microscopy may be indicated for identifying abnormalities in the morphology of the mitochondria and ultrastructure of the muscle cell.

Examination of a small peripheral nerve, usually the sural nerve, may be helpful in the investigation of the peripheral neuropathies.

Recombinant DNA studies With the identification of the specific gene abnormalities in a number of the neuromuscular disorders (**Table 8.2**) DNA studies are becoming important for diagnosis, carrier detection and antenatal diagnosis. In the future, the gene location in even more disorders is likely to be specifically identified.

Duchenne muscular dystrophy (DMD)

This is the commonest muscular dystrophy, with X-linked recessive inheritance and an incidence of 1:3000 male-born infants. The age of onset is within the first five years of life. There is symmetrical and initial selective weakness of the pelvic and pectoral girdles (**8.14**), hypertrophy of the calves (**8.15**) relentless progressive weakness, with loss of ambulation usually by eight to 12 years (**8.16**). Selective atrophy of pectoralis major and brachioradialis is particularly evident. Associated features include the development of contractures and thoracic deformities, cardiomyopathy and variable intellectual impairment. Life expectancy is into the late teens or early 20s, and death is usually through respiratory failure.

The serum creatine kinase is markedly elevated and the muscle biopsy virtually pathognomonic, showing progressive changes with time (**8.17–8.20**)—degenera-

TABLE 8.2 Neuromuscular Disorders & Molecular Genetics

1. Duchenne muscular dystrophy
   Becker muscular dystrophy — Xp21.2

2. Spinal muscular atrophies — 5q11 – q 13
   Long-arm X-chromosome

3. Dystrophia myotonica — 19q 13.2 – 13.3

4. Malignant hyperthermia — 19q 13.1

5. Central core congenital myopathy — 19q 12 – 13.2

6. Charcot–Marie–Tooth
   HMSN I (a) — chromosome 17 p12 – p 11.2
   HMSN I (b) — chromosome 1q 21 – 23

7. Fascioscapulohumeral dystrophy — 4q35

8. Mitochondrial encephalopathies — several mutations and deletions of mitochondrial DNA

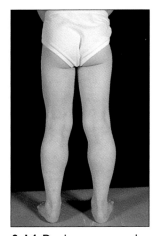

8.14 Duchenne muscular dystrophy: hypertrophied calves and thighs in an 8-year-old boy.

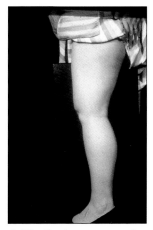

8.15 Duchenne muscular dystrophy: hypertrophied calf and thigh muscles in a manifesting female carrier of Duchenne muscular dystrophy.

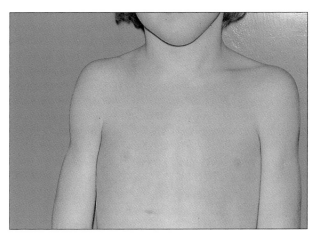

8.16 Duchenne muscular dystrophy: wasting of muscles around the shoulder girdle and particularly triceps humerus.

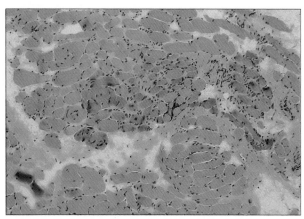

8.17 Duchenne muscular dystrophy: H&E staining showing variation in fibre size with some hypertrophied fibres.

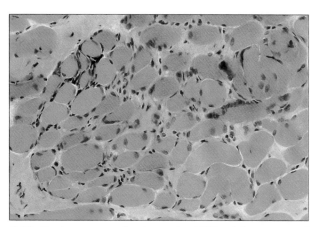

8.18 Duchenne muscular dystrophy: H&E staining: groups of degenerating fibres.

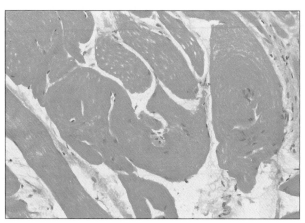

8.19 Duchenne muscular dystrophy: H&E staining: hypertrophied fibres with whorling of fibre splitting.

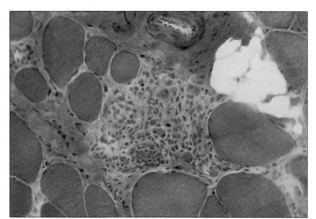

8.20 Duchenne muscular dystrophy: modified trichrome showing increase in connective tissue and adipose tissue, and focal infiltration of mononuclear cells.

tion and regeneration, variation in fibre size with large hyaline fibres, internal nuclei, and proliferation of adipose and connective tissue. Absence of dystrophin staining differentiates the problem from Becker dystrophy. The gene location is at Xp21 and specific probes have identified an intragene deletion in over 60 % of patients with DMD. This finding and other recombinant DNA techniques are of great importance in determining the carrier status of female relatives and in prenatal diagnosis.

Management of the child with DMD consists of encouraging ambulation and standing for as long as possible and prevention of contractures (**8.21**) by passive stretching. It is imperative to avoid immobilisation with acute illness or injury, as it can result in a rapid and permanent deterioration in the child's physical condition. Ambulation can be prolonged with the use of calipers (**8.22**). Scoliosis often develops and becomes progressive, especially once the child is chairbound. This can be

prevented by the use of spinal supports and the child maintaining the standing position (**8.23**) for part of the day in calipers or a standing frame. Progressive scoliosis (**8.24**) is an indication for surgical fixation of the spine (**8.25 and 8.26**). In the later stages, nocturnal ventilatory insufficiency may occur, characterised by daytime headaches, irritability, lack of concentration and somnolence. This can be helped by nocturnal assisted ventilation.

Becker muscular dystrophy (BMD)

BMD is an X-linked recessive form of muscular dystrophy which has a similar clinical pattern and inheritance as DMD, but is milder with a slower and more variable rate of progression. The majority of cases have an onset between five and 15 years of age, though some may not

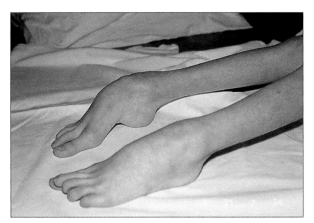

8.21 Duchenne muscular dystrophy: severe equinus deformities developing in a 15-year-old boy with DMD.

8.23 Duchenne muscular dystrophy: standing frame to enable standing for varying periods of time.

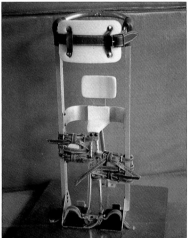

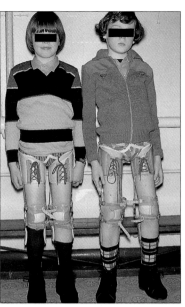

8.22 Duchenne muscular dystrophy: two brothers with DMD in full-length callipers to help maintain their upright posture.

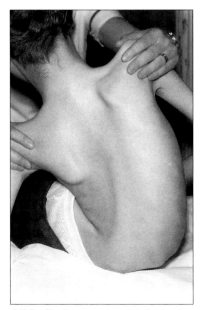

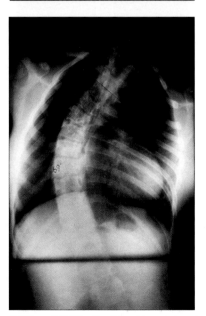

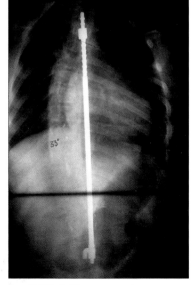

8.24 Duchenne muscular dystrophy: severe scoliosis developing in a 12-year-old boy with DMD.

8.25 and 8.26 Duchenne muscular dystrophy: (**8.25, left**) x-ray to demonstrate severe scoliosis, which is partially corrected (**8.26, right**) after spinal stabilisation operation

present until adult life. The usual clinical features consist of proximal muscle weakness and prominence of calf muscles. Progression is slow, with inability to walk occurring after the age of 16 years and death is at an average age of 42 years (range 23 to 63 years) (**8.27–8.29**).

The serum creatine kinase is markedly elevated as in DMD. The muscle biopsy shows variable dystrophic changes with features of degeneration and regeneration, variable loss of muscle fibres, proliferation of adipose and connective tissue. Staining for dystrophin is patchy, unlike DMD where dystrophin is absent. The gene location is similar to that of DMD at Xp21.

Management consists of prevention of fixed deformities by passive stretching and promotion of activity, with the use of calipers in the later stages if required.

Emery–Dreifuss muscular dystrophy

This is an X-linked muscular dystrophy which is clinically distinct from the Duchenne and Becker type and presents in late childhood or adult life. The muscle weakness and functional disability is mild and only slowly progressive (**8.30 and 8.31**). It is characterised by rigidity of the spine with limited neck and trunk flexion

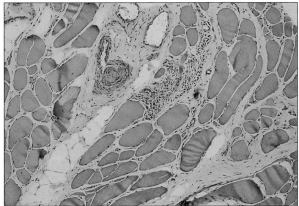

8.27 Becker's muscular dystrophy: H&E staining showing focal fibre degeneration and proliferation of endomysial connective tissue.

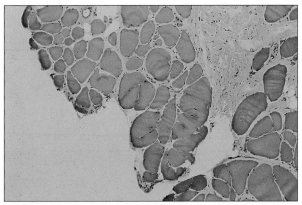

8.28 Becker's muscular dystrophy: H&E staining—hypertrophied fibres showing fibre splitting.

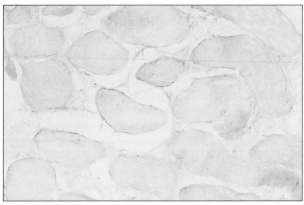

8.29 Becker's muscular dystrophy: dystrophin staining showed patchy membrane staining.

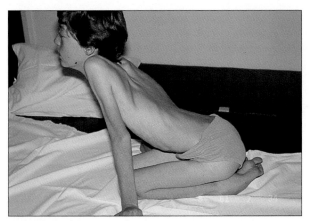

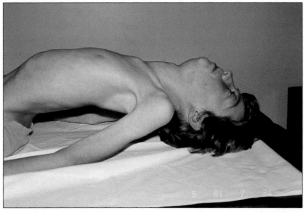

8.30 and 8.31 Rigid spine syndrome: marked rigidity of lumbar and dorsal spine with marked contractions of neck extensor muscles. Muscle weakness was minimal, and the condition was not inherited.

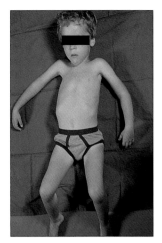

8.32 Muscular dystrophy: autosomal recessive with cerebral hypomyelination. Marked weakness and contractures of proximal and distal muscles in a 6-year-old boy.

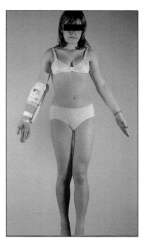

8.33 CT brain scan of boy in **8.32** shows extensive hypomyelination in both cerebral hemispheres.

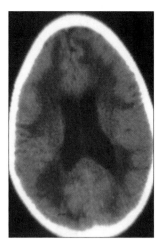

8.34 Muscular dystrophy—autosomal recessive: 12-year-old girl with some proximal limb girdle weakness, hypertrophied quadriceps femoris muscles, very tight tendo-achilles and raised serum creatinine kinase of 684 units.

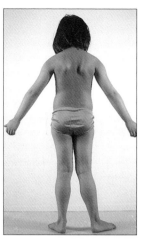

8.35 Muscular dystrophy—autosomal recessive: 8-year-old girl with progresssive proximal limb girdle weakness, hypertrophied calf and thigh muscles. Serum creatinine kinase 1630 IU/l. Chromosomes 46XX and muscle biopsy changes of a dystrophic process.

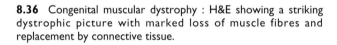

8.36 Congenital muscular dystrophy : H&E showing a striking dystrophic picture with marked loss of muscle fibres and replacement by connective tissue.

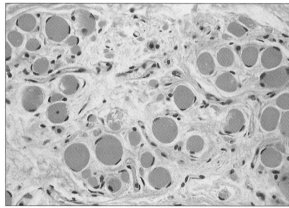

and flexion contractures of the elbows. Muscle wasting is prominent in the upper arms and lower legs. Cardiac involvement with arrhythmias may be life-threatening and may need a cardiac pacemaker.

Serum creatine kinase shows slight to moderate elevation. Muscle biopsy shows mild dystrophic changes and foci of atrophic fibres resembling denervation. The gene has been located to Xq28.

Congenital muscular dystrophy

This term is used for a heterogenous group of children (**8.32–8.35**) who present at birth or early childhood with hypotonia, weakness and contractures of various muscles. The condition tends to remain relatively static or show only slight progression, though some may show functional improvement with time. Some cases show marked mental retardation (Fukuyama type), and some have mental retardation, hydrocephalus and ocular abnormalities (Santavouri type).

The serum creatine kinase is normal or mildly elevated. Muscle biopsy shows variable changes associated with a dystrophic process. The muscle biopsy often appears worse than the clinical picture would suggest, and should not be used as an index of severity of the disease (**8.36**). The condition is autosomal recessive in inheritance, although some cases may be sporadic.

Management consists of active physiotherapy to encourage mobility and stretching of contractures. Surgical correction of residual deformities may be required. Death is usually from respiratory failure.

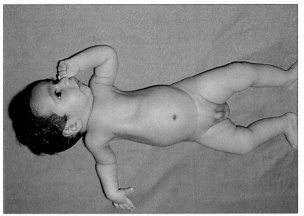

8.37 Spinal muscular atrophy (Werdnig–Hoffman) Type I: Severe proximal wasting, marked chest deformity due to weakness of intercostal muscles and hypotonia, with thighs in abduction.

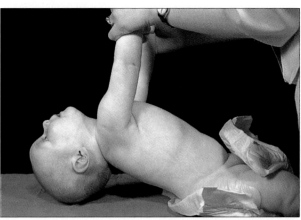

8.38 Spinal muscular atrophy (Werdnig–Hoffman) Type I: 5-month-old infant with marked weakness of neck muscles.

Limb girdle dystrophy

An autosomal recessive disorder, presenting usually in the second or third decade. It consists of progressive muscular weakness and atrophy, usually first appearing in the pelvic girdle musculature. Its progression is variable but usually slow. The syndrome is poorly defined, and may be mimicked by other disorders, such as Becker dystrophy, spinal muscular atrophy, or mitochondrial disorders.

The serum creatine kinase may be elevated. Muscle biopsy shows variable dystrophic changes. Management consists of promoting ambulation and physiotherapy to prevent the onset of deformities.

Fascioscapulohumeral dystrophy

An autosomal dominant condition with onset from early childhood to adult life. It is characterised by weakness of facial and shoulder girdle muscles with later involvement of pelvic and anterior tibial muscles. The course is usually mild and slowly progressive with a normal life span. Those with very early onset may have marked progression with loss of ambulation before their teens.

The serum creatine kinase may be normal or mildly elevated. Muscle biopsy shows variable pathological changes from focal atrophic changes to dystrophic features or variability in fibre size, splitting of fibres, internal nuclei and proliferation of connective tissue.

Spinal muscular atrophies (SMA)

The spinal muscular atrophies are a group of genetically determined disorders in which there is progressive degeneration of the anterior horn cells of the spinal cord. There is progressive weakness and wasting of skeletal muscles. The wasting is usually symmetrical and more severe proximally than distally. Its various forms in childhood can be classified as:

• Severe (infantile onset) SMA (Werdnig–Hoffman disease)
• Intermediate SMA
• Mild (juvenile onset) SMA (Kugelberg–Welander disease)

Most cases of SMA are autosomal recessive in inheritance and the gene location is on chromosome 5q12-14. Occasional cases of chronic SMA are autosomal-dominant, with the gene location being unknown.

Severe SMA (Werdnig–Hoffman)

This is the most severe form of SMA, with onset *in utero* or within the first few months of life. It is characterised by marked limb and axial weakness and hypotonia, normal facial movements, poor head control, sucking and swallowing difficulties, costal recession and diaphragmatic breathing (**8.37 and 8.38**). Anti-gravity power in hip flexors is absent. Intellectual function is not affected. The child is prone to respiratory infections and 95 % of affected children die before 18 months of age. Management is mainly supportive, with treatment of respiratory infections and suction of pharyngeal secretions.

Intermediate SMA

It presents usually between six and twelve months of age, with development appearing normal in the first few months of life so that the child is able to sit unsupported. Weakness of legs and truncal muscles becomes prominent, so that standing is not achieved (**8.39**). Tendon jerks are usually absent or diminished. Fasciculations may be observed in the tongue, but facial muscles are spared. Many cases show little progression, and some

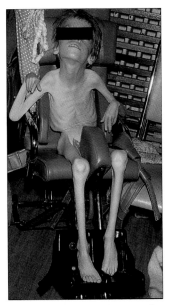

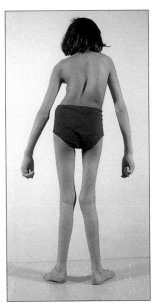

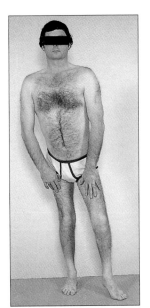

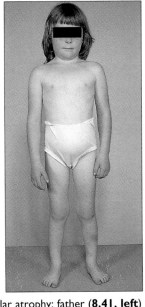

8.39 Spinal muscular atrophy Type II: severe proximal and distal muscle wasting in an 8-year-old boy.

8.40 Spinal muscular atrophy: girl aged 11 years with proximal and distal muscle wasting and developing early spinal scolisosis.

8.41 and 8.42 Spinal muscular atrophy: father (**8.41, left**) and daughter (**8.42, right**) with chronic spinal muscular atrophy (autosomal dominant). Father demonstrating marked wasting and weakness of neck muscles.

may show functional improvement. Scoliosis is common and may lead to cardiorespiratory complications. Management consists of prevention of scoliosis by early spinal bracing or later by surgical fusion of the spine. A standing frame or calipers may be used for the early achievement of a standing position, and ambulation helped by the use of appropriate orthoses.

Mild SMA (Kugelberg–Welander)

The disease begins after infancy and before adult life. Muscle weakness is predominantly proximal, affecting legs more than arms with resulting impairment of walking and running abilities (**8.40–8.42**). Hypertrophy of the calf muscles may occur. Weakness usually remains static and survival into adult life is the rule, and many have a normal life span. Management consists of encouraging activity and maintaining ambulation by the use of suitable calipers if necessary, and the early treatment of respiratory infections.

Investigation of the spinal muscular atrophies reveals the serum creatine kinase to be normal or slightly elevated, and electromyography shows features of denervation and re-innervation. Muscle biopsy shows large-group atrophy, with variable clusters of enlarged fibres in the more chronic cases (**8.43–8.45**). Recombinant DNA studies may help in carrier status and antenatal diagnosis.

Inflammatory myopathies—polymyositis (PM)/dermatomyositis (DM)

The onset of these disorders is usually insidious and may be present two to 52 weeks before the diagnosis. Weakness usually starts in the legs and progresses to arms, and muscle pain and aching is common. Weakness may progress to involve neck flexors and truncal muscles. The classical rash of DM is a violaceous discolouration of the eyelids (**8.46**) and an erythematous eruption over the malar area and extensor surface of the joints (**8.47**), especially the fingers. General malaise with fever is also common.

Involvement of other organs is rare and can occur at any time in the disease. Ulceration of gastrointestinal mucosa with melaena, skin ulceration, albuminuria and other signs of renal involvement, and cardiac murmurs and pericardial friction rubs, may also occur. Calcification of muscle or subcutaneous tissue (**8.48**) is another complication.

Diagnosis is mainly clinical with supportive evidence. The ESR and serum CK may be normal. EMG may show a myopathic picture with fibrillation potentials suggestive of denervation. Muscle biopsy (**8.49–8.51**) may be normal or show areas of necrosis of varying severity, but the extent of muscle involvement

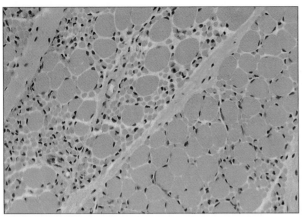

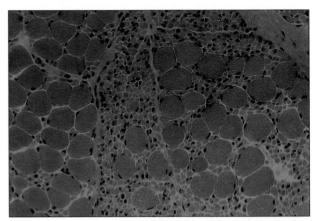

843 and 8.44 Spinal muscular atrophy: biopsy shows a typical picture of SMA with large-group atrophy and a number of enlarged fibres. **8.43 (left)** H&E section. **8.44 (right)** Gomori trichrome.

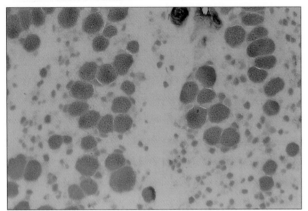

8.45 ATPase pH 4.3. This shows atrophy of both type I and type 2 fibres with selective hypertrophy of type I fibres.

in the biopsy correlates poorly with the clinical picture.

Treatment is with corticosteriods: prednisolone, 1–2 mg/kg/day is the initial treatment of choice. The dose can be reduced and changed to alternate day therapy, once a clinical response has been attained.

Treatment usually should be continued for one to two years at the lowest maintenance dose. Children who do not respond to corticosteroids may require immuno-suppressant therapy with azathioprine or cyclosporin. Supportive measures with physiotherapy are important to prevent the development of contractures.

Myasthenic syndrome

Myasthenia is characterised by abnormal fatiguability after repeated or sustained muscle activity and by improvement with rest or the administration of anti-cholinesterase drugs. Although the majority of cases are found in young adults, 20 % have an onset before the age of 20. Various clinical syndromes of defective transmission at the neuromuscular junction in infancy and childhood have been described; the commonest clinical problems are as follows:

Transient neonatal myasthenia   A transient disorder occurring in 12 % of infants born to myasthenic mothers and related to transplacental passage of maternal antibody to acetylcholine receptors (AChR). Maintenance therapy is directed at providing support of respiration and feeding until the weakness spontaneously remits.

Congenital myasthenia   This occurs in infants born to non-myasthenic mothers. Symptoms are present at birth or soon afterwards. The myasthenia is usually mild with a static or slowly progressive course. Antibodies to AChR are absent. Inheritance is thought to be autosomal-recessive.

Juvenile myasthenia   This is similar to adult myasthenia of the autoimmune type and has a high titre of AChR antibodies.

Clinical features in these disorders commonly include ptosis and weakness of extraocular muscles (**8.52 and 8.53**), together with weakness of other muscle groups. Diagnosis is based on demonstrating fatiguability of muscles after repetitive stimulation of peripheral nerve at 4–10 Hz and the response to intravenous edrophonium (Tensilon). Treatment of juvenile myasthenia includes use of anticholinesterases, corticosteroids, thymectomy and plasmapheresis (*see* **Table 8.3**). All cases should be screened for thymoma, and thymectomy performed where it is found or where medical treatment brings poor control.

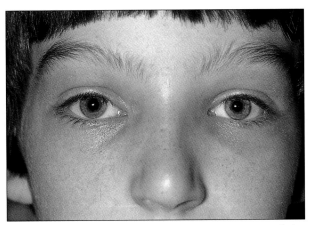

8.46 Dermatomyositis: heliotrope rash present around the eyes.

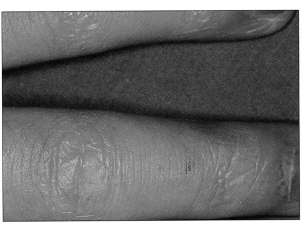

8.47 Dermatomyositis: redness and scaling of the skin over interphalangeal joints.

8.48 Dermatomyositis: late stage. Calcinosis of subcutaneous tissues around the knee joint.

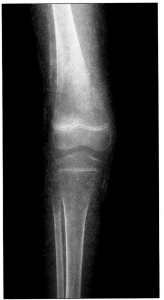

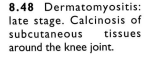

8.49 H&E mononuclear inflammatory cells are both perivascular and interstitial.

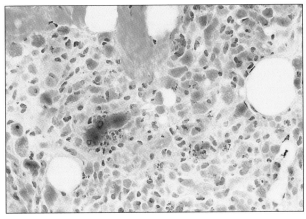

8.50 Areas of necrosis and degenerating muscle fibres.

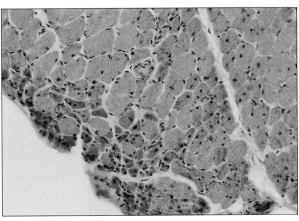

8.51 Perivascular atrophy.

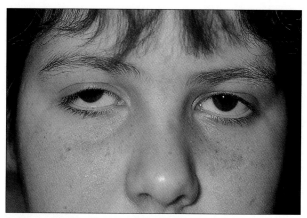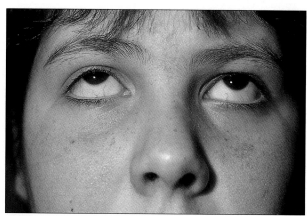

8.52 and **8.53** Teenage girl with myasthenia gravis. Failure to maintain upward gaze with the emergence of ptosis (**8.52, left**) following sustained effort (**8.53, right**).

Myotonic disorders

The cardinal feature of these syndromes is myotonia, a state of delayed relaxation after a sustained contraction. It is best demonstrated by slowness of relaxation of hand grip or by percussion over the tongue or peripheral muscles. On EMG, the myotonia manifests as spontaneous bursts of high-amplitude, high-frequency discharges with gradual waning (**8.54**).

Myotonia congenita This includes the autosomal dominant (Thomsen's disease) and more common autosomal recessive (Becker) varieties (**8.55–8.58**). The condition begins early in life, with widespread myotonia resulting in a generalised painless stiffness, increased by rest and cold and relieved by exercise. There is generally diffuse muscle hypertrophy.

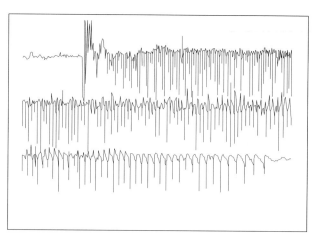

8.54 EMG showing sustained high-frequency myotonic discharge with gradual waning.

Dystrophia myotonica Although the disorder is more prominent in adults, it is also seen in children, resulting in mild facial weakness, distal wasting, and weakness and myotonia of hand grip. Intellectual impairment of varying degree is common. The myotonia rarely causes a problem. In a small number of cases, myotonic dystrophy presents in the neonatal period with marked hypotonia, facial diplegia and feeding difficulties. A history of reduced foetal movement *in utero* is common. The inheritance of myotonic dystrophy is autosomal-dominant and is located on chromosome 19q13.3. In the congenital syndrome, the mother is always affected by the disorder (*see* Chapter 18 for section on imprinting) (**8.59–8.63**).

Metabolic myopathies

In this group of disorders, a single enzyme deficiency leads to symptoms of muscle disease. This may lead to a presentation in early life as a floppy infant, later with muscle weakness or with cramps on exercise. The main categories are the glycogen-storage disorders, and the mitochondrial and lipid-storage myopathies.

Glycogen disorders These disorders result from a hereditary deficiency of some of the enzymes involved in the synthesis or breakdown of glycogen. In three (myophosphorylase deficiency, phosphofructokinase deficiency (**8.64–8.67**) and acid maltase deficiency), the muscle involvement is the sole or predominant manifestation. In two (brancher and debrancher enzymes deficiency), muscle involvement occurs but hepatic involvement is the predominant feature. Glycogen storage disorders are considered in more detail in Chapter 13.

Lipid disorders Oxidation of fatty acids is a major source of energy for skeletal muscle, particularly during prolonged low-intensity exercise or during periods of fasting, when glycogen stores become depleted. Two disorders of muscle lipid metabolism have been identi-

TABLE 8.3 Treatment of Myasthenia Gravis

1. **Anticholinesterase agents:**
   — Neostigmine is relatively short-acting, lasting 2–3 hours with rapid onset of action.
   — Pyridostigmine has slower effect and longer duration of action, lasting 3–5 hours.

2. **Plasmapheresis:**
   Useful in acute fulminant myasthenia and in preparation of severely affected patients for thymectomy.

3. **Immunosuppressant therapy:**
   —Corticosteroid therapy on an alternate-day schedule is effective but reserved for severe cases because of its well-known adverse effects.
   —Azathioprine is also effective, and, when given with prednisolone, allows the dose of the latter to be reduced more rapidly than when steroids are given alone.

4. **Thymectomy:**
   Results in a significant and lasting improvement in many patients and is probably the treatment of choice in children because of the possible adverse side effects of long-term anticholinesterase or immunosuppressant therapy. For children, it significantly increases the remission rate up to 67 %.

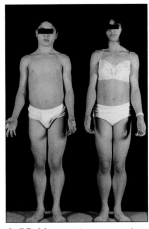

8.55 Myotonia congenita: (autosomal recessive): brother and sister with marked hypertrophy of muscles with myotonic hand grips and characteristic EMG changes of 'dive bomber' myotonic discharges.

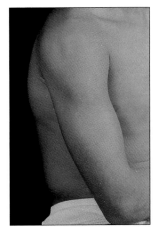

8.56 Myotonia congenita (autosomal recessive): percussion myotonia of right deltoid of boy in previous slide.

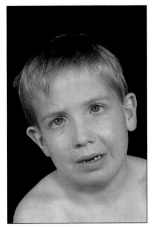
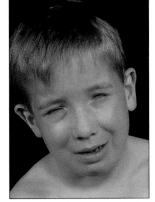

8.57 and 8.58 Myotonia congenita: to demonstrate the myotonia of the orbicularis oculi and the difficulty of opening the eyes after closing them tightly.

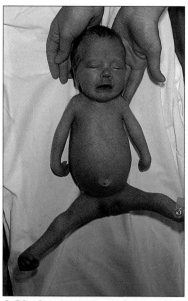

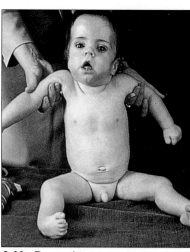

8.60 Dystrophia myotonica in a one-year-old child with facial weakness and equino deformities of feet.

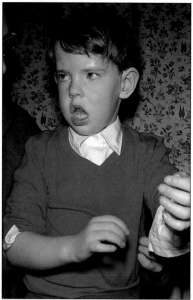

8.59 Severe congenital dystrophia myotonica with distal arthrogryposis in a newborn at 32 weeks' gestation.

8.61 Dystrophia myotonica: 8-year-old boy with marked facial weakness and moderately severe learning disabilities.

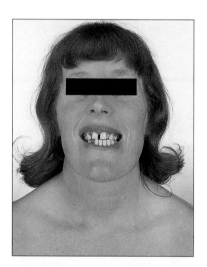

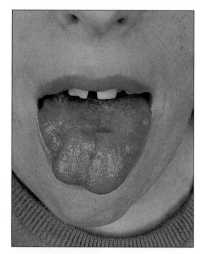

8.62 and 8.63 Dytrophia myotonica: mother of infant with congenital dystrophia myotonica, previously undiagnosed but demonstrating (**8.62, left**) facial weakness and (**8.63, right**) percussion myotonia of tongue.

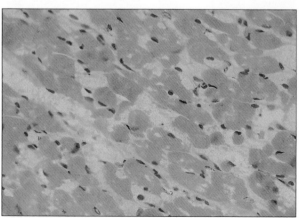

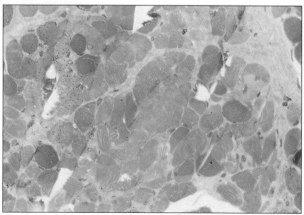

8.64 Glycogen storage disease: fatal infantile—deficiency of phosphofructokinase: H&E staining shows rather disrupted fibres with some vacuolation.

8.65 Glycogen storage disease: fatal infantile—deficiency of phosphofructokinase: PAS staining shows increase in staining in sarcolemmal area.

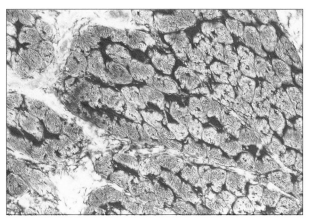

8.66 Glycogen storage disease: fatal infantile—deficiency of phosphofructokinase: epoxyresin: semi-thin section shows fibres containing subsarcolemmal areas that have a ground-glass appearance .

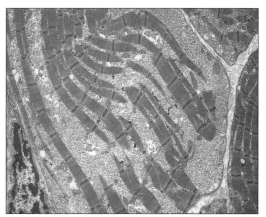

8.67 Glycogen storage disease: fatal infantile—deficiency of phosphofructokinase: EM—showed marked accumulation of normal glycogen particles beneath the sarcolemmal and between myofibrils.

fied—carnitine palmityl transferase (CPT) deficiency and carnitine deficiency. These enzymes are essential for the transport of fatty acids into the mitochondria.

Mitochondrial myopathies A group of disorders associated with abnormalities of mitochondrial function and structure within muscle. Myopathy may be the major manifestation of this disorder or may be part of a widespread multisystem disorder (mitochondrial encephalomyelopathies). Disorders of mitochondrial function may be classified by means of the biochemical defect:

1. Defect of transport: includes carnitine palmityl-transferase and carnitine deficiencies.

2. Defects of substrate utilisation: deficiency of pyruvate carboxylase, pyruvate dehydrogenase complex and defects of beta-oxidation.

3. Defects of Kreb's cycle.

4. Defects of oxidation—phosphorylation coupling—including Luftt's hypermetabolic myopathy.

5. Defects of respiratory chain: deficiency of complex I –V either singly or in combination.

There is great heterogeneity in the clinical presentation of the mitochondrial disorders (**8.68–8.70**). Even the pure myopathies vary considerably in age of onset, distribution of weakness, severity and course. Usually, mitochondrial disorders are multisystem, resulting in a constellation of symptoms and signs; they are also considered in more detail in Chapter 13, but three main recognised syndromes include:

Kearns–Sayre syndrome (KSS): onset before 20, ophthalmoplegia, pigmentary retinopathy, plus one of the following: heart block, cerebellar syndrome, CSF protein above 100 mg/dl.

MELAS: mitochondrial encephalomyelopathy, lactic acidosis and stroke-like episodes.

MERRF: myoclonic epilepsy with 'ragged-red fibres' which are seen on muscle biopsy.

Muscle biopsy abnormalities may consist of the presence of strongly reacting, more granular fibres, with oxidative enzyme reactions (SDH and NADH stains) (**8.71**) or the disrupted red staining 'ragged-red fibres' with Gomori trichrome stain (**8.72**). Electron microscopy may identify abnormal morphological changes of the mitochondria. Biochemical testing of the muscle biopsy will identify the specific abnormality (*see* Chapter 18 for comment on the inheritance of these disorders).

Familial periodic paralyses

These are dominantly inherited disorders characterised by episodes of flaccid weakness, during which the patients are either hypo- or hyperkalaemic. The primary disorder is a membrane abnormality which is due to increased permeability to either sodium or potassium. The attacks last from hours (hyperkalaemic) to days (hypokalaemic). The weakness may be localised or generalised. The cranial and respiratory muscles are generally spared, except in severe episodes. Rest, following a period of prolonged exercise, tends to bring on the weakness of muscles, although continued mild exercise may abort attacks. Cold may also bring on an attack. In the hypokalaemic variety, a meal with excess carbohydrate may also precipitate an attack. Myotonia is often seen in the hyperkalaemic variety.

Treatment in the hypokalaemic form consists of oral potassium chloride supplements in an acute attack and the avoidance of high carbohydrate meals.

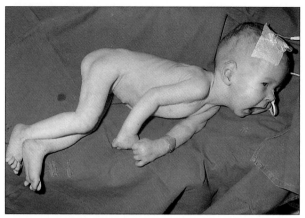

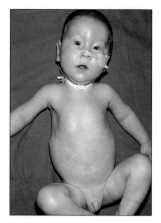

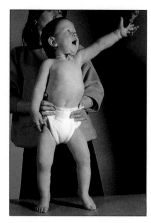

8.68 Congenital mitochondrial myopathy: six weeks old. Severe proximal and distal weakness, severe swallowing diffi-culties and respiratory arrest. Needing prolonged assisted ventilation for first four months.

8.69 Congenital mitochon-drial myopathy: 6-month-old infant with permanent tra-cheostomy tube and increase in muscle power.

8.70 Congenital mitochon-drial myopathy: 14 months of age. Standing with mini-mal aid and able to lift arms above shoulder height.

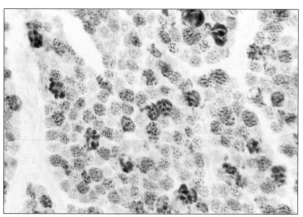

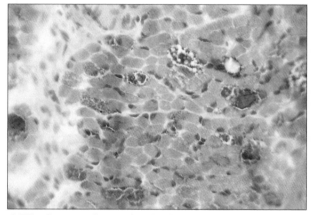

8.71 Congenital mitochondrial myopathy: muscle biopsy NADH stains showing coarse granulation and accumulation of abnormal mitochondria.

8.72 Congenital mitochondrial myopathy: muscle biopsy. Modified trichrome.

Acetazolamide 125–250 mg daily may help in prevent-ing attacks.

Treatment of acute attacks of the hyperkalaemic form consists of oral glucose, 2 gm/kg body weight plus 10–20 IU crystalline insulin subcutaneously. Interval therapy consists of a diet rich in carbohydrate and use of diuretics such as acetazolamide or chlorothiazide to pro-mote a kaliuresis.

Hereditary motor sensory neu-ropathy (HMSN)

This group of disorders includes diseases previously referred to as peroneal muscular atrophy, Charcot –Marie–Tooth disease, Roussy–Levy syndrome and Déjérine–Sottas disease. It is characterised usually by a slowly progressive symmetrical disorder, in which the peripheral neuropathy, predominantly motor in type, is associated with foot deformities, particularly pes cavus. It is inherited as an autosomal-dominant or -recessive trait, and in most cases the neuropathy progresses over several decades so that mobility is usually preserved into middle age.

On the basis of clinical, genetic, electrophysiological and histological evaluation, HMSN can be classified as follows:

HMSN Type I A demyelinating hypertrophic neuropa-thy, usually transmitted as an autosomal dominant, although autosomal-recessive inheritance has been described. Gene localisation is on chromosomes 1 and 17 (**8.73–8.76**).

HMSN Type II A neuronal type with similar inheritance pattern to Type I but gene location unknown.

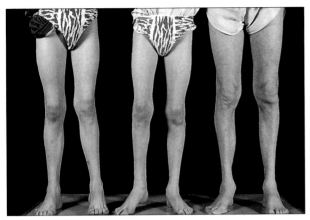

8.73 Hereditary motor and sensory neuropathy Type I (autosomal dominant): father and two sons with this condition demonstrate wasting and weakness, most marked below the knees.

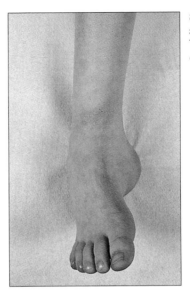

8.74 Hereditary motor and sensory neuropathy Type I: pes cavus deformities.

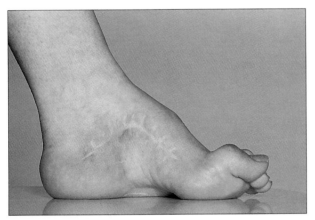

8.75 Hereditary motor and sensory neuropathy Type I: clawing of toes.

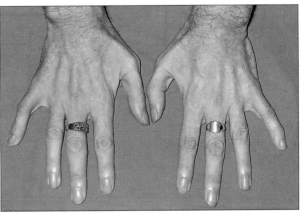

8.76 Hereditary motor and sensory neuropathy Type I: wasting of intrinsic hand muscles.

HMSN Type III Déjérine–Sottas disease with autosomal recessive inheritance.

The clinical features of HMSN Type I and II are similar, and the division is made on the basis of electrophysiological and pathological findings. In HMSN I, nerve conduction velocities are markedly reduced (less than 38 m/sec) and nerve biopsy shows evidence of demyelination and remyelination. In HMSN II, conduction velocities are greater than 30 m/sec and nerve biopsy shows axonal degeneration. Distal wasting and weakness in the lower limbs, and to a lesser extent in the distal upper limbs with mild distal sensory loss, may be observed. Foot deformities with high arches, pes cavus and hammer toes are common and may be the only recognised feature in apparently unaffected members of a family known to carry the trait. It is important to perform nerve conduction studies on both parents as well as the child.

Foot deformity can be a major disability and require adapted shoes. Orthopaedic correction should be deferred into the teens. Shortening of the tendo-achilles consequent upon weakness can be prevented by passive exercise.

HMSN III (Déjérine–Sottas) is autosomal recessive in inheritance. The disorder is much more severe and is present from infancy or early childhood. Motor development is delayed and never becomes normal. In addition to distal weakness in the lower limbs, proximal and truncal weakness is present. In the early teens, distal upper limb weakness develops. The peripheral nerves are palpably enlarged. Most children are wheelchair dependent by their late teens. The CSF protein is often raised, the motor nerve conduction velocities are very slow and sensory nerve action potentials usually absent. Nerve biopsy reveals prominent segmental demyelination and onion bulb formation.

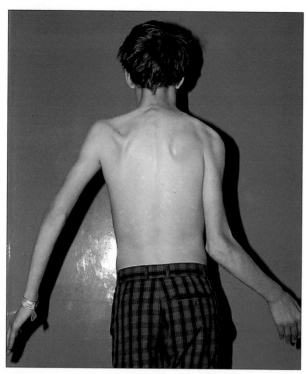

8.77 Bilateral acute brachial neuropathy (neuralgic amyotrophy): 9-year-old boy with a 3-week history of severe pain in the shoulder girdle associated with marked wasting of muscles around the shoulder girdle, inability to elevate arms and winging of both scapulae. CT myelography demonstrated no abnormality. EMG revealed acute denervation changes in muscles around the shoulder girdles.

Acute inflammatory polyradicu-loneuropathy (AIP)—Guillain–Barré syndrome

This syndrome involves an acute symmetrical ascending paresis of sub-acute or acute onset, starting in the legs and moving upwards to involve the trunk and upper limbs, often causing a marked flaccid quadriplegia. Weakness is often more severe proximally than distally and respiratory muscle involvement may be life-threatening. Bulbar involvement may also occur and facial palsy is common. There may be associated sensory symptoms and also at times evidence of autonomic dysfunction. The evolution of the weakness may occur over a variable period of a few days to a few weeks, followed by a process of recovery which may be slow and continue over several months.

The CSF shows a characteristic picture of raised protein without increase in cells, but in the early stages the CSF may be normal. The neuropathy is of the demyelinating type and may be confirmed by very slow motor nerve conduction velocities, though this feature may sometimes be absent in the early stages of the disorder.

The aetiology is obscure but may have an immunological basis. There is often a preceding infection, usually respiratory or gastrointestinal. Treatment is supportive. If respiratory embarrassment occurs, ventilatory support may be necessary. In severe cases that are progressing, plasmapheresis particularly in the early stages has been shown to be beneficial. Corticosteroid therapy is not indicated. High-dose intravenous immunoglobulin in a dose of 0.4 g/kg/day for five days is an effective therapy and will probably replace plasmapheresis in children. The overall prognosis in children is usually good and the majority show full recovery, though some may be left with residual weakness.

Brachial neuritis (Neuralgic amyotrophy)

A disorder characterised by the development of shoulder pain of sudden onset, usually lasting several days or weeks, followed by long-term weakness of the shoulder girdle or arm muscles or both (**8.77**). Most are affected unilaterally, although some may be affected bilaterally. The aetiology of the syndrome is unknown. It frequently follows exercise of the affected limb, an infectious illness, and/or immunisation. Clinical features consist of muscle weakness, wasting and sensory loss in the shoulder or limb, depending on the roots or nerves involved. The commonest affected root is C4, but sensory loss is often minimal. The neurological examination is otherwise normal. Prognosis is good and nearly all cases show full recovery, although the period of recovery may be protracted over two years or so.

Bell's palsy

Sudden paralysis of one side of the face can occur at any age (**8.78**). The disorder often begins with pain in the mastoid region or ear for a day or so, followed by weakness of the face. The weakness is usually maximal in a few hours but progression may continue for a few days in some cases. The upper and lower facial muscles are affected, resulting in impairment of eye closure and drooping of the side of the mouth, causing some slurring of speech.

The condition commonly follows an upper respiratory tract infection. Prognosis in children is good, with 80 % recovering completely in the six months after onset. Prognosis is less good if onset of recovery is delayed for more than three weeks, but recovery may continue for as long as six months. Treatment with steroids, either in the form of prednisolone 1 to 2 mg/kg/day, or ACTH in a reducing dose for a period of five days is advocated by some, if given in the first 72 hours after onset; scientific evidence to support this prac-

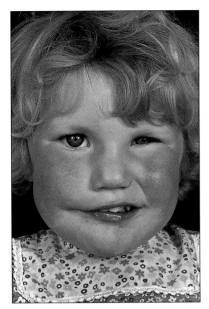

8.78 Right facial weakness (Bell's palsy) demonstrating weakness of both upper and lower face.

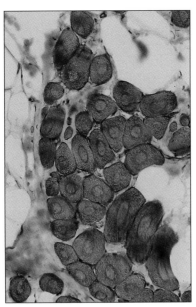

8.79 Central core disease: Type I fibres showing loss of staining with PAS.

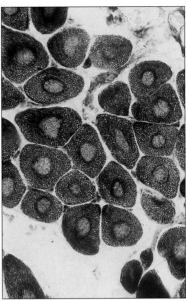

8.80 Central core disease: the cores are unreactive with NADH-TR.

tory tract infection. Prognosis in children is good, with 80 % recovering completely in the six months after onset. Prognosis is less good if onset of recovery is delayed for more than three weeks, but recovery may continue for as long as six months. Treatment with steroids, either in the form of prednisolone 1 to 2 mg/kg/day, or ACTH in a reducing dose for a period of five days is advocated by some, if given in the first 72 hours after onset; scientific evidence to support this practice is not available. As the majority of children will improve spontaneously, the use of steroids is debatable.

An association between Bell's palsy and coarctation of the aorta has been described: the blood pressure should be measured in all children. Sarcoidosis should be suspected where the paresis is bilateral. Melkersson's syndrome is a dominantly inherited cause of recurrent facial paresis seen in association with facial oedema and a 'scrotal' tongue; there is variable penetrance. Clinical assessment should always pay particular attention to the presence of deafness and cerebellar ataxia which would suggest the presence of a cerebellar-pontine angle space-occupying lesion. In cases of delayed recovery, the presence of a stapedial reflex is a very good prognostic sign.

Congenital myopathy

This is a group of inherited muscle disorders characterised by specific changes in muscle structure that can be demonstrated by the application of histochemical techniques and electron microscopy. Clinically, these children present in a non-specific manner either with the floppy infant syndrome or later with muscle weakness. The only reliable way of establishing the diagnosis is by muscle biopsy. Some of the congenital myopathies have certain characteristic features and may be suspected clinically. Individual disorders have differing modes of inheritance and are considered below:

• *Central core disease:* autosomal dominant. It is characterised pathologically by central areas within muscle fibres which are devoid of the normal histochemical reactions for oxidative enzymes (**8.79 and 8.80**), myophophorylase and glycogen. The clinical features are hypotonia from birth or early infancy, facial and proximal limb weakness and skeletal deformities. This disorder is associated with a susceptibility to malignant hyperthermia, so great care is indicated when surgery is carried out.

• *Multicore disease:* autosomal recessive. Muscle fibres show multiple areas devoid of enzyme activity. Muscle weakness is variable and usually non-progressive (**8.81**).

• *Nemaline myopathy:* autosomal recessive or dominant. Histologically, multiple, small, rod-like particles, thought to represent Z-band proteins, are present within most muscle fibres (**8.82–8.84**)

There are three clinical presentations:

111

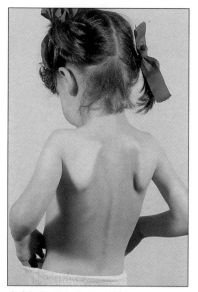

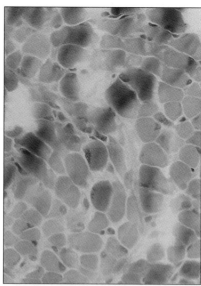

8.81 Congenital multicore myopathy: 4-year-old girl with marked winging and weakness of shoulder girdle muscles.

8.82 and 8.83 In nemaline rod myopathy, characteristic aggregates of rod (red in colour) are best seen in in the Gomori trichrome stain (**8.82, left**), and are easily overlooked on routine H&E staining (**8.83, right**).

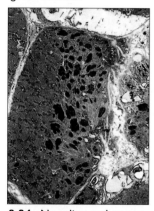

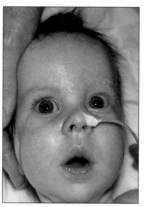

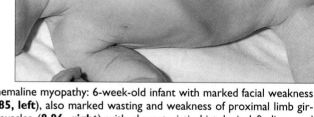

8.84 Nemaline rod myopathy: electron micrograph shows degeneration and loss of structure in the fibres with numerous rectangular dense rods.

8.85 and 8.86 Congenital nemaline myopathy: 6-week-old infant with marked facial weakness and swallowing difficulties (**8.85, left**), also marked wasting and weakness of proximal limb girdle muscles and intercostal muscles (**8.86, right**) with characteristic histological findings and death at four months of age.

recessive and dominant.

The principal feature is the presence of a large proportion of muscle fibres with central nuclei, surrounded by a relatively clear zone of sacroplasm which contains glycogen granules, increased numbers of mitochondria and lipid vacuoles, but in which myofibrils are absent (**8.89 and 8.90**). Clinically, the disorder may present in infancy and progress rapidly to death from cardiopulmonary failure by the age of 18 months. In others, the disability may run a milder course and not present till later life. Ptosis and ophthalmoplegia are frequently found.

• *Congenital fibre-type disproportion:* autosomal dominant and recessive (**8.91 and 8.92**). The histology demonstrates an excessive disparity of size between Type 1 and 2 muscle fibres in the absence of other obvious histological abnormalities. This disorder may present in infancy with hypotonia and muscle weakness which may be mild or severe.

8.87 and 8.88 Congenital nemaline myopathy: (**8.87, left**) marked weakness of nuchal and proximal limb girdle muscles in a 7-year-old girl. (**8.88 right**). Weakness of facial muscles and micrognathia also evident.

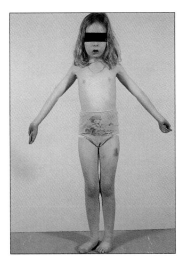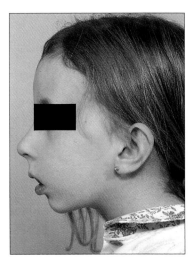

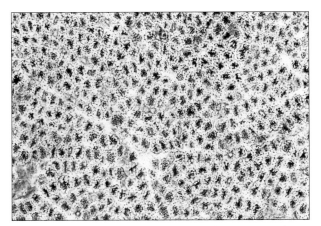

8.89 Centronuclear myopathy: the NADH reaction shows aggregation of enzyme activity in the fibre centres.

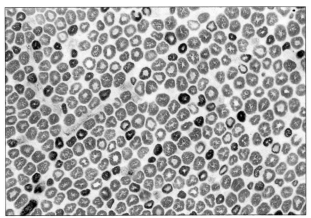

8.90 Centronuclear myopathy: the ATPase shows central areas devoid of staining.

8.91 Congenital fibre type disproportion: 9-year-old girl with mild weakness investigated earlier for 'failure to thrive' and very slim musculature.

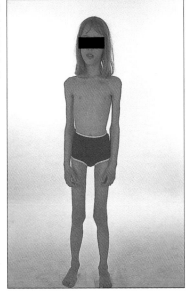

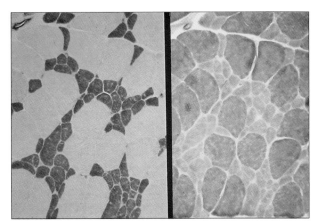

8.92 Congenital fibre type disproportion: histological changes on muscle biopsy show type I fibres to be small on NADH and ATPase staining of muscle biopsy.

Chapter 9: Vascular Disease

Michael A. Clarke, James Leggate, W. St. Clair Forbes

Traumatic causes of intracranial haemorrhage

- Extradural haematoma
- Subdural haematoma
- Intracerebral haematoma
- Sub-arachnoid haemorrhage

Extradural haematoma

Head injury is the commonest cause of death in children between the ages of one and fourteen. Death is due to haematoma formation and associated diffuse cerebral swelling. Haematomas may also form in the subdural space, as well as within the cerebral parenchyma (*see* below).

Extradural haematoma (**9.1**) occurs in approxiamtely 8 % of children admitted to hospital with head injury. Extradural haematoma is not seen as frequently with skull fracture as it is in adults. Nonetheless, over 95 % of children under two (Leggate *et al.*, 1989) will have an associated skull fracture. The source of the bleeding in children, in contrast to adults, is not to a great extent related to fractures across the lines of the middle meningeal arteries: in 50 %, extradural haematomas are seen to arise from venous bleeding, and in a sizeable number from bone fracture margins themselves (**Table 9.1**). This latter factor may account for the increased fre-

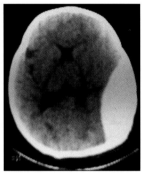

9.1 Extradural haematoma—note biconvex haematoma crossing parietal occipital suture line. Little mass effect seen as suture widely opened and thin pliable skull prevents pressure build-up.

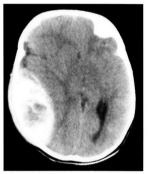

9.2 Extradural haematoma in an 8-month-old child. Note similar size to **9.1**, but with increased mass effect with shift of the midline. Note central low density or 'lucent swirl' indicative of active bleeding.

quency of the prolonged lucid interval between trauma and recognition of the haematoma in the infant compared to the adult.

In the very young infant, the haematoma may present with anaemia or shock before any symptoms or signs of raised intracranial pressure are recognised. More commonly, presentation is with a deterioration of conscious level, seizures and the emergence of focal signs.

As a sizeable proportion of the child's circulating blood volume may be lost, management of these haematomas depends on expert anaesthetic care and resuscitation prior to evacuation of the haematoma. Active bleeding is often seen at the time of the CT scan and is known as a 'lucent swirl' (**9.2**). Early recognition prior to neurological deterioration and evacuation of the haematoma with haemastasis remains the treatment of choice. Where the child is operated on with a Glasgow Coma Scale Score of 9 or more, a good outcome can be expected in over 90 % (**9.3 and 9.4**). Where deterioration of conscious level has progressed to a Coma Scale

TABLE 9.1 Extradural Haematoma in Infants	
Mid-meningeal artery	42.5 %
Bone	27.5 %
Dura	7.5 %
Unknown	22.5 %

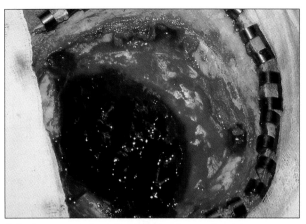

9.3 Intraoperative photograph of extradural haematoma. Bone margin and dural surface can be seen.

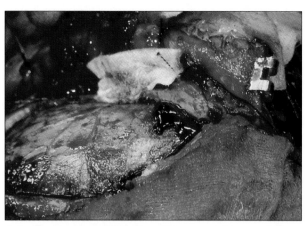

9.4 Dural surface of **9.3** after clot removal. Note underlying middle meningeal vessels.

TABLE 9.2 Extradural Haematoma in Infants: Location of Haematoma

Parietal or temporal	7.5 %
Parieto-occipital	12.5 %
Temporo-occipital	7.5 %
Post-fossa	5 %

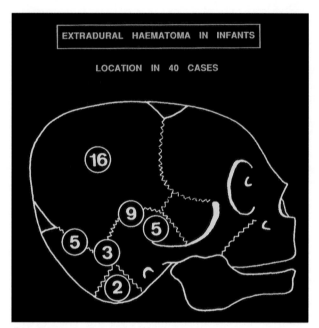

9.5 Location of extradural haematoma.

Score of 8 or less, the mortality and morbidity is much higher. The presence of a suture line, and its supposed adherence of the underlying dura, does not, however, prevent the spread of extradural haematomas across skull-plate bones, and it is not uncommon for sizeable extradural haematomas to cross one, or even more, suture lines (**9.5**) (*see also* **Table 9.2**).

Where extradural haematomas are situated in the posterior fossa, they typically present late and have a poor outcome because of acute deterioration, usually associated with respiratory or cardiovascular failure. Treatment of these haematomas, as for the supra-tentorial collections, comprises decompression, haemostasis and resuscitation.

Subdural haematomas

Subdural haematomas may be acute or subacute. When acute, they are related to trauma. The average incidence of subdural haematomas in children with head injuries is approximately 5–8 %, and is considerably less frequent than that found in adults. Non-accidental injury (NAI) typically produces traumatic subdural haematomas, often associated with some subarachnoid bleeding, which reflects the shearing nature of the injury, produc-

Practice Point 9.1

Suspect non-accidental injury when skull fractures are:

- Occipital
- Wide (greater than 5mm)
- Multiple
- Growing
- Depressed
- Non-parietal
- Complex configuration
- Involving more than one bone

9.6 and 9.7 Skull fractures in NAI. Occipital fractures (arrowed) are to be viewed with suspicion as are those which are multiple, of complex configuration, depressed, wide (> 5 mm) or growing, non-parietal or involving more than bone.

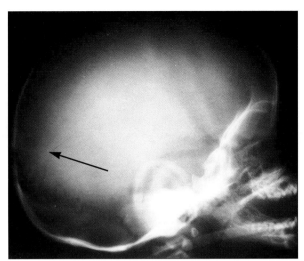
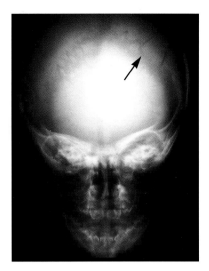

TABLE 9.3 Neurosurgical Features of Non-Accidental Injury

- Cephalhaematoma
- Retinal haemorrhage
- Skull fracture
- Diffuse axonal injury (D.A.I.)
- Intracerebral haemorrhage
  — Subarachnoid
  — Subdural

ing tearing of the cortical bridging veins and laceration to the cerebral cortex itself. Inter-hemispheric acute subdural haematomas, together with evidence of contusion or damage to the front of the corpus callosum or around the tectal plate area of the mid-brain, are pathognomonic features of NAI (*see* **Practice Point 9.1**). Whilst radiological and clinical features may suggest NAI as a cause, these are non-specific, and a wider differential diagnosis must always be entertained. Intracranial haemorrhage due to NAI must be differentiated from birth trauma, accidental injury, and spontaneous bleeding. The history needs to be viewed in the light of family circumstances. The site, age and nature of the bleed will aid diagnosis, as will the character of any attendant skull fracture (**Table 9.3**).

Symptoms can be insidious in onset (*see* below), and within the first three or four weeks of life, birth trauma remains a likely culprit, even after an apparently atraumatic delivery. Haemorrhagic disease of the newborn can present with subdural haemorrhage, emphasising the importance of a platelet count and clotting screen at any age.

The usual presentation is with acute encephalopathy, coma and seizures, and frequently evidence of cerebral anoxia and haemorrhage are found together. An acute onset of symptoms is most likely to reflect a recent bleed. A rebleed may cause confusion in this respect. Although this is most likely to occur within a week or two of the initial haemorrhage, rebleeding may be delayed for some weeks. A gradual onset of symptoms with accelerating head growth and a filling fontanelle would indicate the time of onset to be more remote.

Retinal haemorrhage is an important and common sign in child abuse. Sezen (1970) found retinal haemorrhage in 14 % of newborns, though only 2.6 % persisted for two to three weeks. Aron *et al.* (1970) found the incidence in children subjected to NAI to be 90 %, and that they could last for several years.

The CT scan appearance may help time the bleed if the haemaglobin concentration in peripheral blood is known (*see* below).

Herpes simplex encephalitis may cause a fulminant, necrotising encephalitis, with frank haemorrhage in the sub-arachnoid space and brain parenchyma. A prodromal illness is seen in 40 %, but the fact that fever may be seen in nearly 60 % of children with subdural haemorrhage adds to the diagnostic dilemma. The viral illness is more likely to be associated with a rise in the ESR and acute phase proteins.

Non-ambulant children are top heavy and commonly injure their heads when they fall from high surfaces. External injury to other parts of the body is rare. Subdural haemorrhage is exceptionally rare in falls of up to 60 inches on to a firm surface. Where NAI is the cause of haematoma formation, there are commonly associated injuries to the skeletal system and other organs. The skull fracture in NAI is likely to be multiple (**9.6 and 9.7**), of complex configuration, depressed, wide (> 5mm) or growing.

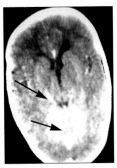

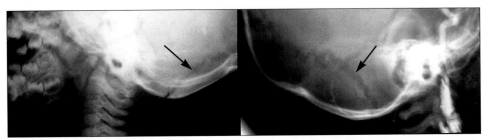

9.9 Posterior fossa extradural haematoma with widening of the lamboid sutures (arrowed) in an infant. X-ray on right taken 11 days after x-ray on left.

9.8 'Goblet' sign (arrowed) seen with compression of the tentorial notch draining veins.

NAI presenting with solely neurological manifestations is often the most dangerous form of NAI, frequently associated with persisting and severe neurodevelopmental handicap.

Where possible after early recognition of subdural haematoma, the treatment consists of craniotomy, with removal of as much as is possible of the subdural haematoma. Where there is massive associated underlying cerebral oedema and shift in relation to the size of the haematoma to be removed, then it may be more appropriate sometimes for radial incisions to be made in the dura and the clot to be released over an area of the brain, without formally opening the dura. The avoidance of the need to open the dura can often contain the underlying swollen brain. Having evacuated all, or as much as is practical, of the haematoma, the underlying brain damage and subsequent cerebral oedema will require treatment. The subject of measurement and control of intracranial pressure is reviewed in Chapter 7.

Chronic subdural haematoma

This is seen typically only in younger children, and is usually due to trauma, often of a relatively minor nature, although the question of NAI must always be considered in children in whom chronic subdural haematomas are identified (*see* above). The presentation is often related to the development of intracranial hypertension as a direct result of the collection. Seizures may also be a manifestation of these collections, and in the younger infant the development of macrocrania may also reflect an underlying collection. In some cases, as in acute subdural haematoma, the presence of retinal subhyaloid haemorrhages may accompany these collections, although it is by no means certain these reflect the raised intracranial pressure rather than the type of injury involved in producing such haematomas.

The collections may often assume isodense CT scan characteristics, and if these collections are bilateral, then the lateral mass effects of each collection may be negated by the other, and in such circumstances it is possible to misdiagnose this condition. The presence of compressed perimesial cisterns and of crowding of the tentorial notch (**9.8**) is often the only radiological sign of bilateral hyperdense subdural haematomas. There is often sulcal widening and distortion of the underlying gyral pattern, suggestive of a process akin to atrophy.

Treatment is required when there is illness due to increased pressure, or accelerated head growth with splaying of the sutures (**9.9**). It consists of aspiration or drainage of the collection, either by intermittent percutaneous tapping, using a spinal needle and entering through either the sutures or through the lateral margins of the anterior fontanelles. The placement of a drain into the subdural space through a single burr hole can also be used to release the pressure on the underlying brain and allow redevelopent of the brain tissue by removal of the mass occupation effect of the subdural haematoma. The presence of blood within the collections or old clot may give some indication as to the length of haematoma formation in relation to any specific events in the child's life. The majority of cases will resolve either by subdural draining or by intermittent tapping. Where this method fails to resolve the haematoma, then a subdural peritoneal shunt may be needed to allow normal development of the underlying brain. A very high protein concentration in the fluid may preclude this approach to treatment. The use of craniotomy for removal of the membrane for chronic subdural haematoma may be used as a last resort.

Where the collection of fluid has communicated with the subarachnoid space, resulting in a collection of clear CSF density fluid, then the treatment remains that of external drainage or internalising the drainage in the form of a subdural-peritoneal shunt.

Intracerebral haematoma is seen in less than 3 % of paediatric head trauma. It is most commonly seen in pre-

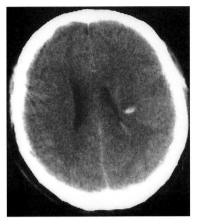

9.10 Diffuse shearing head injury—petechial haemorrhage. Oedema and haemorrhage at right periventricular region.

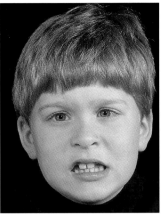

9.11 Recovery following shearing head injury: left VI nerve palsy and left lower quadrant facial hypokinesia (upper motor neurone VII).

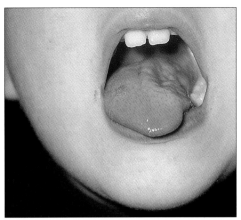

9.12 Recovery following shearing head injury: left haemiatrophy of tongue due to lesion of left XII cranial nerve.

mature babies, where it is found in the germinal matrix in the peri-third ventricular region following traumatic delivery or in association with grade III or IV intraventricular haemorrhage.

Treatment consists of removal of the mass effect by haematoma drainage and is indicated where there is deteriorationin the neurological status of the child or continuingenlargement of the haematoma. Outcome, including the incidence ofepilepsy, is not significantly altered by the timing of the drainage procedure.

Sub-arachnoid haemorrhage most commonly is the result of trauma; other pathologies are reviewed below.

Neuroradiology in trauma

The introduction of computerised tomography (CT) has had a profound impact on the early assessment and diagnosis of head injuries. CT should be the initial imaging modality when significant brain injury is suspected, in order to define the nature and severity of the injury.

Cerebral oedema The cause of brain swelling has been attributed to increased cerebral blood volume and the subsequent development of cerebral oedema. The CT findings are:

(1) A slight increase in the density of the brain, which may be due to the addition of increased blood. The density returns to normal with the resolution of oedema and decreased blood flow.

(2) Absence or compression of the lateral and third ventricles and perimesencephalic cisterns.

The changes of ventricular size may be more apparent on review of serial CT examinations as the ventricles are normally small in the paediatric age group.

Contusion The initial post-injury CT appearance of contusion is:

(1) An area of increased density, higher than surrounding brain due to the extravasated blood.

(2) Low density of the swollen brain substance, producing a non-homogeneous appearance (**9.10**).

There is associated mass effect, which increases because of oedema at the site of the contusion, and becomes maximal between the third and the sixth days after injury. Further bleeding at the site of the contusion results in the formation of a contusional haematoma. The combination of oedema fluid and haemorrhagic tissue produces an area of variable density ranging from hypodense to hyperdense.

Shearing injuries The areas most commonly involved are the corpus callosum, septum pellucidum, medullary pyramids, third ventriclar region and deep white matter (**9.11 and 9.12**). The CT findings are:

(1) Bilateral cerebral swelling with cisternal and ventricular compression, eccentric haemorrhage in the corpus callosum, sub-arachnoid haemorrhage and the absence of specific focal mass lesions.

(2) Small focal areas of haemorrhage, less commonly identified, adjacent to the third ventricle or within the white matter of the cerebral hemispheres.

(3) Atrophic enlargement of the lateral ventricles and focal areas of decreased density within the cerebral white matter appear two to three weeks after injury.

Intracerebral haematoma Acute intracerebral haematomas are most commonly found in the frontal and temporal lobes. They are commonly associated with contusions. Multiple lesions may be present. The CT appearance is of a well-defined area of increased density within the brain parenchyma, associated with mass effect and surrounded by a zone of lower density representing macerated tissue and oedema. The development of haematomas may be delayed, occurring during the first 48 hours after injury and usually associated with a poor prognosis. The size and density of haematomas will gradually decrease with time.

Sub-arachnoid and intraventricular haemorrhage accompanying an intracerebral haematoma are readily detected on CT.

Acute subdural haematoma The haematoma may be located over the convexity, and tentorium, in the middle or posterior cranial fossae or within the interhemispheric fissure. Location of a subdural haematoma within the posterior fossae is more common in children than in adults. CT appearance of an acute subdural haematoma is a crescentic concavo-convex lesion located against the calvarium laterally, and the cerebral cortex medially. The density of the haematoma will vary with its age and is of greater density than the surrounding brain parenchyma in the acute phase. The shape of the subdural haematoma may be modified by the presence of extensive parenchymal damage. Acute interhemispheric subdural haematomas are common in childhood, especially in abused children. Associated skull fractures are infrequent.

The density of the subdural haematoma decreases with time, approximating to that of brain (isodense lesion) two to four weeks after injury, and becomes hypodense approximately three to four weeks after the episode of trauma. The rate of this change depends on the haemaglobin concentration; the higher the concentration, the slower the resolution.

Extradural haematoma Extradural haematomas may be arterial or venous in origin. These haematomas are uncommon in infants and children. The CT appearance is of a well-defined biconvex (lenticular) lesion which is hyperdense in relation to the surrounding brain. The firm dural attachment to the inner table of the skull limits peripheral expansion of the haematoma, thus accounting for the convex medial margin. The degree of associated mass effect and midline shift is usually proportionate to the size of the collection, unlike the subdural haematoma.

Non-accidental head injury Subdural haematoma is the commonest abnormality in this syndrome. In the majority, it is located in the posterior (parieto-occipital) portion of the interhemispheric fissure on either side of the falx, at the site of drainage of the cerebral veins attached to the superior sagittal sinus. A similar appearance is produced by an interhemispheric sub-arachnoid haemorrhage, which is also a common finding in cases of NAI. The parafalcine collection is almost certainly the result

of shaking. Cerebral swelling, either focal or diffuse, can be found in over 60 % of patients. Occasionally, the effects of very severe hypoxic injury can be seen when CT shows a diffuse reduction in attenuation of the cortical grey matter, but with preservation of the grey matter in the basal ganglia region, cerebellum and brainstem. In those that survive, marked gross cerebral atrophy and ventricular dilatation develops rapidly, which reflect irreversible brain damage. Intracerebral haematoma and contusion are equally common, with or without evidence of a skull fracture.

The CT scan indicates much more severe and diffuse general atrophy than would be expected to have developed in an older child or adults after a similar insult, and children over the age of five have a better prognosis than younger children or infants.

Non-traumatic intracranial bleeding

• Arterio-venous malformation
• Tumour
• Aneurysm
• Coagulopathies

Aneurysm, arterio-venous malformation (AVM), caroti-co-cavernous fistula and vein of Galen aneurysms (**9. 13 and 9.14**) (arterio-venous shunts) are the common non-traumatic causes of intracranial bleeding in children. The source of bleeding is most often attributable to an AVM, with slightly under one third being due to aneurysm and a slightly lesser proportion to abnormalities not demonstrable neuroradiologically (*see* below).

During early cerebral circulation development, thin-walled channels connect the arterial elements of the developing brain's vasculature to the venous elements. Persistence of these thin-walled channels with numerous inter-connections is reflected in the typical intracerebral AVM. Whilst the large majority of these lesions are quiescent for many years, the possiblity of rupture of the thin-walled vessels persists. The resulting haemorrhage is less easily controlled than where thick-walled muscular vessels are involved. The typical configuration of the haemorrhage is in a V-shaped appearance, with the apex pointing medially to the ventricular cavity. The anatomical location of the AVM either superficly (**9.15**), or deep (**9.16 and 9.17**) within the cerebral cortex and white matter, and the location of the malformation in relation to the eloquent areas of the brain, will all determine the nature or consequence of the bleed. Typically, the clinical course of such a haemorrhage is for repeated bleeds with progressive neurological deterioration with each successive bleed. The intracerebral haematomas

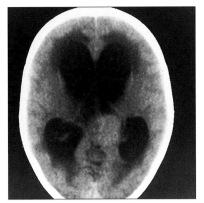

9.13 Vein of Galen aneurysm: unenhanced scan shows obstructive hyprocephalus with periventricular lucency.

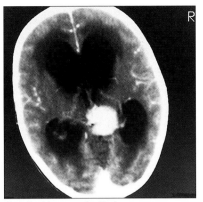

9.14 Vein of Galen aneurysm: enhanced scan shows aneurysmal dilatation of straight sinus with obstruction to junction of third ventricle and aqueduct.

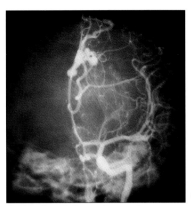

9.15 Small frontal arteriovenous malformation: note feeding I vessel from peri-callosal artery.

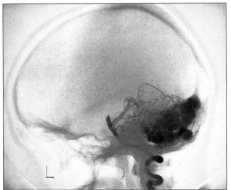

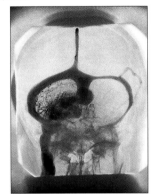

9.16 and 9.17 Subtracted angio-gram views of right cerebral hemisphere arteriovenous malformation from the posterior inferior cerebellar artery and the superior and anterior inferior cerebellar arteries (**9.16, left**). The high flow through this malformation is causing retrograde venous flow up into the superior saggital sinus (**9.17, right**).

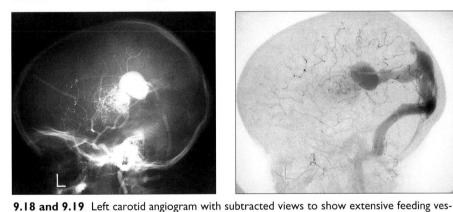

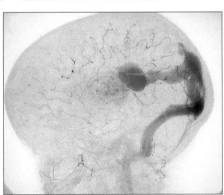

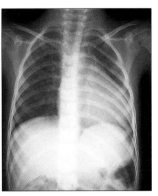

9.18 and 9.19 Left carotid angiogram with subtracted views to show extensive feeding vessels of the vein of Galen malformation predominantly from the anterior artery together with the branches of the anterior cerebral and middle cerebral circulation. Note the shunt and frontal access device tubing *in situ*. On these subtracted views the extensive venous drainage via the straight sinus through the torcula to the sigmoid sinus is clearly seen.

9.20 Chest x-ray of patient with vein of Galen aneurysm demonstrating mild cardiomegaly but without signs of high-output cardiac failure.

from an AVM appear to dissect through the white matter fibres rather than disrupting them, and in such a way, even very large intracerebral haematomas may result in near-normal neurological recovery, which is unusual with a haematoma formed by rupture of an aneurysm.

Typically, AVMs will present either with haemorrhage or epilepsy, either in isolation or together with evidence of surrounding brain ischaemia with resulting loss or deterioration of function of that portion of the brain. Epilepsy is the most common presentation in children, and an AVM should always be considered in a child with both migraine and epilepsy. In severe cases, high-output heart failure may be noted, but this is more typically seen in other conditions, such as vein of Galen aneurysms (**9.18–9.20**).

The presence or absence of an intracranial bruit in a

young child is of no help in determining whether an arterial malformation is present. Many young children have bruits transmitted to the skull from flow in the carotid or subclavian vessels.

The leptomeningeal angiomatosis associated with Sturge–Weber syndrome is not associated with intracranial haemorrhage.

Surgical excision of these lesions remains the main aim of treatment, but the risk should be carefully weighed. Treatment may be conservative if the perceived risk of surgery is too high, or stereotatic radiotherapy may be given using the 'gamma knife' or focused radiotherapy using a linear accelerator. The natural history of AVM is not clearly understood, making comparision of any technique to the natural history difficult. With a small-sized (less than 2 cm diameter) AVM in a non-eloquent area and with only superficial venous drainage (**9.21**), surgical excision can be achieved with minimum morbidity and mortality. Surgical removal may not cure epilepsy, but seizure type and frequency may be ameliorated. Post-operative angiography is usually carried out to ensure that total removal of the malformation has been completed and no nidus remains. Success depends on the size of the AVM, the extent of the venous drainage and whether this is superficial or deep, and the number of feeding arterial vessels.

The use of interventional radiology is often considered where surgically unressectable lesions are identified after investigation. The use of particle techniques with gel sponge inserted through directed catheters, or the use of pellets or other substances, can result in obliteration of the nidus of the AVM. The use of the glues is controversial, and complications relating to adhesion of the catheter with the nidus of the AVM are well reported. Nevertheless, interventional neuroradiology has a significant role to play in the management of AVMs.

Certain AVMs that have presented with proven subarachnoid haemorrhage or intracerebral haemorrhage may not be shown on angiography. Such lesions are known as 'occult' malformations and usually represent malformations which have destroyed themselves at the time of the haemorrhage.

In childhood, aneurysms are rare and more common amongst older children. Presentation is similar to arterio-venousmalformation, with rupture leading to subarachnoid haemorrhage, with subsequent development of meningismand, depending on the site of the bleed, associated with neurological dysfunction.

The treatment consists of occlusion of the aneurysm sac, either by obliteration of the lumen via intravascular-radiological techniques utilising wire coils, or balloon embolisation (**9.22–9.27**). Alternatively, occlusion of the neck of the sac can be achieved by the application of a stainless steel non-ferrous magnetic aneurysm clip (**9.28**).

Neuroradiology and intracranial haemorrhage

Role of CT

- As a screening procedure to confirm the presence or absence of cerebral abnormalities.
- To demonstrate haemorrhage.
- To determine if other associated intracranial abnormalities are present.

Angiography is mandatory for precise anatomical delineation and characterisation of the abnormality prior to treatment, and also to demonstrate associated abnormalities, e.g. aneurysms.

CT of intracerebral haemorrhage A fresh intracerebral haematoma appears as a region of increased density, which depending on its size, may exert considerable mass effect. There is usually little surrounding oedema, since bleeding dissects through cerebral tissue, but athypodense 'halo' is frequently seen. The protein component of haemaglobin is the main determinant of attenuation, the iron in haemaglobin having little contribution. In the case of anaemia, the CT detection of haemorrhage may be difficult. The hyperdense lesion becomes isodense after seven to ten days following the absorption of the clot. A ring enhancement pattern after intravenous contrast is seen at this stage, and can persist for up to six months. With the clot retraction, there is a decrease in the associated mass effect. Eventually, a well-defined area of low density may be seen at the site of the haematoma.

MRI of intracerebral haemorrhage Acute haematomas (less than three days old) yield rather non-specific MRI features. The long T1 and T2 relaxation timeso f fresh blood are shared by infarct, tumour and oedema. After three days, the T1 time shortens and signal intensity increases. This is explained by the oxidation of haemaglobin to methaemoglobin, a paramagnetic substance, which influences T1 relaxation time. The long T2 relaxation time persists, but this pattern of a short T1 and long T2 relaxation time for chronic haematomas is more specific. Acute haematomas have a central area of hypointensity on T2-weighted images due to deoxyhaemoglobin formation.

CT in sub-arachnoid haemorrhage CT provides a non-invasive means of demonstrating blood in the sub-arachnoid space, and may obviate the need for a diagnostic lumbar puncture. The CT appearances may reflect the severity of the initial bleed and the patient's subsequent pre- and post-operative course can be monitored for complications. However, a normal cranial CT examina-

9.21 (left) Small-frontal arteriove-nous malforma-tion: superficial draining vein to superior saggittal sinus (*see also* **9.15**).

9.22 (right) CT: aneurysm of left intracranial artery.

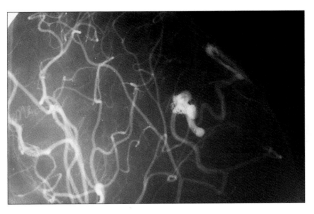

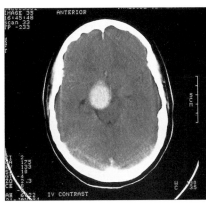

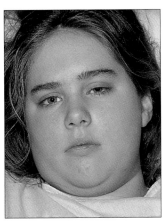

9.23 Patient with left third nerve palsy.

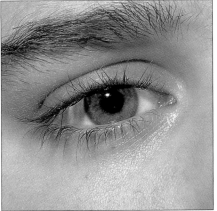

9.24 and 9.25 Close-up showing normal right eye (**9.24, left**) and ptosis in dilated pupil of left eye (**9.25, right**).

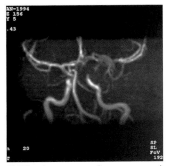

9.26 Aneurysm demonstrated by angiography.

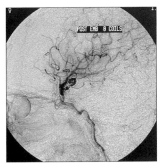

9.27 Obliteration of lumen by wire coils.

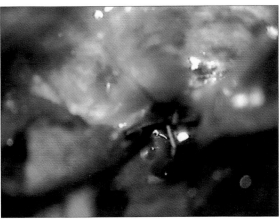

9.28 Intraoperative photograph of clipping of internal carotid posterior communicating artery aneurysm.

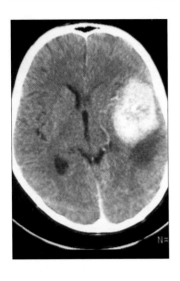

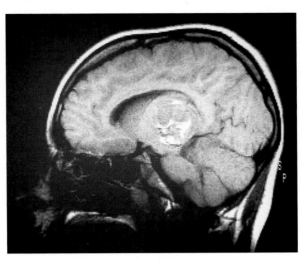

9.29 (left) Arteriovenous malformation on CT scan. Note prominent draining vessel.

9.30 (right) Arteriovenous malformation of thalamus on MR scan. Note flow void in prominent draining vessels.

tion in a patient with a suspected sub-arachnoid haemorrhage in no way excludes the diagnosis. Complications of sub-arachnoid haemorrhage such as re-bleeding,cerebral ischaemia, secondary to vasospasm and the subsequent development of hydrocephalus can all be detected on sequentialCT scanning.

Arteriovenous malformation (AVM) The commonest location is supratentorial, mostly cortical but often with deep extensions. They are most frequent in the middle cerebral artery distribution, but any cerebral artery may be involved (**9.29**). They not uncommonly occur in the brainstem. On the plain CT scan the unruptured AVM will show serpiginous densities due mainly to prominent draining veins. Low-density areas may also be identified following previous bleeds or infarcts. Tubular calcification within the vessel wall and punctate dystrophic calcification may also be indicative of an arterio-venous malformation. There may be an associated mass effect due to the presence of the AVM. Following contrast enhancement, most AVMs will demonstrate abnormal enhancement. Associated features such as intraventricular haematoma, intraventricular haemorrhage, ventricular compression, ipsilateral ventricular enlargement and hydrocephalus will also be demonstrated.

MRI is of great value in the diagnosis of vascular malformations (**9.30**), and is particularly useful in those lesions close to the midline where the relationship to adjacent structures can be accurately assessed. Those in the infratentorial compartment are also well shown. The flowing blood within theAVM contributes a poor signal leaving a 'signal void'. The T2-weighted spin echo sequence is the most helpful in visualising venous malformations. MR can be helpful in showing the presence of the old haemorrhage because of its hyperintensity on both T1-weighted and T2-weighted associated with hypointensity to haemosiderin effects.

Aneurysms Arterial aneurysms are rare in childhood. Aneurysms as small as 2 to 3 mm in diameter may be demonstrated using intravenous contrast-enhanced thin-section axial CT. Angiography normally shows only that part of an aneurysm in continuity with the circulation, whereas CT will show both the patent lumen and any co-existing mural thrombus, so as to reflect the true size of the lesion more accurately. Following rupture of an aneurysm, the hyperdensity of sub-arachnoid blood persists for about one week, after which the cerebrospinal fluid becomes isodense with adjacent brain. The distribution of intracranial bleeding, especially when intraparenchymal, can often point to the location of the aneurysm or at least lateralise it. Complications of a ruptured aneurysm such as intraventricular haemorrhage, hydrocephalus and cerebral ischaemia due to vasospasm can be detected on CT and MR. There is a correlation between the CT and MR findings in sub-arachnoid haemorrhage and the prognosis following a bleed.

Angiography in AV malformations and aneurysms Angiography is usually undertaken just prior to surgery, the timing of which depends on the patient's clinical condition. Surgery is directed towards the prevention of recurrent haemorrhage. Angiography demonstrates the dilated feeding arteries and draining veins, and will demonstrate the rapid circulation in AVMs. The precise size, shape and neck ofthe aneurysm will be demonstrated on angiography, which may also demonstrate the presence of arterial vasospasm.

Mycotic aneurysms These may be secondary to congenital heart disease withseptic emboli, cavernous sinus thrombophlebitis, osteomyelitis of the skull, and meningitis. These are most-commonly situated along the more distal arteries: they may rupture causing intracerebral or sub-arachnoid haemorrhage.

Vein of Galen aneurysm (*see* **9.16–9.19**)   The CT appearances are of:

(1) A sharply defined mass, rounded or triangular in configuration, of increased density. This is situated in the midline in the region of the vein of Galen. The mass shows homogeneous enhancement.

(2) A triangular complex of straight sinus and torcula herophili in continuity with rounded mass.

(3) Hydrocephalus resulting from compression of the third ventricle or acqueduct by the malformation.

(4) Calcification may be seen in the wall of the malformation, although this is rare in infancy but occurs in up to 50 % of cases in adolescence. CT will also readily disclose thrombosis or calcification within the malformation itself. In early cases, angiographic evaluation is essential for demonstrating the feeding arteries and the venous drainage.

Ultrasound has been used to detect the abnormality *in utero* and in the neonate.

Cavernous haemangiomas   CT shows a well-defined hyperdense lesion which enhances, often poorly, and which may contain flecks of calcification. There is no appreciable mass effect but there may be associated haemorrhage. The CT findings are not specific. The MR findings of a cavernous haemangioma are more specific.

Abnormalities of cerebral vasculature

Moya moya disease   The term 'Moya moya', an angiographic appearance, means "something hazy, like a puff of smoke drifting in the air" in Japanese. These appearances result from the development of an abnormal vascular network at the base of the brain and are due todevelopment of collateral vessels following recurrent thrombosis of basal arteries. It may present as repeated stroke or as progressive motor and intellectual deterioration. Neuro-surgical techniques to bypass stenosed arteries have met with varying success. There is evidence of abnormal sympathetic and trigeminal innervation of cerebral vasculature, but the cause of the disorder is unknown.

Aneurysms may be present in association with fibromuscular hyperplasia (**9.31 and 9.32**) or dysplasia. Fibro-muscular hyperplasia is a non-atheromatous stenotic disease of arteries, usually affecting the extracranial internal carotid artery and the proximal intracranial portion. This leads to the development of a basal collateral circulation similar to that seen in Moya moya disease. Angiography reveals the 'string of beads' appearance of the artery. Treatment of FMH consists of antiplatelet drugs to prevent microemboli, and in extreme cases, the use of extracranial to intracranial anastamosis, using the superficial temporal artery to anastamose to branches of the middle cerebral artery.

Another putative cause of cerebro-vascular disease in childhood is a congenital abnormality of the internal carotid artery (loops and kinks), where elongated and angulated internal carotid arteries have been found in children who have had angiography but no symptoms of ischaemia.

Stroke

Hemiparesis of acute onset is the commonest presentation of stroke in childhood. The commonest cause is probably vascular thrombosis and the commonest site the internal capsule.

In most cases, no specific cause is found. It is probable that even the transitory or permanent hemiparesis of acute onset that may follow prolonged hemiconvulsions (sometimes febrile) have a vascular rather than a neural aetiology.

Congenital hemiparesis is also presumed to have a vascular aetiology. Most of these are attributable to second trimester intra-uterine events (*see* Chapter 11 for more detail). A history of ante-partum haemorrhage is sometimes obtainable, but most often there is no evidence of an episode of vascular insufficiency in either the pre-or perinatal period.

The commonest vascular site of all strokes in child-

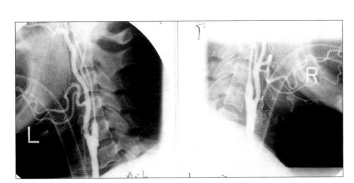
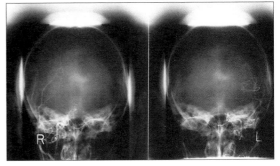

9.31 (left) and 9.32 (right) An example of fibro-muscular hypoplasia with absence of the internal carotid circulation bilaterally.

hood is the terminal carotid middle cerebral artery or its branches and in particular the lenticulo-striate branches supplying the internal capsule.

Presentation is usually typical of vascular aetiology with an acute onset. The stroke is due to intercerebral haemorrhage with rupture and bleeding into the sub-arachnoid space. Headache and meningism may be prominent symptoms. This sequence is usually the result of a ruptured arterio-venous malformation.

Headache may also occur as part of complex migraine (*see* below) presenting with hemiparesis, but is not prominent in other causes of stroke in childhood. An acute hemiplegia complicates acute childhood exanthemata (chickenpox, measles etc.). No vascular pathology can be demonstrated on angiography, and *in-situ* thrombosis is the likely aetiology. Both immunological theories involving immune complex deposition on arterial walls or disordered trigeminal and sympathetic innervation have been invoked as possible mechanisms.

Angiography is unwise in the acute phase of hemiparesis as vasospasm may worsen infarction. Cranial CT can also be normal in the very early stages of cerebral infarction, but may show low attenuation. It is rarely visible if the internal capsule is involved, but may be more easily seen if cortex and subcortical white matter are involved, as in middle cerebral artery thrombosis. After 10 days to two weeks, clear areas of low attenuation may be evident in the internal capsule. Healing is by gliosis.

Most children with acute hemiplegia without identifiable cause show good recovery, but all warrant full investigation. Recurrence is exceptionally rare.

Migraine and stroke

Stroke has been reported to recur in relation to migraine and particularly complicated migraine episodes. The aetiology is cerebral infarction. The prognosis for stroke and migraine is usually good but, as with all cases of stroke in childhood, thorough assessment and investigation are needed.

Children most at risk are those with focal neurological symptoms which may commence as an aura or during the headache phase or after the headache (*see* Chapter 4).

Distinction from complex migraine is by observation of the rate of recovery. Focal neurological symptoms in the context of classical migraine should resolve within 24 hours, but may persist for up to seven days.

Infarction may involve any of the cerebral and retinal vessels, and has rarely been reported to occur in a different vascular territory to that evident from the symptomatology of the aura. Long-term aspirin treatment should be considered in such children if investigation reveals increased platelet adhesiveness still present one month after the episode, although the efficacy of this approach

is not proven.

Alternating hemiplegia is a progressive disorder occurring in infancy and young children. Presentation is recurrent hemiplegia (not always alternating) and headache. There is progressive intellectual and motor deterioration. The cause is unknown; there is a possible relationship with migraine or other cerebrovascular disorders in childhood, and the treatment of choice is with calcium channel blockers.

Identifiable causes of stroke in childhood

Hypertension must always be considered.

Mitochondrial cytopathies may present with stroke. In this group of disorders, there is often no clear relationship between a specific mitochondrial abnormality and a specific clinical presentation. Mitochondrial encephalopathy with lactic acidosis and stroke-like episodes (MELAS) is one recognisable syndrome. Not all children have raised serum lactate and may have raised CSF lactate when serum lactate is normal. Biochemical investigation may require provocative testing. Tissue biopsies with *in vitro* chemical analysis and mitochondrial DNA analysis are invariably necessary if such disorders are suspected. There is no effective treatment but there are important genetic implications and antenatal diagnosis may be possible.

Other metabolic disorders to consider include homocystinuria and transcarbamylase deficiency.

Vascular occlusion in sickle cell disease may lead to cerebral infarction and encephalopathy. Treatment requires rehydration, direction and prevention of hypoxia and exchange transfusion.

Congenital disorders leading to hypercoagulability (protein C deficiency, antithrombin 3 deficiency) are very rare but identifiable causes of stroke in childhood.

Cerebrovascular disease associated with systemic disorders

Cyanotic congenital heart disease predisposes to cerebral infarction resulting from arterial venous thrombosis or embolism.

Venous thrombosis presents acutely with seizures, stroke and raised intracranial pressure, and results from hyperviscosity. This is most commonly seen in the context of severe gastro-enteritis, or following the intra-cranial spread of middle ear infection. Cerebral abscess must also be considered.

Mitral valve prolapse is common but its role in causing stroke is uncertain. Children with mitral valve prolapse as the only abnormal finding and stroke have been reported.

9.33 (left) Ultrasound showing vegetations on the mitral valve (arrowed).

9.34 (right) Mouth ulceration in Behçet's disease.

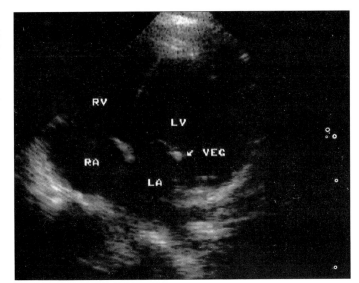

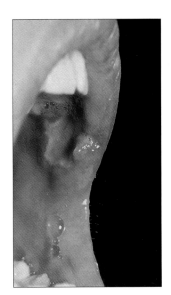

Embolic stroke results from right to left shunts, bacterial endocarditis or emboli (**9.33**) from prosthetic valves (*see* mycotic aneurysm above).

Cerebral infarction may also follow cardiac surgery using bypass. It is likely that air embolism is not the cause in most cases.

Intracranial haemorrhage as the manifestation of systemic disease may occur in factor IX deficiency, or less frequently actor VIII deficiency. This is a real risk, especially in the younger child. The role of trauma is uncertain.

Intracranial haemorrhage may complicate leukaemia (or its treatment) and idiopathic thrombocytopenic purpura, but the riskis not high. Vitamin K deficiency can cause all types of intracranial haemorrhage.

Focal signs and seizures are frequent in bacteraemia and microbacterial meningitis, especially when the diagnosis is delayed; the presumed pathology is an infectious arteritis; severe meningitis is more appropriately described as a meningoencephalitis.

Auto-immune disease and associated vasculitis only rarely produces central nervous system symptoms in childhood. Systemic lupus erythematosis (SLE) is rare in infancy but older children (over 10 years) account for up to 20 % of the reported cases. Visual disturbance, paraesthesiae, weakness, depression and irritability may all be noted. Confirmation of diagnosis is sought from the presence of antinuclear antibodies (dsDNA-extractable nuclear antigen, antiocardiolipin and other phospho-lipids). Evidence of complement consumption (low C3and C4) via immunofluorescent studies on skin biopsy is supportive evidence (IgG, C3 and C4 skin deposits are seen in 75 % of patients with SLE).

Symptoms of central nervous system sarcoidosis reflect a local vasculitis. It is usually seen in later childhood and may also present as an aseptic meningitis. There may be associate duveitis, skin rashes (erythema nodosum or plaques) or adenopathy. The erythrocyte sedimentation rate is raised and there may be eosinophilia, hypercalcaemia and hypergammaglobulinaemia. Typically, the chest x-ray shows hilar adenopathy. Diagnosis may be confirmed by means of the Kveim test and angiotensin-converting enzyme is positive in 80 %.

Behçet's disease is a rare disorder with typical skin lesions and ulceration of mucous membranes (**9.34**). Along with mouth and genital ulceration, there may be iritis, uveitis and accompanying erythema multiforme or nodosum; pustular or papular lesions may also be present, particularly at the site of venopunctures. Meningoencephalitis may develop between one and 11 years after diagnosis, with the emergence of cranial nerve involvement, pyramidal signs and abnormal CSF and EEG. There may ultimately be a good prognosis.

The aetiology of steroid-responsive relapsing encephalomyelitis has yet to be defined, but there is value in viewing it as an auto-immune phenomenon. Presenting featuresare with fever, meningeal irritation, impairment of consciousness and various neurological signs with prominent rhombencephalic involvement. Relapses may follow non-specific viral infection. It is steroid-responsive and generally has a favourable outcome; early recognition may allow unnecessary investigations to be avoided.

Polyarteritis nodosa (*see* **Table 9.4**) occurs in older children, and angiography reveals segmental narrowing and microaneurysmal dilatation.

Neuroradiology and cerebrovascular occlusive disease

The majority of cerebrovascular accidents in children are due to thrombotic occlusion of the intracranial arteries, primarily in the middle cerebral artery distribution or the extracranial portion of the internal carotid artery. The basilar arteries are less frequently involved.

The role of CT in ischaemic infarcts is:
(1) To differentiate between acute haemorrhage and infarction.
(2) To exclude other pathology.
(3) To monitor the recovery.

CT in ischaemic infarcts

It is important to be familiar with the patterns of appearance of cerebral infarction in order not to make diagnostic errors, particularly when the appearances are atypical. Difficulties are most likely to arise in the early period after a stroke, when most typical changes expected on CT have not had a chance to develop. Thus, scanning within 24 hours may be quite normal or show only vague low attenuation areas. Alternatively, if the infarction affects a large volume of brain, there may be considerable swelling and mass effect, simulating a neoplasm. Even in these patients it is probably not wise to enhance the scan unless there is a real clinical doubt about the diagnosis which will affect immediate management, and this is unusual. It is better to wait for a period and repeat the study. If contrast is given at an early stage then a non-ionic medium is indicated. The situation can be further complicated because patterns of enhancement at this stage can be quite confusing and again can simulate the appearances of tumours. The diagnosis can be confirmed by follow-up examination.

The CT appearances of vaso-occlusive infarcts are first evident between 24 and 48 hours after the onset of symptoms. Initially there is a focal, poorly-defined hypodense area whichinvolves the cortex and white matter. The low density is due to intracellular oedema and tissue necrosis. The hypodense area is confined to the

TABLE 9.4 Diagnostic Criteria for Polyarteritis Nodosa

Major findings:

Renal	—	Raised creatinine, or low GFR
Musculoskeletal	—	Myalgia, arthralgic, tenderness
Neuroradiology	—	Aneurysm or occlusion of visceral arteries
Biopsy	—	Small- or medium-sized artery with necrosis and granulocytes in artery wall

Major findings:

Cutaneous	—	Livedo reticularis
Gastrointestinal involvement	—	Loss of >5 % body weight
Constitutional symptoms	—	
Peripheral neuropathy	—	
Central nervous system disease	—	
Hypertension	—	(diastolic BP > 95 % for age)
Cardiac involvement	—	
Lung involvement	—	
Acute phase reactants	—	
Hepatitis B surface antigen	—	

— Diagnosis established by one major and four minor criteria (after Ozen, *et al.*, 1992).

vascular supply area of the occluded artery. The lesion becomes more sharply delineated as oedema increases by the third to fourth day, with increasing hypodensity. Density increases after seven to 10 days with subsiding oedema. The mass effect is minimal during the first 24 hours of onset, but is maximal by the fifth day. This gradually subsides and is usually absent after the third week. During the second week, irregular and isodense bands appear within the low-density areas mostly in grey matter, producing a gyral-type configuration. They are due to the hyperaemia following improved collateral circulation and new capillary ingrowth.

Between the fourth week and the third month, the hypodense area becomes more clearly defined with ipsilateral ventricular dilatation. The low-density area may resolve or may develop cystic change with a density equivalent to CSF. In some cases, sulcal enlargement may be the only abnormality.

The vast majority of infarcts display contrast enhancement 14 to 21 days after the ictus. Enhancement is maximal duringthe third week; thereafter it decreases rapidly and is unusual after the second month. Enhancement is due to breakdown of the blood-brain barrier, new capillary growth and luxury perfusion.

The appearances of contrast enhancement may simulate those of tumour or abscess. Mass effect is usually absent when contrast enhancement occurs in an infarct and the lesion usually has a vascular distribution. Follow-up CT scans will help to exclude tumours and abscesses.

Contrast enhancement should not be carried out routinely in cases of infarction.

The role of angiography in ischaemic infarcts

Angiography is required in the following:
(1) Extracranial occlusive disease.
(2) Intracerebral occlusive disease such as vasculitis.
(3) Moya moya disease.

Haemorrhagic infarction

Is usually a further complication after the onset of embolic infarction. CT displays a band-like region of mild or moderately increased density, with ill-defined margins assuming the gyral configuration of the cortex. The surrounding cortex is hypodense. Following intravenous contrast, the area of infarction will develop increased density without enhancement of the area of haemorrhage.

Moya moya disease

The CT appearances of:
(1) Parenchymal areas of hypodensity due to ischaemia.
(2) Cerebral atrophy.
(3) Haemorrhage which may have intraventricular, sub-arachnoid or basal ganglionic location.
(4) Curvilinear densities in the region of the basal ganglia representing parenchymal collateral vessels.

MRI in ischaemic infarcts

The earliest onset of signal changes varies from 30 minutes to six hours. The signal changes are due to post-infarction oedema which causes a hypointense signal on T1-weighted images and hyperintense signal on T2-weighted images. These changes increase for the first 24 hours. Of the two parameters, T1 and T2, prolonged T2 (hyperintense signal) seems to be the more sensitive marker of infarction. Multiplanar imaging permits the identification of a single abnormality in a vascular territory. Ventricular compression and sulcal effacement are readily detected. Loss of grey/white matter differentiation occurs in both new and old infarction. Infarct contours become more sharply marginated with time. In addition, the diagnosis of vessel occlusion can be made with MR by noting a persistently increased or isointense signal within the appropriate vessel. The dating of infarcts by MR is unreliable as with CT. A chronic infarct consisting of either gliosis or porencephaly can be confidently diagnosed: hypointense on T1 and hyperintense onT2, similar to CSF. MR can distinguish a haemorrhagic cortical infarct from both a purely ischaemic infarct and from an intraparenchymal haematoma.

Chapter 10: Cerebral Tumours

James Leggate, W. St. Clair Forbes

Tumours of the central nervous system (CNS)

Central nervous system (CNS) tumours, the second commonest cause of malignancy, may be intracranial or intraspinal in childhood. The intracranial group are supra- or infratentorial; the intraspinal group may be extradural or intradural. The intradural tumours may be extramedullary or intramedullary (**Table 10.1**). The intraspinal tumours are dealt with in more detail in Chapter 17.

Histological classification according to the cell of origin can be useful in determining prognosis. Outlook also depends on the anatomical site: an astrocytoma within the cerebellar hemisphere is regarded as a benign lesion, whilst an astrocytoma of the brain stem may prove to be rapidly fatal (**Table 10.2**) (**10.1–10.6**). The main cell types found in childhood CNS tumours are astrocytoma, primitive neuroectodermal tumour (PNET), cranopharyngioma, ependymoma, germ cell tumour, ganglioglioma, choroid plexus tumour, meningioma and pineocytoma. The most common are the astrocytoma and PNET, save for the posterior fossa where astrocytomas, PNETs and ependymomas have equal incidence.

TABLE 10.1 CNS Tumours in Childhood

Intracranial	—	Supratentorial
		Infratentorial
Intraspinal	—	Intradural
		Extramedullary
		Intramedullary
	—	Extradural

TABLE 10.2 Cell Type: W.H.O. Classification of Paediatric CNS Tumours

Glial	—	Astrocytic
		Oligodendroglial
		Ependymomal
		(Ependymoma)
		Choroid plexus
		Glioblastoma multiforme
		Mixed
Neuronal	—	Ganglioma
		Gangliocytoma
		Neuroblastoma
PNET		(Primitive Neuroectodermal Tumour)
		— Medulloblastoma
		— Medulloepithelioma
Pineal cell tumours		
		— Pineocytoma
		— Pineoblastoma

Throughout the CNS, tumours tend to be more common in males with the exception of ependymomas and optic nerve gliomas which are more common in females. The overall incidence of tumours within the nervous system ranges from 2–5 cases per 100,000 population, a consistent finding throughout the populations of Africa,

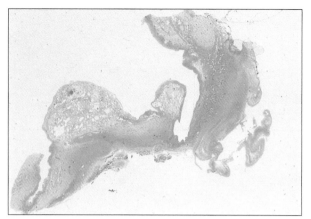

10.1 Pilocytic astrocytoma in posterior fossa. H & E sections show tumour nodule with microcystic areas attached to the wall of the large cyst.

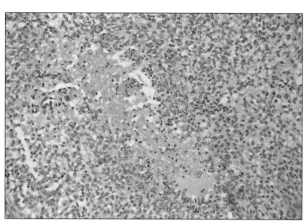

10.2 Medulloblastoma. H & E shows a highly cellular tumour with a fine fibrillated background.

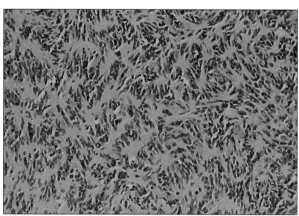

10.3 H & E medulloblastoma showing Rosette formation.

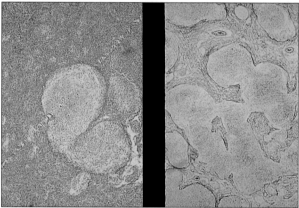

10.4 H & E and reticulin staining showing a desmoplastic medulloblastoma with reticulin-free islands and globules.

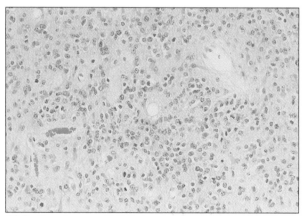

10.5 Ependymoma H & E showing ependymal rosettes with small central lumen.

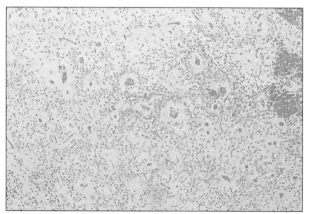

10.6 H & E showing another characteristic with formation of perivascular pseudo rosettes.

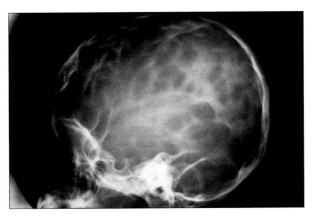

10.7 Copper beating on lateral skull x-ray showing the effects of raised intracranial pressure.

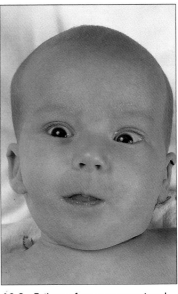

10.8 Failure of up-gaze associated with raised intracranial pressure.

TABLE 10.3 Signs and Symptoms of Supratentorial Tumours in Children

Infants	Children
Failure to thrive	Headaches
Rapid head growth	Nausea/vomiting
Vomiting	Deteriorating vision

Japan, Asia, Europe and North America (Dohnmann and Farwell, 1976).

Although the incidence of overall tumour occurrence is constant, the tumour types vary between the different countries. Astrocytomas of the cerebellum and PNET's are more common in Europe and North Africa, whereas craniopharygiomas are more frequently seen in Japan.

From the time of Cushing (Cushing, 1927), it has always been said that the majority of childhood intracranial tumours are to be found within the posterior fossa, but more recently a study from the Children's Hospital of Philadelphia demonstrated that only 40 % were to be found within the posterior fossa, 5.5 % within the spinal cord and 54 % in the supratentorial compartment.

Clinical features

CNS tumours may present with:
• Loss of function of normal neural tissue.
• Symptoms due to obstruction of CSF pathways.
• Distant endocrine effects.

In the supratentorial compartment, mass effect from the tumour may produce symptoms and signs of raised intracranial pressure (**10.7 and 10.8**). In the infant prior to suture fusion, symptoms such as headache cannot be appreciated, and failure to thrive with vomiting, signs of raised intracranial pressure with suture separation and bulging of the fontanelle may be the predominant clini-

cal presenting features. In the older child, headaches, especially in the early morning associated with nausea and vomiting, also with diminished visual acuity are commonly the early signs of raised intracranial pressure (**Table 10.3**). Neurological dysfunction will depend upon the site. Within the optic pathway, tumours (usually astrocytomas) will produce early changes in visual acuity and in visual fields, whilst pineal region tumours together with tumours within the sella and parasella regions may produce delayed puberty or even precocious puberty. Tumours within the pineal region may present with features attributable to the obstruction of CSF outflow from the back of the third ventricle. In these respects, tumours in this region may be silent until they present with acute obstructive hydrocephalus.

Within the posterior fossa, tumours may present with lateralising cerebellar signs including nystagmus, ataxia, diplopia, head tilt and cranial nerve dysfunction (**10.9 and 10.10**) as well as more subtle cerebellar hemisphere signs, such as dysdiadochokinesis. Tumours within the posterior fossa will often, by distortion of the fourth ventricle or the inferior aspect of the aqueduct, cause CSF outflow obstruction with resultant hydrocephalus and intracranial hypertension. Although unusual, some posterior fossa tumours may present with sleep apnoea and with signs of posterior fossa intracranial tension with hypertension of the systemic blood pressure and bradycardia.

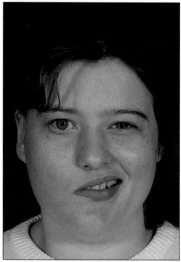

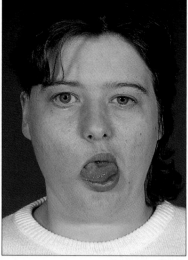

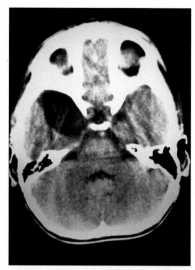

10.9 and 10.10   Seventh (**10.9, left**) and 12th cranial nerve palsy (**10.10, right**) in young girl with posterior fossa tumour.

10.11   Right sylvian fissure arachnoid cyst with "temporal lobe agenesis".

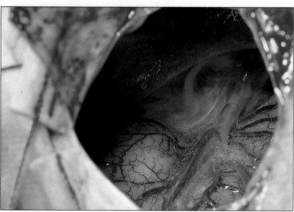

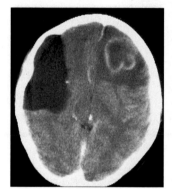

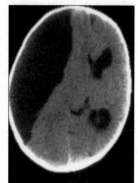

10.12   Operative site after membranectomy for temporal fossa arachnoid cyst showing vessels of sylvian fissure lying deep in the operative field.

10.13   Arachnoid cyst: post-contrast CT of large left fronto-temporal non-enhancing CSF collection. Note bulging of over-lying cranial vault and coincidental right frontal abscess.

10.14   Large arachnoid cyst on axial CT showing mass effect.

Clinical signs

The presence of a focal neurological sign, such as a uni-lateral sixth or seventh nerve palsy, nystagmus, gait ataxia, diminished visual acuity, papilloedema, pupillary assymmetry, failure of upgaze, and unilateral hemipare-sis may all be signs of intracranial tumours. The pres-ence of a monoparesis or spastic tetra/paraparesis in the presence of a torticolis or scoliosis may well be seen on examination of a child with a spinal tumour.

Conditions imitating CNS tumours

Arachnoid cysts

These are benign cysts which probably represent a developmental anomaly involving splitting of the arach-noid membrane (**10.11**), a pinch-cock like mechanism then allowing ballooning of the cyst as CSF enters but is unable to leave. They are most often seen as an inciden-tal finding but occasionally may cause neurological dys-function through local pressure effects. Treatment, when needed is by drainage, marsupialisation and shunting as indicated (**10.12**).

The arachnoid cyst shows characteristic appearances on CT and MR of CSF. These are well-defined lesions of CSF imaging characteristics and does not exhibit con-trast enhancement. The cyst may have a straight inner margin representing the cyst attachment with the arach-noid membrane. Lesions over the cerebral convexity usually have a biconvex or semi-circular configuration (**10.13 and 10.14**).The cysts may be either supratentorial of infratentorial. The commonest site is the sylvian fis-sure followed by the posterior fossa. Suprasellar arach-noid cysts may enlarge and obstruct the foramen of Monro and also extend into the lateral ventricles (**10.15 and 10.16**).

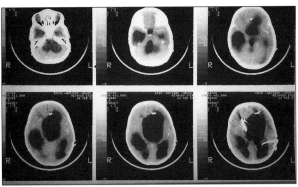 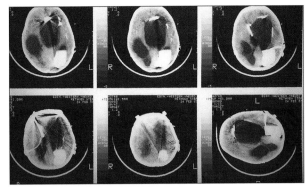

10.15 and 10.16   Suprasellar arrachnoid cyst before (**10.15, left**) and after (**10.16, right**) intraventricular contrast.

Benign intracranial hypertension: pseudotumour cerebri

This is a rare condition of childhood of unknown aetiology. An association with chronic middle ear disease has been noted as has its association with some drug therapy, notably steroids. Headache and diplopia due to a lateral rectus palsy is the most common presentation. The vast majority of children with the condition have papillodema which is relatively rare in other causes of raised intracranial pressure. The condition is usually self-limiting and without sequel, but the prolonged raised pressure does put the child at risk of optic atrophy. Monitoring of visual acuity and the possibility of blind spot enlargement leading to scotoma is advisable.

Diagnosis is one of exclusion. The CT scan can be normal but very often shows the appearances of diffuse cerebral oedema with ventricles of small size. The lumbar puncture usually shows normal CSF but the pressure is measurably raised (it is important to keep the head in a neutral position).

There have been no good controlled trials of therapy. Lumbar puncture readily reduces pressure and brings short-term symptomatic relief. Treatment with Dexamethosone and diuretics has also been tried. Where the raised pressure is long term and persistent, lumbo-peritoneal shunting has been used with good results. The condition can relapse and remit in up to a third of those involved.

Investigations

Neuroradiology and intracranial tumours

CT is the primary and most useful investigation for cerebral tumours. Plain radiography is reserved for further clarification of a CT abnormality in the calvarium, skull base or as part of surgical planning. Angiography has a similarly limited role and may be used to assess tumour vascularity as in the case of meningiomas or in haemangioblastomas. CT has a high sensitivity for detecting tumours in the supratentorial compartment but has a lower specificity. MRI has advantages in terms of high contrast sensitivity, multiplanar imaging and absence of ionising radiation. MRI is superior in the detection and subsequent management of tumours in the brain stem, middle and posterior cranial fossae and where CT interpretation is hindered by the presence of artefact. MRI has a superior sensitivity over CT, although tumours which do not show any substantial increase in T1 or T2 relaxation times can be difficult to detect. Fortunately, the majority of these tumours are large and exert mass effect. Gadolinium (DTPA) may be used as a contrast agent in order to increase the sensitivity.

Cerebral infarction and radiation necrosis are major causes of diagnostic confusion.

In the pre-term and term infant, tumours may be diagnosed using ultrasound. These examinations should be supplemented by means of CT or MRI for further assessment of the tumour site, margins and vascularity.

Role of imaging in cerebral tumours (*see* **Table 10.4**, overleaf)
• Diagnosis.
• Surgical planning.
• Monitory following therapy.
• Detection of complications following treatment.
• Late assessment.

CT signs of brain tumours
• Attenuation changes.
• Enhancement characteristics.
• Mass effect as determined by the distortion of adjacent normal structures and/or midline shift.
• Presence of oedema.

The abnormal attenuation is due to:
1) The physical properties of the tumour tissue itself or due to calcific, and haemorrhagic, necrotic or cystic changes within it.
2) Reactive peritumoural intracerebral oedema.
3) Ischaemic changes caused by the involvement of cerebral vessels either by a tumour or by compression between the tumour or the displaced vein and the falx or tentorium. Periventricular CSF oedema results in a periventricular hypodensity on CT (**10.17**) or increased signal on the T2-weighted MR image, is seen secondary

TABLE 10.4 Imaging Intracranial Tumours

Ultrasound	Useful in neonates.
Plain x-rays	Of limited value.
Angiography	Can be useful in pre-op tumour evaluation and embolisation.
CT	Pre- and post-IV contrast.
MRI	Greater sensitivity and specificity. May need IV Gadolinium DTPA.

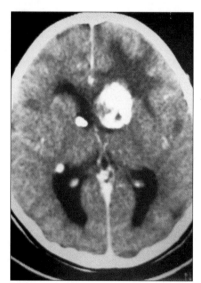

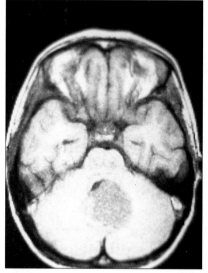

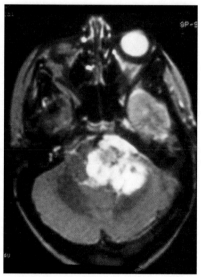

10.17 Giant cell astrocytoma at foramen of Monro with associated peritumoural oedema and heterogeneous enhancement with contrast.

10.18 and 10.19 Axial MR scan of posterior fossa before (**10.18, left**) and after (**10.19, right**) intravenous Gadolinium DTPA contrast medium to show medulloblastoma.

to the relatively rapid onset of ventricular obstruction, and may be seen in the presence of a tumour mass.

Favourable prognostic signs on imaging include well-defined cysts, smooth enhancing mass lesions, minimal surrounding oedema, minimal mass effect, cortical situation and location in the non-dominant hemisphere.

Unfavourable prognostic signs include poorly defined tumour margins, oedema, large size, heterogeneous enhancement, contralateral extension, extension to the middle and posterior cranial fossae and CSF seeding.

MR signs of brain tumours   The MR features are non-specific ranging from hypointense to iso/hyperintense on T1-weighted sequences (depending on whether tumoral haemorrhage has occurred) to iso/hyperintense on T2-weighted images. Enhancement with Gadolinium DTPA occurs in similar circumstances to contrast enhancement in CT (**10.18 and 10.19**). Peritumoral oedema is recognised as increased signal on T2-weighted sequences. The presence of tumoral calcification may not be recognised on MR scanning or seen as areas of signal void. MR has a slightly higher accuracy in tumour detection than CT and has a superior specificity. MRI is superior to CT in tumours of the brain stem, middle and posterior cranial fossae.

Infratentorial tumours

MRI has advantages over CT and is especially valuable in demonstrating midline and deep-seated lesions (**10.20 and 10.21**). It defines the tumour extent more accurately and provides greater detail about cystic or necrotic areas. It demonstrates the extent of tumour infiltration into the brain stem more accurately and will determine more pre-

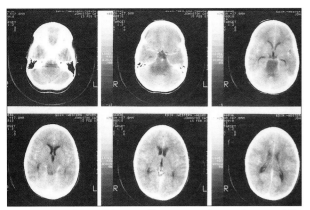
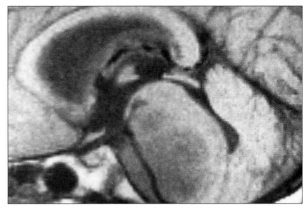

10.20 and 10.21 CT scan of brainstem glioma showing diffuse low-density appearances (**10.20, left**). On MR scanning, by comparison, the low density is seen to lie anteriorly within the brainstem, which is grossly swollen extending from the upper medulla through to the mid-brain (**10.21, right**).

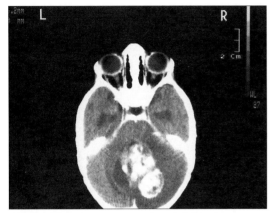
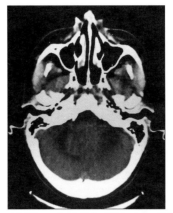

10.22 CT scan appearance of medulloblastoma.

10.23 and 10.24 CT before (**10.23, left**) and after (**10.24, right**) i.v. contrast.

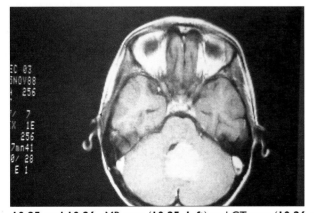
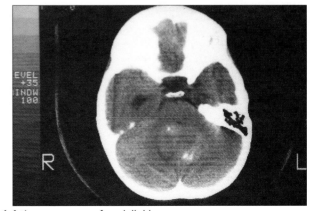

10.25 and 10.26 MR scan (**10.25, left**) and CT scan (**10.26, right**) appearances of medulloblastoma.

cisely the origin of a tumour.

The medulloblastoma on CT will frequently appear uniformly hyperdense and less often isodense or of mixed density (**10.22**). They are rarely hypodense. Typically, they are large, round to oval, well-defined, non-calcified and midline masses, situated in the inferior vermis behind the fourth ventricle. Contrast enhance-

ment occurs in almost all, and is typically homogeneous (**10.23 and 10.24**). Tumours arising within the cerebellar hemisphere or extending from the midline into the hemisphere will be detected. Brainstem compression and infiltration are more accurately identified on MRI (**10.25 and 10.26**). CT and preferably MRI will demonstrate CSF seeding which is usually manifest as intense lepto

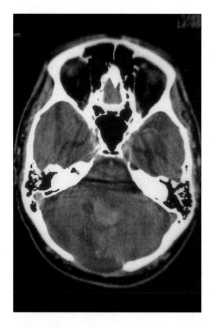

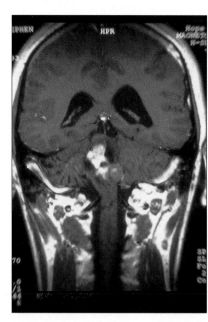

10.27 (left) Brain stem astrocytoma: axial CT scan showing extension posteriorly. Note craniectomy defect.

10.28 (right) Brain stem astrocytoma: coronal MR showing cystic components.

meningeal enhancement in the basal cisterns, Sylvian fissures and suprasellar cistern. Infrequently, parenchymal metastases from medulloblastoma are detected at the grey and white matter interface of the cerebral hemispheres, often in the frontal regions. Myelography/MRI scanning of the spine is required to detect intraspinal metastases. The majority are intradural/extramedullary lesions.

The cerebrellar astrocytoma is demonstrated on both CT and MRI usually as a large cystic lesion with contents above that of CSF with an enhancing mural nodule . Solid astrocytomas are usually round, lobulated and well defined. Their imaging characteristics are variable relative to brain and they show variable patterns of pathological enhancement, which may be ring-like, dense, homogeneous or faint. Calcification is not a feature of astrocytomas but maybe seen in medulloblastomas (uncommonly) and ependymomas. In the typical cystic tumour with an intratumoural nodule, the imaging characteristics rarely pose a diagnostic problem.

The ependymoma most commonly arises from the floor of the fourth ventricle. The imaging appearances of ependymoma tumours are variable. The majority are isodense on CT with variable patterns of enhancement. Calcification is seen in 50 % and the presence of a calcified mass within the fourth ventricle should lead to the diagnosis of an ependymoma. CT/MRI/myelography is used to demonstrate the presence of CSF seeding both intracranially and into the spinal canal (**10.29 and 10.30**).

Brainstem glioma

This is a neuroectodermal tumour arising in the brainstem or the lip brain and may involve the posterior thalamus or upper cervical cord. These gliomas usually occur between the ages of six and eight years with an equal instance in males and females. MRI, rather than CT, is

the method of choice (**10.27 and 10.28**) for diagnosing these tumours and demonstrating their extent. The sagittal and coronal sections are best for delineating the extent of involvement, especially inferior extension through the foramen magnum. The axial plane is helpful in detecting brainstem asymmetry, alterations in brainstem size and exophytic tumour extension into the lateral cisterns, e.g. cerebellopontine angle cistern. Sagittal MRI is superior to CT in differentiating brain-stem glioma from intraventricular ependymas and midline vermian astrocytomas, both of which may secondarily involve the brainstem. On T1-weighted images, the brainstem glioma is homogeneous, hypointense and appears well demarcated from normal adjacent brain. Rarely, haemorrhage into the tumour produces focal areas of high signal on T1-weighted images. Tumoural cysts are identified by their hypointensity when compared with the solid tumour. Exophytic tumour is hypointense but can be differentiated from CSF. On T2-weighted images the tumour is typically homogeneous and hyperintense in signal. Rarely, small focal areas within the tumour may remain isointense. The T2 hyperintensity of the tumoral cyst is greater than that of the solid tumour. Exophytic tumour also appears hyperintense on T2-weighted images. These tumours show variable enhancement following Gadolinium DTPA.

On CT, these tumours display variable attenuation characteristics and may or may not show contrast enhancement. The tumours are usually detected by the expansion of the brainstem which results in posterior displacement of the fourth ventricle and compression of the surrounding cisterns. The basilar artery is often displaced anteriorly and laterally. Calcification within the tumour is rare.

Hydrocephalus occurs less frequently and later than with other posterior fossa masses.

MRI and CT therefore assist in the prognosis and in planning surgical or radiation treatment. Calcification

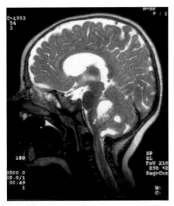

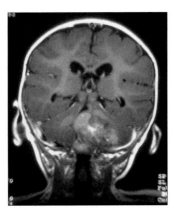

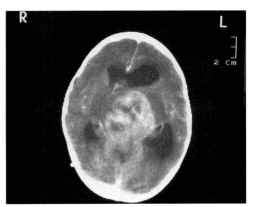

10.29 Posterior fossa ependy-moma. Sagittal MRI T2W.

10.30 Coronal TIW post-i.v. Gadolinium. Heterogenous mass with multiple cystic areas—displacing brainstem to right with moderate hydrocephalus.

10.31 PNET. CT post-i.v. contrast. Enhancing post-fossa tumour extending through tentorium into third ventricle and basal ganglia, causing hydrocephalus.

may develop within the bran-stem following radiation therapy, and may be large enough to produce areas of signal hypointensity.

Supratentorial tumours

Hemispheric tumours

The commonest tumours are astrocytomas, primitive neuroectodermal tumours (PNET) and ependymoma (**Table 10.5**).

The astrocytoma presents on CT and MR as large masses, usually cystic with a medially situated mural nodule. A solid tumour is less frequently found. The most frequent sites, in decreasing order of frequency are: 1) The temporal lobe, where cystic tumours are twice as common as cystic masses; and 2) The frontal lobe, where solid tumours are twice as common. The most common CT feature is a low-density lesion which usually enhances. On MR, the lesions are hypo- to isointense on T1-weighted images, and hyperintense on T2-weighted images. The calcification may be present, and is readily detected on CT and less frequently on MR as areas of signal void.

The primitive neuroectodermal tumour (PNET) usually occupies the deep white matter where it presents a varied appearance on imaging (**10.31**). It is characteristically well-defined and may be hypodense, isodense or hyperdense with calcification in over 50 % ofcases. Cyst-like areas may be present and MR scanning will detect intratumoural haemorrhage. Contrast enhancement may be homogeneous or patchy. Seeding into the CSF pathways may be seen in 50 %.

The imaging features of ependymoma are not diagnostic, and considerable difficulty may arise in distinguishing it from PNET, which also shows calcification with the same frequency (50 %). These tumours may occasionally be intraventricular.

Choroid plexus papilloma

Most cases occur under the age of five years and there is a male preponderance. The lateral ventricle is the commonest site, followed by the fourth and third ventricles in order of frequency. Malignant change may occur. The CT features (**10.32**) are of a homogeneous isodense or hyperdense mass showing smooth, well-defined lobulated margins. There may be focal areas of calcification within it. The tumour exhibits intense homogeneous enchancement following contrast administration (**10.33 and 10.34**). However, there may be central hypodense areas indicating necrosis. The mass typically engulfs the choroid plexus. Hydrocephalus is common at presentation due to over-production of CSF and obstruction. On MR (**10.35**), the signal characteristics are heterogeneous due to focal calcification. The lesion may be iso- to hypointense on T1-weighted images and iso- to hyperintense on T2-weighted images. Intense enahancement with Gadolinium DTPA occurs.

TABLE 10.5 Supratentorial Astrocytoma

Males: Females   2:1
Peak at three years
Cystic or solid
Grade I-IV, Glioblastoma multiforme
     Anaplastic
Prognosis—histology
     —Site
     —Surgical resection
DXT and chemotherapy

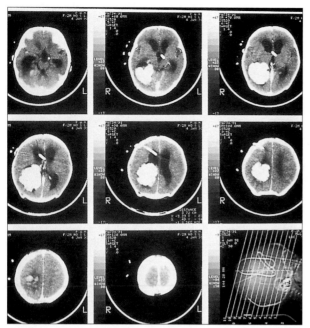

10.32 CT scan post-i.v. contrast of lateral ventricular choroid plexus papilloma with associated hydrocephalus.

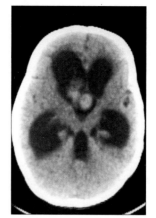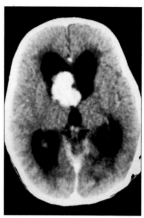

10.33 and 10.34 Choroid pexus papilloma: CT scan appearances before (**10.33,left**) and after (**10.34, right**) contrast.

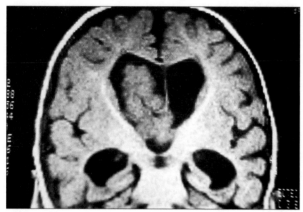

10.35 MR scan of choroid plexus papilloma. Note associated hydrocephalus.

Suprasellar region tumours

The most common tumours are:
- Craniopharyngioma
- Optic nerve glioma
- Hypothalamic glioma
- Teratoma
- Germinoma
- Pituitary adenoma

Hydrocephalus secondary to obstruction either at intraventricular foramen level or at the posterior end of the third ventricle and aqueduct results in increased intracranial pressure.

Craniopharyngioma

These tumours constitute a spectrum of solid and cystic tumours mainly occurring in the suprasellar sub-arach-noid space, with some extending into the sella or third ventricle. Calcification is extremely common, occurring within 70 to 80 % of cases. CT is preferable for demonstrating the calcificatiron (**10.36**). The tumour usually presents on CT as a hypodense or isodense lesion with calcification. Rarely, the tumour may be hyperdense, due to the increased protein content outweighing the low density of the cholesterol within the cyst. Contrast enchancement may occur in the more solid tumours or around the rim of the cystic lesion. Either CT in the axial and coronal planes or MR in the coronal and sagittal planes (**10.37 and 10.38**) should be used in the pre-operative and post-operative assessment of these patients. On MR, variable signal characteristics are demonstrated depending on the contents of the cyst. The features are further complicated by haemorrhage into the cyst and by the associated solid mass and calcification. A more proteinaceous cyst has longer T2 relaxation than solid tumours.

Optic nerve and hypothalamic glioma

Optic nerve glioma may present as either a unilateral or bilateral orbital mass. When bilateral optic nerve gliomas are present, the diagnosis of neurofibromatosis should be considered (**10.39**). This slow-growing tumour can arise anywhere along the optic tracts,from the orbit to the occiptial lobes. MRI (**10.40**) is more sensitive than CT in differentiating optic nerve glioma from dural ectasia, which is identified as a prominent dilated sub-arachnoid space surrounding a normal or small optic nerve. Within the orbit, the coronal and axial projections best demonstrate involvement of the optic nerves, whereas involvement of the chiasm may require imaging in the sagittal plane as well. Optic radiation involvement

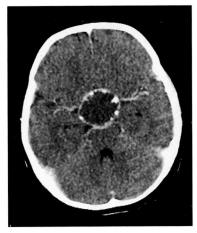
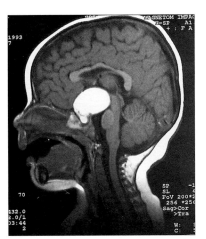
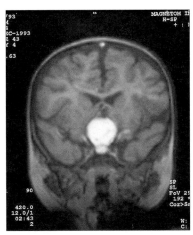

10.36 CT scan of craniopharyngioma showing ring calcification.

10.37 and 10.38 Sagittal (**10.37, left**) and coronal (**10.38, right**) MR scan appearances of craniopharyngioma in infant with involvement of the pituitary fossa as well as the suprasellar region by tumour.

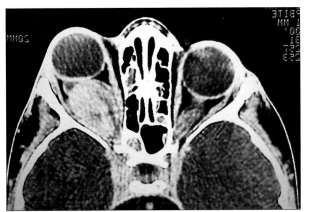
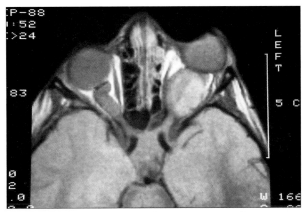

10.39 and 10.40 Optic nerve glioma on CT scan (**10.39, left**) and (**10.40, right**) MR scan. Note involvement of optic nerve up to optic nerve foramen with sparing of optic chiasm.

(**10.41**) is clearly identified in the axial plane. Within the orbit, the signal intensity of an optic nerve tumour is variable on T1- and T2-weighted sequences. Cystic areas are readily distinguished from solid tumours. However, the majority of tumours are solid and mildly hypointense or isointense on T-weighted sequences. On a T2-weighted sequence, the solid tumour is hyperintense. Chiasmatic tumours are predominantly solid and display either hypointense or isointense signal on T1-weighted images. On T2-weighted images the tumour is moderately hyperintense, making differentiation of tumour and surrounding CSF difficult at times. Infiltrative involvement of the optic radiations result in focal or diffuse high signal in the distribution of the optic tracts. MRI is more sensitive than CT in detecting posterior optic tract infiltration. MRI is the method of choice for long-term follow-up.

The hypothalamic glioma appears on CT as a large amorphous mass in the floor of the third ventricle and suprasellar cistern and is of low attenuation. Intense, often homogeneous enhancement follows contrast administration. On MRI, the tissue characteristics of a

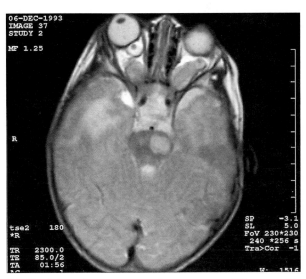

10.41 Bilateral optic nerve glioma seen on MR scan with involvement of optic tracts and radiation as well as gliomatous changes seen within mid-brain, typical of Von Recklinghausen's disease (neurofibromatosis type 1).

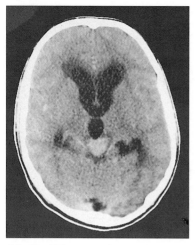

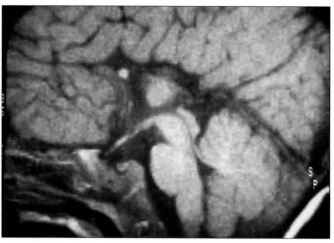

10.42 CT scan of pineal region tumour with associated obstructive hydrocephalus.

10.43 Pineal region tumour seen on MR scanning without hydrocephalus.

hypothalamic glioma are similar to those of a chiasmatic glioma. Differentiation of this tumour from a chiasmatic glioma is often difficult on CT. Demonstration of a normal, uninvolved chiasm on MR suggests the diagnosis of a hypothalamic glioma. However, in the presence of a chiasmatic infiltration by a hypothalamic glioma, differentiation of the two on MRI is not possible unless orbital or optic tract tumour is present.

Pineal region tumours

This group includes germinomas, teratomas, pineocytomas, pineoblastomas. They are diagnosed on CT by their attenuation characteristics pre- and post-contrast medium administration and by the type of calcification, if any.

Germ cell tumours are the most common. Germinomas are typically high-attenuation lesions on CT (**10.42**), showing uniform enhancement, and may contain a variable amount of calcification. Synchronous or asynchronous development of a second lesion in the hypothalamus and suprasellar region is frequent. Teratomas have heterogeneous attenuation with little enhancement but marked calcification engulfing normal pineal calcification. Pineocytomas are iso- or hyperdense with nodular enhancement with no abnormal calcification. Pineoblastomas show increased attenuation and marked enhancement. The pineoblastomas may be associated with retinoblastomas.

MRI is effective in demonstrating the pineal region tumours (**10.43**). There is the advantage of multiplanar imaging especially in the sagittal plane. However, small areas of calcification will not be detected, though the larger areas can be inferred by areas of signal void. The MRI characteristics of primary pineal cell tumours overlap considerably. However, the presence of fat and a cyst of a T1-weighted image suggests the diagnosis of a ter-

atoma. Solid tumours are predominantly hypointense on T1-weighted images and are hyperintense on T2-weighted sequences.

Other investigations

Where germ cell tumours are considered a possible diagnosis, blood serum levels of beta HCG (human chorion gonadatrophin) and alphafetoprotein are estimated prior to surgery. These markers where raised, alter the management of such tumours from one of surgery to chemotherapy and radiotherapy. In such circumstances, even in the presence of raised serum markers, it may be considered advisable to carry out a stereotactic biopsy to confirm the histology.

Treatment

In all tumours of the CNS, management is aimed at confirmation of the tumour histology, combined where appropriate with removal of as much of the tumour as is possible without deterioration in the neurological state of the child. Where total excision is not practicable or safe, or where the tumour itself is inaccessible to direct surgical extirpation, then radiotherapy and/or chemotherapy is used to arrest the disease process and where possible to reverse it. The use of CT- or MR- guided stereotactic biopsies (**10.44–10.50**) has enabled the surgeon to offer a much increased chance of histological confirmation of a tumour type with minimal risk to the child. The procedure can be performed within the brain stem itself with negligible risk of mortality and minimal risk of morbidity. The use of the ultrasonic surgical aspirator has minimised the need for traction, and suction dissection technique on intracranial and intraspinal tumours reduces the risk of damage to surrounding normal nervous struc-

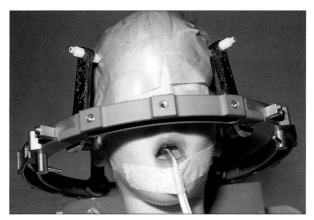

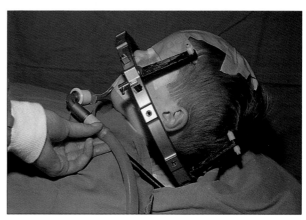

10.44–10.50 Stereotactic biopsy showing the following: **10.44 and 10.45** Base ring attachment.

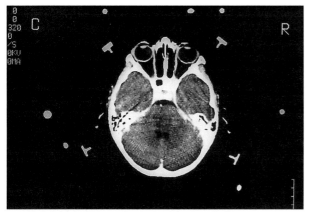

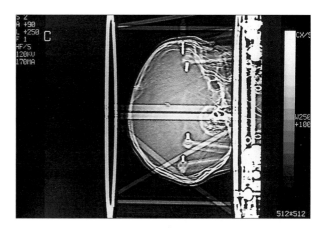

10.46 and 10.47 Scan co-ordinates and target.

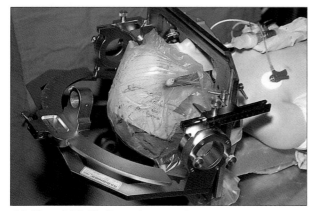

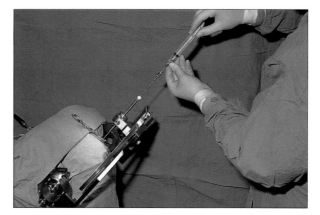

10.48 and 10.49 Operative procedure.

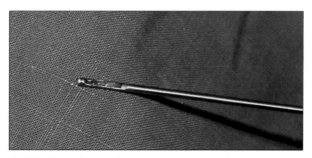

10.50 Operative specimen.

tures. Within the spinal cord and in the supratentorial compartment, the use of laser technology to aid the dissection of tumour margin from surrounding normal neural tissue has increased the likelihood of achieving a total surgical removal of some benign tumours which would otherwise prove to be inaccessible to conventional surgical instruments.

Radiation therapy

Ionising radiation is either used as an adjunct to surgical therapy, as with astrocytomas of the cerebral hemispheres or as the primary treatment in certain types of tumour, such as with germinomas of the pineal region.

Where radiation therapy is given as an adjunct to surgical removal of a tumour, the choice of local or craniospinal access radiation therapy will be determined by the histological nature of the tumour involved. In astrocytomas of the cerebral hemispheres, local radiotherapy is all that is necessary, whereas in other tumours whole craniospinal access irradiation therapy is given. These are tumours where seedling spread throughout the CSF pathways is known to occur, such as in supratentorial PNET, certain pineal region tumours, and, in particular, medulloblastomas of the posterior fossa.

The damaging effects of irradiation therapy on the developing CNS is well recognised. This may occur acutely from the toxic effect of the radiation or there may be a delayed encephalomyelopathy due to a vasculitis. The clinical presentation will depend on the site, and dose of the irradiation and the age of the child when the treatment was given; children below the age of five years are particularly vulnerable. Intellectual impairment, with a mean drop in IQ of between 16 -20 points reported in some studies, hypothalamic pituitary damage with resultant loss of growth and endocrine disturbance, damage to the visual pathway, increasing ataxia and cerebellar dysfunction and, in the case of spinal tumours, neurological deterioration have all been described.

Normal doses of radiation therapy range from between 3000–5000 rads, (30–50 Gray), and to the cranio-spinal access from between 2000–3500 rads (20–30 Gray). Failure of radiation therapy to improve outcome following surgical debulking or removal of certain tumours and reported side effects has led to the continuing assessment, usually through multicentre trials, of chemotherapy in the treatment of tumours of CNS.

Chemotherapy

Various agents have been used in the treatment of central nervous system tumours (*see* **Table 10.6**). These include vincristine, methotrexate, procarbazine, vinblastine, cis-platinum and the nitrosoureas (BCNU, CCNU, TCNU). Their benefit is most proven in the treatment of PNETs, and trials have been carried out since the1970s to try to ascertain the optimal drug combination and timing of usage to maximise the beneficial effects of this

therapy. Following Bloom's trials, he demonstrated an improved outcome with adjuvant chemotherapy in children with medulloblastomas (Bloom, Wallace and Herk, 1969), but recently two large studies have failed to show any significant benefit in outcome in those children treated with surgery and irradiation alone compared with surgery, irradiation and adjuvant chemotherapy (Friedman and Schold, 1985). This finding was confirmed by an American study. Criticism of these studies centred on the fact that chemotherapy was given after radiation and that the drugs used were given in small doses and may not be as effective as those more recently developed. In view of this, a further multicentre, multinational trial has commenced, and its results, demonstrating the outcome of children treated by surgery followed by chemotherapy prior to radiotherapy, is awaited with interest. In children with widespread disseminated PNET at the time of initial diagnosis, the use of chemotherapy produces a radical change in the CT or MR scan appearances but the ultimate outcome has yet to be evaluated.

Like radiotherapy, chemotherapy has toxic side effects on the developing brain, and for this reason, these effects are thought to be minimised by delivering the chemotherapy prior to breakdown of the blood-brain barrier which occurs during ionising radiation therapy. In this way, the rationale is to limit the therapeutic agent to that area in which the blood-brain barrieris already destroyed, namely in the tumour bed. Sytemic side effects of chemotherapy are well known and occur in children being treated with tumours of CNS to the same degree as those with solid tumours elsewhere in the body.

Neuroradiology and the effects of radiotherapy and chemotherapy

Radiation damage may result in both early and late effects.The early changes between one week and three months are due to glial cell damage with consequent vasogenic oedema. On CT, these changes are manifest as low-attenuation lesions showing varying degrees of contrast enhancement. The contrast enhancement may persist for several months. In the early stages, there is a varying degree of mass effect. These changes are indistinguishable from tumour recurrence. MRI has not provided specific appearances for radiation changes in the brain with increased sensitivity of local and more generalised increase signal intensity on T2-weighted images. Late radiation effects are demonstrated as low-attenuation areas on CT and hyperintense areas on MR without mass effect, and with no enhancement.

The late effects of combined radiotherapy and chemotherapy may result in multifocal areas of calcification within the parenchyma. This may be both periventricular and parenchymal in distribution with associated generalised cerebral atrophy.

TABLE 10.6 Medulloblastoma

Radiotherapy—SOGy P.fossa—25–35Gy CNS

Chemotherapy—SIOP I and 2
                —CCSG (U.S.A.)
                —U.K. CCSG

Drugs—CCNU, Vincristine, Methotrexate
        —CCNU, Vincristine, Prednisolone

Overall—Surgery and DXT—54 %, 5-year survival; 35–40 %, 10 years alive

Pre-DXT Chemo—? difference
8 in I Chemo—? difference

Adjuvant therapy

Hydrocephalus resulting from tumour mass or secondary to a high CSF protein will need to be treated in a conventional manner by the use of CSF diversionary procedures. The use of shunts in certain tumours is known to produce seedling spread of tumour cells with peritoneal deposits. The majority of astrocytomas in the posterior fossa with obstructive hydrocephalus will require some form of temporary CSF drainage. In children with medulloblastomas, about a third present with obstructive hydrocephalus. They will require a CSF shunt long term, despite release of the blockage by surgical debulking, and it is in these cases that peritoneal seedlings have been reported (Hoffman *et al.*, 1970).

Conclusion

Within the CNS, solid tumours can present in a variety of ways including loss of neuronal function, hydrocephalus and raised intracranial pressure. The aim of therapy is to achieve total tumour removal and, depending on histological type, adjuvant radiotherapy and chemotherapy is then employed to prevent tumour recurrence and to prolong the disease-free interval. All treatment modalities involve damage to the CNS, and these effects must be balanced against the potential benefits when selecting the treatment type. The development of modern technology including the ultrasonic aspirator and laser together with newer imaging techniques has helped the surgeon achieve greater removal of tumour with less cost to the developing child's nervous system.

The development of modern techniques, such as tumour-targetted monoclonal antibodies designed to deliver the chemotherapeutic agent specifically to the cells within the tumour, has undoubtedly given hope for a new direction of tumour therapy. At present, however, cross-reactivity between various cells and these antibodies suggest that the specificity of these techniques can be improved. Future developments will depend on a better understanding of tumour cell biology linked to their histological features.

Chapter 11: Developmental Anomalies of the Central Nervous System

Richard W. Newton, W. St. Clair Forbes

Embryology

The complex structures of the brain and spinal cord develop from the primordial neural tube. The neural tube is formed by the ectodermal layer of the embryonic plate folding up into two parallel longditudinal ridges known as neural folds (**11.1**). This occurs from the second week of embryonic life. The neural folds fuse dorsally, fusion occurring first at the level that would be mid-cervical and proceeding rostrally and caudally. Failure of the neural tube to close completely causes common congenital malformations, the most serious of which leaves dura, vertebral arch and skin missing with the spinal cord exposed (*see* Chapter 12 for a description of hydrocephalus and spina bifida).

The neural crest differentiates from the neural tube ultimately to form a number of important peripheral neuro-ectodermal derivatives: the dorsal root and autonomic nervous system ganglia, the medulla of the adrenal gland, the melanophores (pigment-containing cells in skin) and Schwann cells of peripheral nerve (**11.2**).

Three imperfectly separated expansions appear in the cephalic portion of the closed tube. These are the primary brain 'vesicles', although the fore-brain, mid-brain and hind-brain characteristics of lower forms never appear as such in human central nervous system development (**11.3**). By the fourth week most mature structures can be identified though often only as groups of primitive neuroblast cells. The brain forms three folds, known as the cephalic, pontine and cervical flexures, occurring at mid-brain level at the pons and between the medulla and cord. Only the cephalic flexure remains in the adult. At 27 days the otic and optic vesicles appear and eight days later the olfactory and optic cups. At 41 days the cerebral vesicle with its pontine flexure is taking form at the time the face is fusing. Fibres into the optic chiasma appear at 47 days.

The rhombencephalon differentiates into an anterior-metencephalic and a posterior-myelencephalic portion. The transverse sulcus marks the boundary between the two and becomes the widest part of the fourth ventricle as it later continues.

In the midline dorsum of the neural tube is the thin

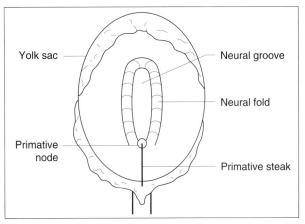

11.1 The amnioembryonic vesicle-ectodermal surface at 22 days.

roof plate and in the midline ventrally the floor plate. There are thickened lateral walls in the midpoint of which is a shallow longditudinal groove, the sulcus limitans. The dorsal part of the wall is known as the alar plate and the ventral part the basal plate. Rapid proliferation of ectoderm has by this time produced many layers to the tube. The cells nearer to the lumen have elongated to give the appearance of a columnar epithelium known as ependyma. A heavily nucleated mid-zone surrounds the ependyma and is known as the mantle. External to the mantle is the narrow, pale, almost cell-free area known as the marginal layer. All these layers are present by the end of the fourth week.

Surrounding mesenchymal tissue becomes highly vascularised, giving rise to the pia mater. This becomes combined with tissue in the ependymal roof of the fourth ventricle to form the choroid tela. Centrally, vessels in the tela invaginate the ventricle to produce the vascular mass known as the choroid plexus (**11.4**).

The mantle layer of the alar plate gives rise to cell bodies which are functionally associated with sensory function, the dorsal grey columns. Whereas the mantle layer of the basal plate forms the cell bodies of motor neurones and the ventral grey columns. The marginal layer is destined to become the cerebral white matter.

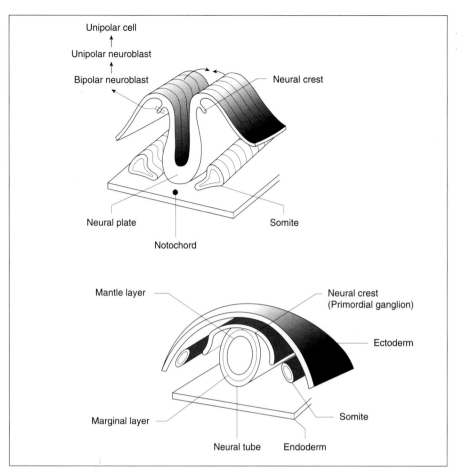

11.2 Development of the neural tube from the neural plate 22 days onwards.

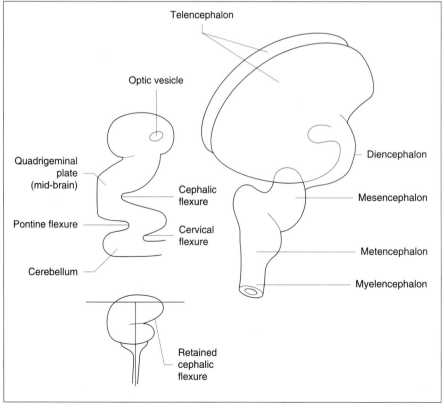

11.3 Embryonic flexures of the brain six weeks onwards.

11.4 Transverse section through human forebrain at 47 days.

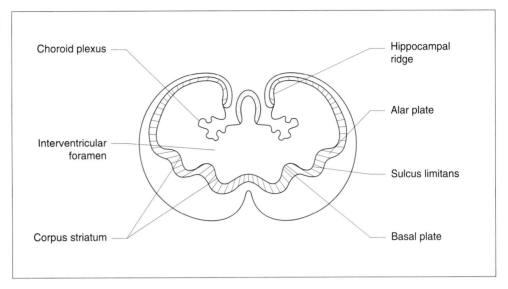

Choroid plexus

Hippocampal ridge

Alar plate

Interventricular foramen

Sulcus limitans

Corpus striatum

Basal plate

The proliferation of cells within the developing brain leads to many distortions. Sensory and motor nuclei tend to be displaced by the growth of the fibre tracts through the region, or by active migration. Nerve cells tend to remain as near as possible to their source of stimulation and when a tendency to displacement occurs, they will migrate in the direction from which the stimuli come. This is known as neurobiotaxis. They migrate by lengthening their axons. This process explains the curious course of many tracts and fibres, best exemplified by the course of the facial nerve. Fibres from the facial nerve nucleus originally lie in the floor of the fourth ventricle but then migrate caudally and dorsally to the sixth nerve nucleus, finally turning ventrally to reach their final position.

The mesencephalon undergoes the least change of any of the cerebral vesicles. The walls thicken significantly, reducing the lumen to a narrow canal, the cerebral aqueduct. The thickened alar section or tectum forms the quadrigeminal plate and its paired superior and inferior colliculi. The ventral portion becomes the larger tegmentum containing the pontine nuclei.

Similarly, the forebrain walls increase in size, reducing the lumen of the neural tube to form the third ventricle. The pia mater invaginates the roof of the third ventricle, forming the choroid plexus. By the tenth foetal week, three main regions can be distinguished: the epithalamus dorsally, the thalamus laterally and the hypothalamus ventrally. The telencephalon begins as a pair of lateral evaginations just behind the rostral limit of the forebrain. It has three principal parts, the neopallium, the rhinencephalon and the corpus striatum. As the hemispheres expand rostrally rising above the forebrain, the roof plate of each side is stretched vertically fusing with the pia to form the choroid plexuses as the pia invaginates the ventricles.

The corpus striatum begins as an enlargement of the floor of the telencephalon just lateral to and below the interventricular foramena. In each of these masses the caudate and lenticular nuclei differentiate. Due to the extensive development of fibres to distant parts of the hemispheres, the internal capsules appear between the thalamus and lenticular nucleus. The rhinencephalon appears as paired swellings on the ventral surface of the hemispheres to form the olfactory lobes.

During the first four months the surface of the hemisphere is smooth. The external grey substance begins to grow faster then the underlying white, resulting in the cortical surface being thrown into the gyral folds. There is mass migration of cells outward from the mantle layer into the relatively cell-free marginal zone. The cortical grey substance tends to lie on the outside of the underlying white matter (**11.5**). This centrifugal movement of neurones occurs along columns of glial cells projecting up to the cortical surface. Differentiation into the six basic cortical layers then occurs. The anterior and hippocampal commissures along with the corpus collosum all originally take their origin from the lamina terminalis representing the most rostral end of the forebrain. With subsequent development and caudal migration their position alters and they represent the main linking fibres between the two hemispheres.

Function of fibre tracts begins with the deposition of myelin sheaths around neurones. Brain myelination begins at about six months of foetal life. It is not fully complete until adolescence. Only fibres in the corpus striatum and the tracts assembling from lower levels are myelinated at birth. Among the last fibres to become ensheathed are the commissures.

Developmental brain disorders

From the foregoing description, it can be seen that there is great scope for a whole range of developmental brain

BRAIN DEVELOPMENT – 4 MONTHS

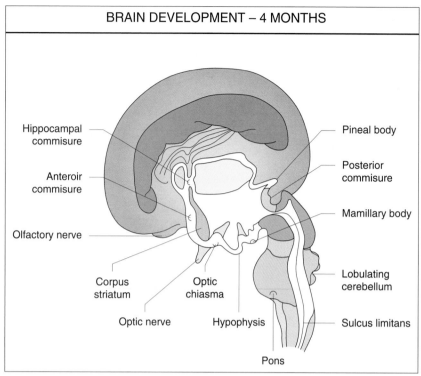

Hippocampal commisure

Anteroir commisure

Olfactory nerve

Corpus striatum

Optic nerve

Optic chiasma

Hypophysis

Pons

Pineal body

Posterior commisure

Mamillary body

Lobulating cerebellum

Sulcus limitans

11.5 Commissure development 4 months.

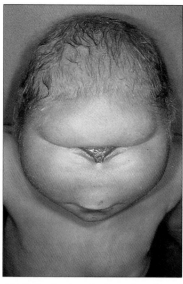

11.6 Cyclopia: single orbit, fused ocular globes.

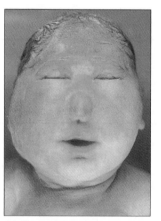
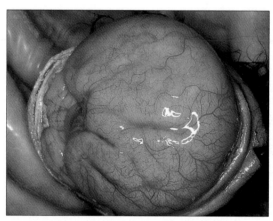

11.7 and 11.8 Cebocephaly: single nostril, marked hypotelorism, holoprosencephaly.

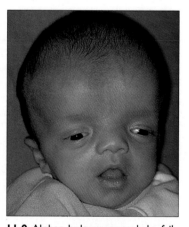

11.9 Alobar holoprosencephaly: failure of cleavage of prosencephalum resulting in facial abnormality, broad forehead, hypertelorism.

disorder if the organisation and migration of neurones is disrupted. The more common disorders are the result of a failure of canalisation in early embryogenesis. Knowledge of the processes that lead to the orderly migration of neurones are as yet poorly understood, but patterns of electrical stimulation and local nerve growth factors are both probably important. Much work needs to be done in identifying relevant biochemical mechanisms and their genetic determinants as well as the possible influence of environmental factors, such as drugs, infection, toxins and irradiation.

In all cases, careful assessment of family predisposi-tion, exposure to environmental factors and clinical pre-sentation needs to be made so that accurate genetic counselling might be given (*see* Chapter 15).

Forebrain abnormalities

Arhinencephaly-holoprosencephaly results from failure of hemispheric cleavage which is often associated with absence of the olfactory tracts and bulbs, and partial fusion of the basal ganglia. The brain forms an undivid-ed monoventricular mass and there is stenosis of the aqueduct of Sylvius. The optic chiasma is atrophic. The associated facial feature is of extreme hypotelorism or

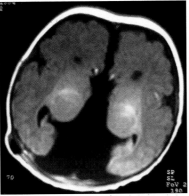

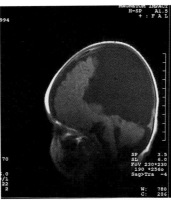

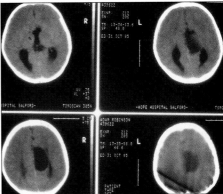

11.10 and 11.11 Lobar holoprosencephaly: MR scan—axial and coronal T1W. Single ventricular cavity with shallow interhemispheric fissure and absent falx, septum pellucidum and corpus callosum. Note rudimentary third ventricle and two thalami.

11.12 Agenesis of the corpus callosum: CT scan. The lateral ventricles are displaced and show characteristic deformity with narrow, elongated frontal horns and ventricular trigones. The third ventricle is large and is herniated between the lateral ventricles.

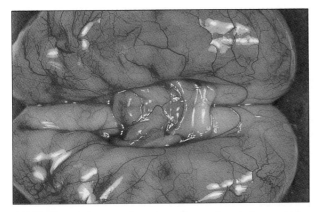

11.13 Partial absence of corpus callosum (posterior commissure only remains).

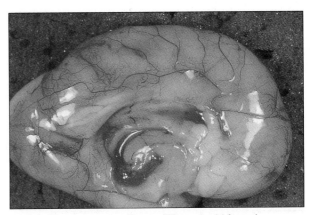

11.14 Absent corpus callosum (20-week-old foetus).

even cyclopia (**11.6–11.11**) with mid-facial hypoplasia and cleft lip and palate. Evidence of hypothalamo-pituitary dysfunction may reflect pituitary hypoplasia . Children with this disorder usually die in early infancy. Most cases are sporadic, although an association with trisomy 13, or deletion of the short arm of chromosome 17 has been reported.

Agenesis of the corpus callosum This is a common condition representing a failure of development of one of the major commissures connecting the two hemispheres. This allows the third ventricle to extend dorsally (**11.12**) towards the interhemispheric fissure and the frontal horns of the lateral ventricles are displaced laterally. The neurones destined to have been callosal fibres migrate caudally, condensed into a thick, longitudinal bundle. There are commonly associated hypoplasias of other neuronal systems and in particular the pyramidal tracts (**11.13–11.15**).

Whereas an isolated agenesis can be found in otherwise perfectly normally functioning people, learning difficulties most frequently accompany the finding. A great majority of cases are sporadic but autosomal recessive,

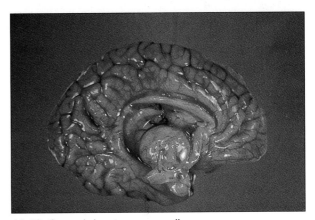

11.15 Control showing corpus callosum.

and X-linked modes of inheritance are also described.

Septo-optic dysplasia This is a rare, sporadic condition resulting from a defect in the septum pellucidum with bilateral optic nerve hypoplasia and pituitary insufficiency.

151

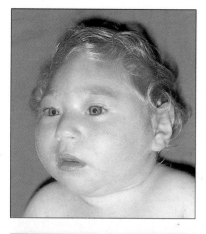

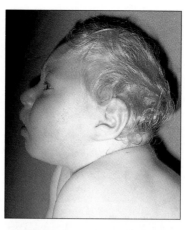

11.16 and 11.17 Familial microcephaly.

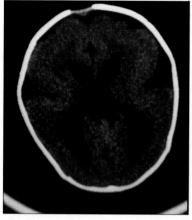

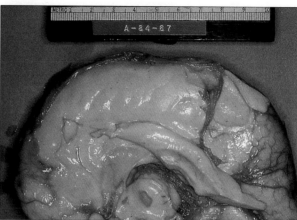

11.18 (left) CT: lissencephaly.

11.19 (right) Lissencephaly seen postmortem in a 17-month-old infant.

Abnormalities of neurogenesis

Microcephalia vera represents an autosomal recessively-inherited condition characterised by marked congenital microcephaly with mental retardation in the absence of any definable dysmorphism (**11.16 and 11.17**). Pathological studies reveal a relatively normal structural appearance of the brain which is smaller in overall size.

Acquired prenatal infections, hypoxic-ischaemic injury, metabolic disorders and chromosomal abnormalities may all be associated with generalised under-development of the brain. Full assessment is always required before genetic counselling is given.

Disorders of neuronal migration

A disturbance in the migration of neocortical neurones occurring before 20 weeks' gestation leads to a number of developmental brain abnormalities.

Lissencephaly (Agyria) In Type I (described by Bielchowsky) the first neurones become situated superficially under the molecular layer rather than forming the fifth and sixth layers of the cortex (**11.18**). A thick diffuse heterotopic band is formed. Due to complete arrest of migration at 12 to 16 weeks' gestation there is an associated heterotopia of the inferior olives. The disor-

der is frequently associated with hydramnios, profound mental retardation and the epileptic encephalopathies of infancy. Associated dysmorphism may lead to the diagnosis of the Miller–Dieker syndrome or the Norman–Roberts syndrome. Chromosomal analysis should be carried out.

Type II lissencephaly (Walker–Warberg or HARD (E) (**11.19**). The acronym refers to hydrocephalus, agyria, retinal dysplasia and occasionally encephalocoele. Neuropathology indicates a progressive disruption of the neuronal migration between 16 and 24 weeks' gestation resulting in abnormality of the meninges, leading to communicating hydrocephalus and vermian agenesis. In some families this may have autosomal recessive inheritance or be due to a persistent viral infection. Fukuyama described a congenital muscular dystrophy in association with this neuropathological disorder as did Walker–Warberg in their muscle–eye–brain disease. Peroxisomal disorders should also be ruled out (*see* Chapter 13).

Heterotopias

The advent of magnetic resonance imaging has led to many more children being identified as having heterotopias as an explanation for the presence of their learning difficulties or seizure tendency (**11.20**). Clearly,

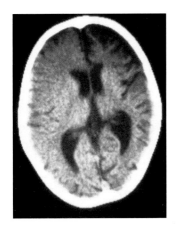

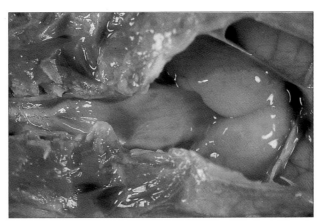

11. 20 (left) Hetero-topia: focal cortical dys-plasia evident on CT scan.

11.21 (right) Dandy–Walker syndrome: cyst wall removed to show absence of cerebellar ver-mis and dilated fourth ventricle.

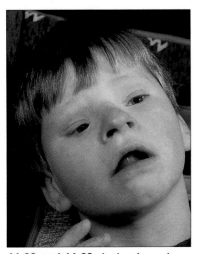

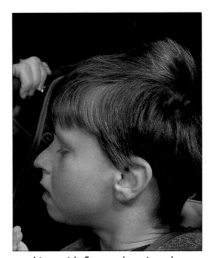

11.22 and 11.23 Joubert's syndrome: dysmorphism with flattened occiput, hyper-telorism, epicanthus and broad nasal tip.

11.24 Joubert's syndrome: cerebel-lar hypoplasia.

focal areas of neuronal migration abnormality may be associated with more widespread subtle abnormality within the brain. At other times, microdysgenesis of this sort may be associated with relatively minor cerebral dysfunction identified on the rare occasions when children with relatively minor problems come to post-mortem following, for example, a road traffic accident.

Cytoarchitectonic studies have demonstrated the rel-ative paucity of dendritic connections between one neu-rone and another, inversion of some cortical neurones or reduction in relative numbers of nerve cells in the pyra-midal tracts, for example.

Cerebellar hypoplasia or atrophy

The Dandy–Walker syndrome involves absence of the inferior two-thirds of the vermis. It is a sporadic condi-tion, but association with Walker–Warberg lissencephaly is also described.

In the Dandy–Walker syndrome, the defect usually occurs between the third and fourth gestational weeks and posterior fossa structures are affected (11.21).

Secondary hydrocephalus commonly develops, although its onset may be delayed by some years. The defect is usually sporadic but may be associated with other cere-bral malformations.

In Joubert's syndrome, there is autosomal recessive inheritance, cerebellar hypoplasia in association with profound learning disability, seizures and episodes of hyperpnoea (11.22–11.24). A small occipital meningo-cele is at times associated with this disorder.

Developmental megalencephalies

Dominantly inherited isolated megalencephalies occur in some families with normal intelligence. There is a well-defined entity with delayed closure of the fontanelles, dissociated motor development and the appearance of communicating hydrocephalus on the CT brain scan (11.25). By the age of two to three years, the CT scan appearance is normal and the children have shown catch-up with their motor development.

Other children with megalencephaly may show sig-nificant learning difficulties, at times associated with

153

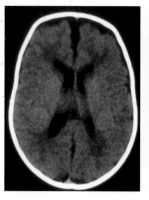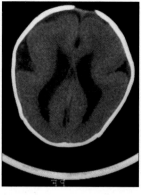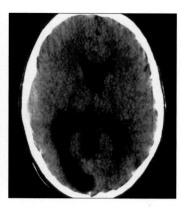

11.25 (left) CT: familial macrocephaly with enlarged CSF spaces in infancy.

11.26 (centre) Pachygyria.

11.27 (right) CT: porencephaly of right occipital lobe.

neurofibromatosis (*see* below). X-linked forms of mental retardation are also described, including the Fragile X syndrome, and appropriate clinical assessment and chromosomal analysis should be carried out in all children with a relatively large head.

Hemi-megalencephaly may be a sporadic finding involving the presence of numerous giant, occasionally multinucleated, nerve cells of neuronal and glial origin in one hemisphere. It may also be seen as a feature of the Linear Naevus Sebaceous syndrome. This involves a facial midline linear naevus sebaceous of Jadassohn in association with partial seizures or infantile spasms, mental retardation and ocular abnormality. Early neuroradiological and electroencephalographic assessment is required as many children benefit from hemispherectomy. The seizures may be controlled by these means and, if surgery is performed early enough, ultimately the remaining hemisphere may restore function to both sides of the body with slow resolution over some years of the resulting hemiplegia and hemianopia.

Microgyria (micropolygyria)

In this group of disorders, a variety of neuropathological change is seen including lissencephaly, pachygyria (**11.26**) and microgyria. The alteration in cortical architecture may be due to a variety of aetiologies, including the peroxisomal disorders, Fukuyama's disease and hypoxic-ischaemic injury dating from 20 to 24 weeks' gestation.

Porencephaly

This refers to a cystic defect in the cerebral hemisphere commonly arising pre- or perinatally from ischaemic or haemorrhagic necrosis. This may arise either through small-vessel disease due to infection or through thrombotic episodes (**11.27**). The result may be a spastic paresis of one or both sides, often associated with learning difficulties but at times with normal intelligence. In its severest form, hydranencephaly and/or multicystic-malacia may result from failure of perfusion of the brain.

Neural tube defects

These are considered in Chapter 12. At times, these also give rise to encephaloceles which may also be formed from the extra-cranial evagination of normally formed brain tissue during the twentieth gestational week, due to the presence of prenatal hydrocephalus. Familial conditions occur, including Joubert's syndrome and Walker's lissencephaly (*see* above).

Neuroradiology of developmental anomalies

A significant number of children with learning difficulties are referred for CT. Many have scans which are normal or have mild cerebral atrophy and the diagnosis can only be further advanced on the basis of biochemical or pathological changes. In a small proportion, imaging may demonstrate quite specific features, allowing a clinical diagnosis to be made before the results of other laboratory tests are available. They are best divided into three groups:

1) Structural damage before, during or after birth.
2) Genetic disorders sometimes associated with identifiable chromosome or abnormalities.
3) Conditions caused by neurodegenerative disorders or metabolic defects.

There is considerable overlap in these groups. The choice of imaging modality depends on the age of presentation and the nature of the abnormality. Ultrasonography, CT scanning and MRI may individually have specific roles or be used in combination.

Role of imaging

The role of imaging is to evaluate:

1) The ventricular system (especially the fourth).
2) The cerebral morphology and the presence of encephalocoeles.
3) The Sylvian fissures.
4) Septum pellucidum.
5) Grey/white matter differentiation.
6) The periventricular strip.

11.28 (left) CT: anterior encephalocoele—evagination of brain through disrupted fronto-ethmoidal bone.

11.29 (centre) Three-dimensional CT of same defect.

11.30 (right) Hydranencephaly: CT scan showing axial section through the level of the lateral ventricles shows large CSF cavity replacing the cerebral hemispheres with severe thinning of the cortical mantle.

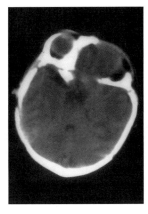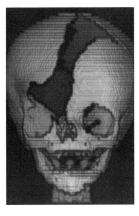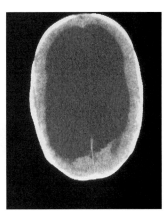

7) The sulci and gyri.
8) The presence of intracranial calcification.
9) The falx cerebri.
10) The size and shape of the cranium, and an assessment of the sinuses.

An evaluation of these signs is used in the assessment of conditions causing structural damage before, during or immediately after birth. These conditions are best considered under the following four groups: disorders of closure, diverticulation and migration, and destructive processes.

1. Closure disorder

Disorders of closure include encephalocoeles, cavum septipellucidi and cavum vergae, agenesis and dysgenesis of the corpus callosum, a Dandy–Walker syndrome, and the Chiari malformations. This group of abnormalities is characterised by abnormalities of the ventricular system and abnormal CSF-containing spaces.

Encephalocoeles may occur within the occipital area, cranial vault, cranial base and fronto-ethmoidal areas **(11.28 and 11.29)**. Occipital location is the commonest and most are associated with Chiari II malformation. Types of encephalocoeles recognised on CT scanning include:

1) Cranial meningocoele (meninges and cerebrospinal fluid).
2) Encephalomeningocoele (brain tissue and meninges).
3) Hydroencephalomeningocoele (brain tissue, a portion of ventricle and meninges).

The bony defects in frontal and ethmoidal encephalocoeles are recognised on axial and coronal CT and the herniated brain tissue within the encephalocoele can usually be visualised on CT. The CT appearances of agenesis of the corpus callosum are characteristic in both the axial and coronal plane.

1) The frontal horns are widely separated in the axial plate and appear narrow in the absence of hydrocephalus.
2) The frontal horns and bodies of lateral ventricles have lateral beaks.
3) The occipital horns may appear dilated in comparison to the bodies of lateral ventricles.
4) The elevated third ventricle is interposed between the bodies of the lateral ventricles, and is usually enlarged.

5) Rarely, an interhemispheric arachnoid cyst may be associated with agenesis of the corpus callosum.

6) Abnormal proximity of the interhemispheric fissure to the third ventricle on contiguous CT or MR sections. This is considered to be a highly reliable feature and has been called the interhemispheric fissure sign of dysgenesis of the corpus callosum.

Lipomas and other fat-containing tumours may be associated with agenesis of the corpus callosum. On CT, lipomas are of low density (minus H values) and appear hyperintense on T1-weighted and T2-weighted sequences on MR. CT may in addition reveal calcification within the lipoma. In the neonate characteristic sonographic features of agenesis can be demonstrated in the axial and coronal planes. Sagittal sections on both ultrasound and MRI show the unique abnormalities of absence of the corpus callosum. The normally prominent corpus callosum is not identified, and vessels of the anterior cerebral-pericallosal arterial system are arranged in an unusual radial fashion. The fat-containing lipoma has a brightly echogenic appearance at sonography.

The Dandy–Walker syndrome and Chiari malformations are considered further in Chapter 12.

2. Diverticulation disorders

Complete or partial lack of separation of the prosencephalon into cerebral hemispheres results in a group of malformations ranging from severe alobar prosencephaly to isolated aplasia of the olfactory bulbs and tracts (see above). CT and MRI scanning demonstrate the spectrum of abnormalities encountered in this group of conditions according to the degree of failure of cleavage.

In alobar holoprosencephaly, the most striking CT and MR feature is the single large ventricle and fused thalamic nuclei. The occipital and temporal horns are absent in the frontal and occipital regions; a peripheral rim of cerebral tissue may be identified. Midline palatomaxillary clefts associated with hypertelorism are common associated features (*see* **11.9**). The differential diagnosis includes hydrocephalus and hydranencephaly (**11.30**). In alobar holoprosencephaly the septum pellucidum, falx

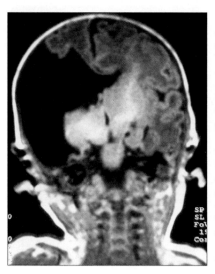

11.31 Schizencephaly. MR scan—coronal T1W. Full thickness cleft with communication between the sylvian subarachnoid space and the right lateral ventricle, pachygyria lining the cleft, absence of the septum pellucidum and single ventricular cavity and marked thinning of the corpus callosum.

cerebri and interhemispheric fissures are absent; in hydranencephaly, the thalami are normal.

In semilobar holoprosencephaly CT and MR demonstrates a single ventricular chamber with partially-formed occipital horns and no sylvian fissures. There is increased cerebral tissue present. The septum pellucidum and corpus callosum are absent and the falx is absent or rudimentary.

In lobar holoprosencephaly the cerebral hemispheres and lateral ventricle are well formed. The lateral ventricles usually have both occipital and frontal horns. Ventricular dilatation is present due to deficient brain substances rather than hydrocephalus. The falx and corpus callosum are better formed but still remain rudimentary whilst the septum pellucidum is absent.

In septo-optic dysplasia, imaging demonstrates absence of the septum pellucidum, dilatation of the lateral ventricles with flattening of the roof of the frontal horns and inferior pointing of the floor of the lateral ventricles, small optic nerves best seen on coronal scanning, and there is dilatation of the chiasmatic and-suprasellar cisterns. Enlargement of the pituitary stalk and infundibulum may be seen when there is associated diabetes insipidus. There is also cortical atrophy with dilated sulci and a diverticular expansion of the optic recess of the third ventricle. This feature is best seen on a T1-weighted sagittal MR section.

3. Disorder of migration and sulcation
In lissencephaly, the CT and MR appearances are of large sub-arachnoid spaces without demonstrable sulci, producing a smooth brain surface, and dilated ventricles. The Sylvian fissures are widened, appearing as deep grooves, with a lack of insular operculisation.

The CT appearance of heterotopic grey matter is that of nodules, usually of the same density as normal grey matter, protruding into the ventricular cavity.

4. Destructive processes
Hydranencephaly is a congenital disorder in which the cerebral hemispheres are replaced by thin sacs which contain cerebrospinal fluid. The cranial vault and meninges are intact. The CT appearances include:

1) A fluid-filled cranium with demonstration of the falx cerebri and tentorium. The falx may be midline or deviated but is usually not thickened.

2) Remnants of the temporal, occipital or subfrontal cortex may be present.

3) Rounded thalamic masses are characteristic. The CT differential diagnosis includes other disorders such as infarction, hydrocephalus, subdural effusions and alobar holoprosencephaly.

In porencephaly, the non-contrasted CT or MRI demonstrates a large, well-defined area of CSF communicating with the lateral ventricles. There is associated hemiatrophy of the ipsilateral ventricle and/or cortical sulci. Thinning or an asymmetry of the cranial vault may also be demonstrated.

Schizencephaly (**11.31**) is a form of porencephaly which is due to arrested growth of the cerebral mantle. The condition is characterised by clefts of CSF density within the cerebral cortex. There may be absence of the septum pellucidum and corpus callosum.

Role of ultrasound in the diagnosis of congenital anomalies

In the pre-term and term infant, sonography is an excellent method of evaluating congenital anomalies. Transducers with multiple focal zones may be needed to image the supratentorial and intratentorial regions optimally in the same patients. The sonographic evaluation of congenital anomalies may be simplified by deciding whether the lesion is anechoic or echogenic and then locating the lesion above or below the tentorium.

Anechoic supratentorial abnormalities   Cranial sonography is indicated in all neonatal spinal dysraphism and also after closure of the spinal defect because hydrocephalus frequently worsens after surgery. Hydrocephalus is readily demonstrated and there may be absence of fenestration of the septum pellucidum, anterior/inferior pointing of the frontal horns, prominence of the massa intermedia and dilatation of the third ventricle. Cephalocoeles, holoprocencephaly, hydranencephaly, arachnoid cyst and an aneurysm of the vein of Galen are also included in this category.

Echogenic supratentorial abnormalities   Echogenic supratentorial abnormalities are typically mid-line defects, the most common of which is agenesis of the corpus collosum. A lipoma of the corpus collosum is demonstrated as a brightly echogenic lesion.

Anechoic infratentorial abnormalities   This group includes the Dandy–Walker malformation, arachnoid cysts, post-haemorrhagic enlargement of the fourth ventricle and cerebellar dysgenesis. Each of these lesions can be successfully differentiated sonographically by careful evaluation of the fourth ventricle.

11.32 (left) Skull x-ray showing cranio-synostosis and saggital suture heaped up (arrowed).

11.33 (centre) Neurofibromatosis: segmental café-au-lait patches.

11.34 (right) Neurofibromatosis: axillary freckling.

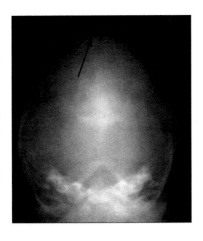

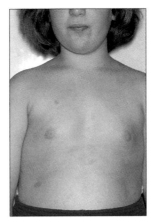

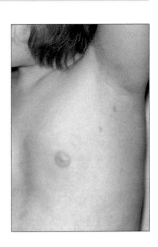

Echogenic infratentorial abnormalities The only echogenic infratentorial abnormality to occur with any frequency is the Chiari II malformation.

Craniosynostosis

Craniosynostosis refers to the absence of one or more sutures separating the membranous bones of the skull. This may be either primary synostosis (present before birth) or secondary craniosynostosis (premature obliteration of one or more sutures). The sagittal and coronal sutures are those most commonly involved. The condition leads to skull deformity and there may be associated learning difficulties, ocular defects and other congenital abnormalitites. Expansion of the skull cannot occur in a direction perpendicular to an involved suture, and thus the shape of the head in untreated cases will account for the sutures involved.

Plain radiographs and CT scanning will reveal the abnormal shape of the cranium and evaluate the fused sutures (**11.32**). The sutures involving the skull base and calvaria are most accurately identified by high-resolution CT scans in both axial and coronal planes. The axial plane is used for all sutures involving the cranial vault except the sagittal suture for which the coronal plane is superior. The developmental changes in sutures and sychondroses occurring with age and alterations in skull tables and diploic space are best demonstrated by CT. The evaluation of patients with syndromes in which the radiographic features are similar, such as Apert's syndrome and craniofacial dysostosis (Crouzon's syndrome), is best achieved by CT which can demonstrate changes in brain, bone and facial soft tissues. Three-dimensional CT reconstructions may have a role in demonstrating the craniofacial abnormalities. CT enables accurate imaging of the deformities involving the calvaria and skull base secondary to craniosynostosis prior to surgical correction.

Treatment is by the creation of an artificial suture by means of a linear craniectomy along the line of the fused suture. The best results are seen when this is done early (before three months of age). This is mandatory where there is total craniosynostosis which would otherwise not allow normal brain growth and lead to impairment.

The neurocutaneous syndromes

With their common ectodermal origin, it is easy to see how skin abnormality might at times reflect associated abnormalities of nervous system development. There are at least 40 conditions involving abnormalites of the nervous system where skin abnormalities make up a recognisable syndrome. Reference will be made to a number of these these in this chapter, although more properly some would belong in the chapter on inherited and metabolic disease (Chapter 13) or a chapter on dysmorphology, and so on. As our knowlege advances on the underlying metabolic basis, classification will become more orderly.

Neurofibromatosis

This represents a spectrum of disorders showing many features, although no one feature or set of features is shared by all of them. The conditions are dominantly inherited with a penetrance which is very variable even within one family. The cutaneous features consist of six or more café-au-lait patches (many people have fewer), axillary freckling and firm nodular neurofibromata, which may be palpable on peripheral nerves (**11.33 and 11.34**). The cutaneous features often become more evident after puberty.

Neurofibromatosis Type I (NF-I) is coded for on chromosome 17. Neurofibromata appear on the course of peripheral nerves including the cranial nerves. They may look unsightly or cause neurological signs if they appear at a site where a peripheral nerve passes through a bony foramen, hence blindness (second nerve) or deafness (eighth nerve) may be a complication. Iris Lisch nodules, optic gliomas and other intracranial astrocytomas are reasonably specific for NF-I. Megalencephaly with learning difficulties and epilepsy is seen in a few. Cranio-facial dysplasia is a relatively frequent feature of NF-I affecting at least 5 % of those involved of all

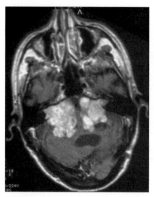
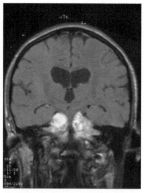

11.35 and 11.36 Neurofibromatosis with bilateral acoustic neuromas. MRI axial **(11.35, left)** and coronal **(11.36, right)** TIW post-Gadolinium. Enhancing tumours in both cerebello-pontine angle cisterns extending into the IAMs.

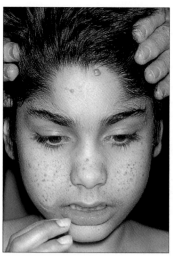

11.37 Tuberose sclerosis: adenoma sebaceum.

ages. This is a progressive lesion with the posterior orbital wall being most commonly affected and the deficit enlarging as the patient gets older. Plexiform neurofibromata may be associated. Vertebral dysplasia may also be present to varying degrees leading to scoliosis. Pseudo-arthrosis can be a major characteristic and makes NF-I the most likely diagnosis. When it is seen in the newborn, it commonly involves the distal portion of one tibia. The severity may range from mild bowing to gross disruption. NF-I accounts for at least 85 % of all NF cases.

Neurofibromatosis Type II (NF-II) is coded for on chromosome 22. This is associated with bilateral acoustic neuromata (**11.35 and 11.36**) presenting with-deafness, and at times a cerebellar pontine angle syndrome with a facial nerve paresis and cerebellar ataxia.

In some families one may see an overlap between the features of NF-I and NF-II. Other associations are phaeochromocytoma, pulmonary hypertension, renal artery stenosis with hypertension and gliomatous change, particularly in the central nervous system lesions. It must be emphasised that most people with this disorder carry no features other than the cutaneous stimata.

Cosmetic disfigurement is the most prominent clinical problem for people with NF-I. Surgical treatment offers the only realistic approach but results are often sub-optimal. Hypertrophic overgrowth of a body segment is seen in a few young people and, rarely, may also need cosmetic surgical intervention.

Congenital and neonatal problems include pseudo-arthrosis, congenital glaucoma and sphenoid wing dysplasia with plexiform neurofibromata.

Early childhood problems include developmental delay, embryonal tumour, progression of specifically located plexiform neurofibromas and the presentation of symptomatic optic gliomas. In the second half of the first decade optic gliomata become more common as do associated learning difficulties with the development of seizures, scoliosis and iris Lisch nodules. The plexiform neurofibromas may worsen. In the second decade all

affected people begin to manifest at least a few cutaneous or subcutaneous neurofibromata, often with puberty, and in this period hypertension and neurofibrosarcomas may declare themselves.

Tuberose sclerosis

Tuberose sclerosis is a dominantly inherited condition with reduced or non-penetrance. The new mutation rate is in the order of 70 %. The prevalence in the community is probably in the order of 1:27,000.

The cardinal features of tuberose sclerosis are facial angiofibromas, subungual fibromas, retinal hamartomas, cortical tubers, subependymal glionodules and renal angiomyolipomas (**11.37–11.43**). The cutaneous features consist most commonly of depigmented patches which fluoresce with ultraviolet light (Wood's light), roughened patches of skin known as chagrin patches, and adenoma sebaceum consisting of the facial angiofibromata in a butterfly distribution on the face. Rhabdomyomata are identifiable in the early weeks on echocardiography but often resolve. Polycystic kidneys may be another feature. More rarely, gingival fibromata, dental enamel pits, and pulmonary lymphangiomyomatosis with pulmonary hypertension are present.

Seizures are the most common presenting symptom in young people with TS and are seen in up to 90 %. All those with significant learning difficulties have seizures. Seventy per cent have seizures in the first 12 months of life, and of those with no seizures in the first five years, intellectual outcome tends to be good.

Those infants presenting with infantile spasms also have developmental delay. Subsequently, children retain a tendency to have seizures, autism, and profound mental handicap.

As in neurofibromatosis gliomatous change can occur in the affected brain. In about 7 %, such a tumour tends to block the outlet of the third ventricle in the second or third decade.

Genetic heterogeneity has been identified with gene locuses for the condition, having been found on 9q and

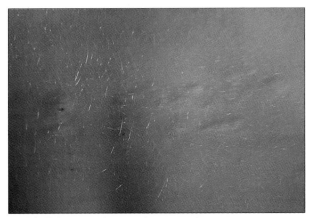

11.38 Tuberose sclerosis: chagrin patch.

11.39 Tuberose sclerosis: depigmented patches.

11.40 (left) Tuberose sclerosis: phakoma.

11.41 (right) Tuberose sclerosis: CT scan—subependymal, calcification and cortical atrophy.

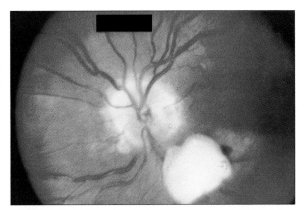

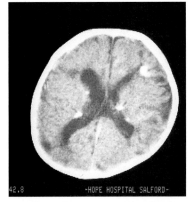

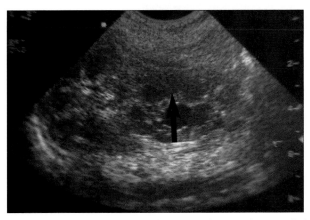

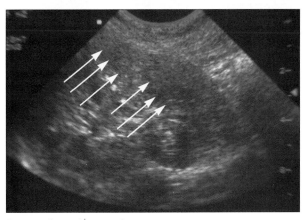

11.42 and 11.43 Tuberose sclerosis: polycystic change in kidney (arrowed) on ultrasound.

11q, with possibly a third at 12q,22-24. Many who carry the gene have stigmata other than the cutaneous features and adequate genetic counselling should involve CT scanning of the head and ultrasound scanning of the kidneys.

Von Hippel Lindau disease

Although there are no skin lesions in this disorder, it is conveniently considered in this section. The cardinal features are retinal and cerebellar haemangioblastomas with occasional involvement of the medulla and spinal cord. Cysts of the kidney, pancreas, epididymis and renal cell carcinomas also occur. Some people develop pheochromocytomas but rarely in childhood. The condition is a dominant with variable expression.

Fluorescein retinoscopy helps define the retinal lesion and disordered capillary permeability often leads to an exudative mound. Other eye abnormalities include glaucoma, uveitis and cataracts.

A cerebellar problem rarely emerges before the age

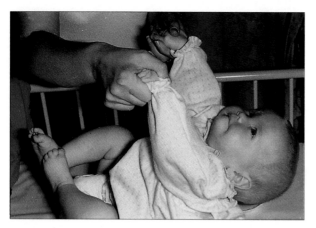

11.44   Gorlin's syndrome: poor axial tone with preserved limb tone may indicate future learning difficulties.

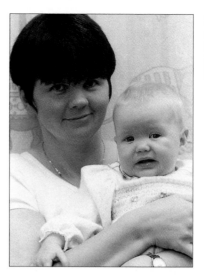

11.45 .Gorlin's syndrome: mother holding daughter with large head and hypertelorism.

of 10 and may not emerge until the sixth decade. The tumours are generally removed with great success though secondary hydrocephalus is a possiblity. The tumours are not radiosensitive.

The retinal lesions are best treated with obliteration of non-macula lesions and all patients should be kept under annual review.

There is no non-penetrance of the disorder. The mutation rate is unkown.

Gorlin's syndrome. The naevoid basal cell carcinoma syndrome

This is an autosomal dominantly inherited condition with complete penetrance and variable expressivity. Typical facies are of macrocephaly, mild hypertelorism and pouting of the lower lip. By the age of 20 or so only about half of those with the condition will have the basal cell carcinoma syndrome (**11.44 and 11.45**). The condition is rarely if ever fatal but the need for continuing resection of the lesions can lead to cosmetic disfigurement. Only 15 % have the naevoid basal cell carcinomas before puberty. Jaw cysts which are odontogenic keratocysts often appear in the first decade but are rarely symptomatic.

Important associated features are severe learning difficulties in about 3 % and the development of medulloblastomas or other rarer sarcomas affecting the many different connective tissue organs of the body. Hypogonadism may be seen in males and fibromas of the ovary are common in females.

Hypomelanosis of Ito

In some families, this is an autosomal-dominant disorder, but in most there is no clear family history. Chromosomal abnormalities including balanced translocation have been described in at least two children. The skin lesion is of linear vorticose or irregular areas of hypopigmentation. These may affect one or both sides of the body and be associated with lesions of the iris or hemi-hypertrophy.

The central nervous system is affected in at least 50 %. Those with seizures in the first year of life are most likely to have a static encephalopathy associated with significant learning difficulties.

The pathology of both skin and brain is very reminiscent of that seen in tuberose sclerosis, neurofibromatosis and in incontinentia pigmenti (*see* below). They are considered the non-specific result of a dysplasia or embryopathy affecting the central nervous system and the skin. Most neuronal migration occurs at between three and six months of gestation (*see* above). At about fifteen weeks' gestation the melanoblasts migrate from the neural crest and mature to melanocytes in the skin. In the sixth month the hair anlage is present, accounting for an association between abnormalities of cerebral cortex and hair. The number, size and pigment content of melanocytes in the basal area of the epidermis is generally reduced and in the brain the signs are of a neuronal migration defect with microcephaly and a rostral displacement.

The disorders of DNA repair
Ataxia telangiectasia

This carries autosomal-recessive inheritance. The cardinal neurological feature is one of truncal ataxia often associated with Cogan's oculomotor dyspraxia. Children are often late to attain their motor milestones but their difficulty with balance and coordination may remain quite mild at least until they reach school age, by which time their abilities are evidently quite different from most others in the class (**11.46–11.49**). After this time, motor performance tends to deteriorate steadily so that by the time the children are in their early teens many of them are confined to a wheelchair. Some of them additionally display choreoathetosis. There are reported

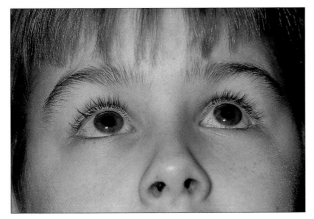

11.46 Ataxia telangiectasia: telangiectasis of sclera.

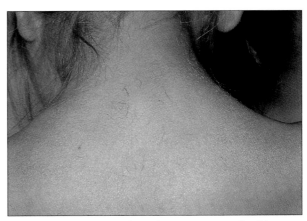

11.47 Ataxia telangiectasia: telangiectasia over shoulders.

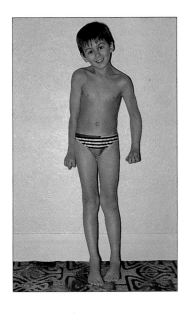

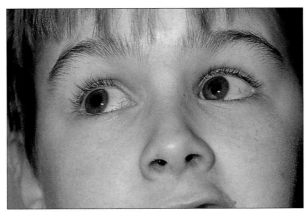

11.48 (left) Ataxia telangiectasia: early clumsiness followed by a less steady gait.

11.49 (right) Ataxia telangiectasia: ocular motor dyspraxia. Here the head moves left. The eyes are left behind and then restituted with a characteristic head flick. Normal vertical eye movement.

cases where the ataxia remains relatively quite mild long into adult life.

The cutaneous feature of the syndrome is the telangiectasis that is most evident from the age of four or five onwards. Then it is most readily seen on the conjunctiva and then subsequently appears over the ear lobes, nape of the neck and top of the shoulders.

An immune paresis principally involving IgA surface antibody also reflects the problem with DNA repair. This manifests itself as a susceptibility to infection and a vulnerability to the development of neoplastic disorders which affect perhaps 10 % of those involved. Acute lymphoblastic leukaemia is one of the most commonly associated conditions and the success of therapy is limited by the vulnerability of tissues to irradiation and chemotherapy.

There also appears to be some limitation of somatic growth. In early childhood, children tend to be on about the tenth centile, but as they enter their teens have often fallen to the third centile or lower. Mental retardation is not generally associated with the condition although the

severe physical disability can hamper academic performance and the early literature suggests that cognitive development may slow a little as time progresses with a fall-off of IQ score. There is, however, no evidence for a dementia.

Before the telangiectasis appears, the condition may be confused with Friedreich's ataxia although there are no signs of loss of posterior column function.

Diagnosis is made on clinical impression and the presence of an immune paresis, particularly a low IgA, and a raised alpha fetoprotein. White cells and skin fibroblasts are unduly sensitive to irradiation and there are now standardised techniques to suggest this which are also useful in detecting the heterozygote state.

Xeroderma pigmentosum

This is also a DNA repair disorder with autosomal recessive inheritance. Its cardinal feature is acute sun sensitivity, often leading in infancy to erythematous and bullous skin lesions. Freckles and hypopigmentation are common, along with dryness, telangiectasis

161

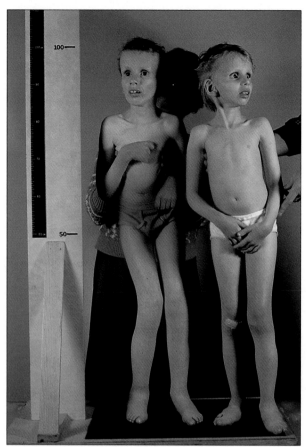

11.50 Cockayne syndrome: small stature, premature aging. Severe learning difficulties, sensori-neural deafness, photosensitive dermatitis.

movement disorder (**11.50**), in addition to spasticity of the lower extremities with flexion contractures.

At birth, babies are of normal size but significant feeding difficulties and subsequent growth failure leads them to become progressively cachetic. At this time they acquire a distinctive facial appearance with a thin prominent nose and zygomatic processes, prognathism, enophthalmos and absent fat. This appearance is usually well developed by the teens, and neurological abnormalities largely resemble those of xeroderma pigmentosum, which may well exist in some young people. Many young people die in their teens in status epilepticus or with malignant hypertension, or renal and pulmonary dysfunction.

Incontinentia pigmenti

As this condition predominantly affects girls, it is thought to be an X-linked dominant condition probably lethal in males *in utero*. The central nervous system is involved in 30 to 50 %. A cerebral dysgenesis leads to delayed development with seizures, spastic paralysis and cerebellar signs in some. The degree of learning difficulty varies greatly. Associated with this there may be a retinal dysplasia leading to a retrolental mass and skeletal and teeth abnormalities.

The skin abnormality is seen in three distinct stages. In the first two weeks of life erythematous, macular, papular, vesicular, bullous or pustular lesions occur proximally in a linear distribution. This is in association with an eosinophilia. In the following two to three weeks pustular, lichenoid, verrucous, keratotic and dyskeratotic lesions occur more distally and as they resolve, often leave areas of atrophied skin. In the third stage, areas of pigmentation appear over a period of some weeks.

Sturge–Weber syndrome

This is a sporadic condition involving a malformation of cephalic-venous microvasculature. There is an abnormality in the growth of the primordial vascular plexus in cephalic mesenchyme as it lies between the epidermis and the telencephalic vesicles in close proximity to the optic cup (**11.51**). This leads in its fullest form to cavernous angioma of the leptomeninges, a facial angiomatous naevus and a choroidal angioma of the eye (**11.52 and 11.53**). The lesion may be unilateral or bilateral and in individual children may affect one or all of brain, eye or skin tissue. The lack of cerebral or ocular symptoms does not preclude them developing at a later date where the facial naevus is present. Sturge–Weber syndrome is not usually applied when neither cerebral or ocular symptoms have appeared.

The port wine-coloured stain on the face is evident at birth and always involves the first division of the trigeminal nerve. Involvement of the skin on that side may be more widespread and there is an association in

and, at times, skin atrophy. Ectoderm around the eye also shows light sensitivity and may lead to blepharitis, iritis or conjunctivitis with keratitis and oedema of the corneum, occasionally leading to ulceration and opacification. Susceptibility to skin neoplasia is very high, and all affected young people should have their eyes and skin inspected weekly for new lesions.

About 20 % have associated neurological problems (a much higher percentage in Japan) and, in its severest form, microcephaly, progessive dementia, choreoathetosis, ataxia and spasticity are seen, along with a progressive peripheral neuropathy. Sensori-neural deafness may also be progressive.

Management is by way of reducing exposure to ultraviolet light as much as possible and the aggressive early treatment of skin cancer.

Cockayne syndrome

This autosomal-recessive condition leads to small stature, severe sun sensitivity, ocular, skeletal and neurological abnormalities. The most common findings are optic atrophy, pigmentary retinal degeneration, cataracts, sensori-neural deafness and an extrapyramidal

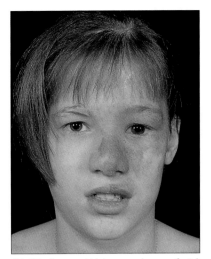

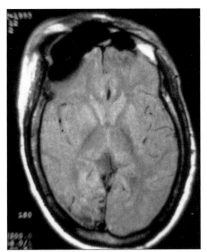

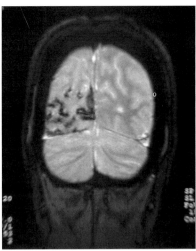

11.51 Sturge–Weber syndrome: facial appearance.

11.52 and 11.53 Sturge–Weber syndrome: MRIs of a proton density axial section (**11.52, left**) and a T2W coronal section (**11.53, right**). The T2W axial image shows large areas of signal void in the right occipital region, indicating the dilated vascular channels of the angiomatous malformation. Note the right heamiatrophy with enlargement of the frontal sinus and thickening of the skull vault. Note: areas of calcification which appear as signal void cannot be differentiated from the angioma.

some with the Klippel–Trenauney syndrome. This syndrome involves angiomatous skin naevi in association with bony hypertrophy, lymphangiomas or varicosities; the genetics are not defined. A bilateral facial naevus does not mean bilateral cerebral involvement. Seizures are seen in up to 90 % of those involved. Abnormal venous return with blood stagnation and hypoxaemia coupled with a high metabolic demand of neurones exhibiting seizure activity often lead to a progressive functional problem. Neurological signs emerge, often starting as a post-ictal paresis contralateral to the cerebral involvement but at times consolidating into a permanent paresis as time goes on. Hemianopias, dysphasias, or quadriparesis may also occur. Where the seizures are intractable and infrequent there are very often associated learning difficulties.

Buphthalmos or glaucoma may accompany a choroidal angiomatous lesion and may be present at birth. Rarely hydrocephalus has been reported but intracranial haemorrhage is exceptionally rare.

In the presence of a facial naevus full radiological assessment of the brain should be carried out with serial CT scanning with contrast to define the extent of the angiomatous lesion. Magnetic resonance imaging offers an even more sensitive technique for this. Intracerebral angioma may become more obvious with the passing of time. Calcification of the lesion becomes prominent. This should be accompanied by a full electroencephalographic assessment of seizure activity.

Management involves regular assessment of ocular pressure. Seizure control is at times difficult to attain. Where the vascular anomalies and seizure discharge is confined to one hemisphere, an early surgical resection of the lesion may offer benefit where the seizures are intractable. The evidence shows that residual handicap is minimised when lobectomy or hemispherectomy is performed in the early weeks with many children surviving with little sign of a hemiparesis or hemianopia. However, exact criteria for this early intervention have yet to be laid down as there are some children in whom a seizure disorder presenting at an early stage stabilises.

Neuroradiology in the phakomatoses

In the phakomatoses, CT and MR scanning are the most useful diagnostic modalities for confirmation of the clinical diagnosis.

Neurofibromatosis

Plain skull films A defect in the posterior superior wall of the orbit is one of the characteristic skeletal features of neurofibromatosis. As a result, the sub-arachnoid space and/or temporal lobe can herniate into the posterior orbit where the constant pulsation of the brain and CSF may enlarge the orbit. Radiographic findings relate to the orbital defect and include hypoplasia of the greater wing of the sphenoid, elevation of the lesser wing of the sphenoid, downward tilting of the floor of the sella, enlargement of the middle cranial fossa and enlargement of the orbit. Hypoplasia of the ethmoid and maxillary sinuses may be detected on plain skull radiograph. An uncommon, but highly characteristic skull defect may be observed in the lambdoid suture, most probably representing a mesodermal defect of the periostium and this is associated with under development of the mastoid bone and air cells on the same side.

CT and MRI scanning Imaging of the brain may show macrocephaly and macrocranium and ventricular dilatation in 32 to 45 % of cases. MRI is more sensitive than CT in the detection of parenchymal changes and suspected intracranial hamartomas in neurofibromatosis. Multiple areas of increased signal on T2-weighted images in patients not exhibiting clinical neurological dysfunction have been demonstrated on MR. Common areas of involvement include the basal ganglia, posterior limb and genu of the internal capsule, external capsule, corpus callosum, thalami, cerebellar peduncle, and brain stem. The areas of increased signal are well demarcated from surrounding brain tissue and demonstrate a lack of mass effect or surrounding oedema. On T1-weighted images they appear isointense to grey matter. Such areas are differentiated from neoplastic involvement by the lack of mass effect, surrounding oedema and clinical manifestation.

Central nervous system neoplasms associated with neurofibromatosis include:
- Optic nerve glioma (the most common)
- Glioblastoma
- Cranial nerve tumours
- Hamartoma
- Meningioma
- Ependymoma
- Astrocytoma

These tumours may be detected on either CT or MRI scanning. Multiplanar MRI has improved the detection of these tumours and has also demonstrated the early and late changes of vasculitis.

Multiple intracranial tumours are not uncommon, particularly eighth nerve tumours and meningiomas. Meningiomas are commonly intraventricular and arise from the choroid of the lateral ventricles where they may be seen as heavily calcified masses on either plain films or CT scanning.

Tuberous sclerosis (including giant cell astrocytoma)

CT is the imaging modality of choice for the diagnosis. The typical CT appearances are:

1) Subependymal nodules which are usually calcified. There is no enhancement of the nodule after contrast administration. In addition to being situated close to the foramena of Monro, they are also sited along the lateral aspects of the lateral ventricles. Hydrocephalus may be present due to occlusion of the CSF pathways.

2) Parenchymal tubers have the same characteristics as subependymal nodules. They may be simulated by calcified arteriovenous malformations which will show contrast enhancement.

3) Intraventricular tumours have a slightly higher density than surrounding brain and will demonstrate contrast enhancement.

Skull radiographs may show characteristic intracerebral calcification and/or cranial vault sclerosis. The calcified subependymal nodules can be seen on CT from as early as two and a half months. The differential CT diagnosis of tuberous sclerosis includes intrauterine infection, Sturge–Weber syndrome, vascular malformation and cerebral heterotopia. Intra-uterine infections such as toxoplasmosis or cytomegalovirus disease frequently result in periventricular calcification. These post-infectious calcifications are usually smaller than the subependymal nodules of tuberous sclerosis and are associated with significant cerebral atrophy and microcephaly. Heterotopic foci are located along the medial ventricular wall and are isodense with brain, whereas the subependymal nodules of tuberous sclerosis are hyperdense and are located along the lateral ventricular wall.

Sturge-Weber syndrome

The hallmark of this abnormality on imaging is the presence of parallel lines (tram lines) of calcification which lie in the superficial layer of the cerebral cortex. These are readily detected on plain films although CT will show the calcification effectively and at an earlier age, and also demonstrates the underlying cortical atrophy that is commonly associated. The CT appearances are characteristic:

1) The gyriform pattern of calcification is well demonstrated. The distribution of the calcification may occasionally be bilateral. Enhancement may be demonstrated in the involved area and may represent the actual malformation or merely a permeability defect off the abnormal vessels.

2) Cortical atrophy is invariably present, either with an enlarged or diminished hemicranium.

Chapter 12: Hydrocephalus and Spina Bifida

James Leggate, W. St. Clair Forbes

Hydrocephalus

Hydrocephalus describes the presence of enlarged cerebral ventricles resulting from an imbalance in the rate of production and absorption of cerebrospinal fluid (CSF) (**12.1 and 12.2**). Traditionally, where the ventricles communicate with the subarachnoid space, the hydrocephalus is known as **communicating** and, where they do not, **non-communicating**. The terms communicating and obstructive may be misleading and have been superseded by the subdivision of hydrocephalus into:
• Intraventricular obstructive hydrocephalus
• Extraventricular obstructive hydrocephalus.

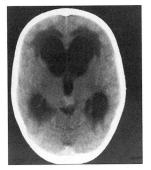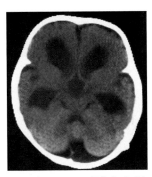

12.1 and 12.2 CT scans showing obstructive (**12.1, left**) and communicating (**12.2, right**) hydrocephalus. Note lesion on left at the level of the aqueduct with triventricular enlargement.

Incidence

The overall incidence of hydrocephalus without spina bifida varies between countries and ranges from 1.2 to 15 cases per 10,000 births. In the United Kingdom, the incidence of both hydrocephalus and spina bifida is decreasing.

Clinical signs

Recently, antenatal diagnosis and management of hydrocephalus has been possible with the use of ultrasound (**12.3 and 12.4**). The placement of ventriculo-amniotic shunts through the maternal uterine wall has been tried. The presence of other associated anomalies, as well as the practical difficulties of shunting at this stage, have led to disappointing results to date.

The signs and symptoms produced by hydrocephalus in children vary according to age. The cranial sutures remain patent up to the age of 15–18 months. This allows the expansion of intracranial contents without the rapid rise in intracranial pressure seen when the skull sutures have fused. Plotting head growth on head cir-

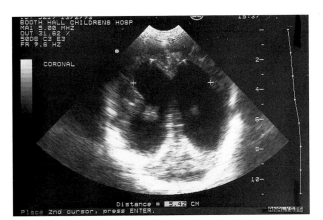

12.3 Ultrasound demonstrating enlargement of the ventricles with bifrontal ventricular horn diameter of 5.42 cms.

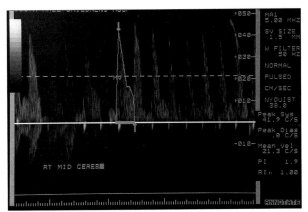

12.4 Ultrasound demonstrating flow pattern in left middle cerebral artery with resistance index of 1.22.

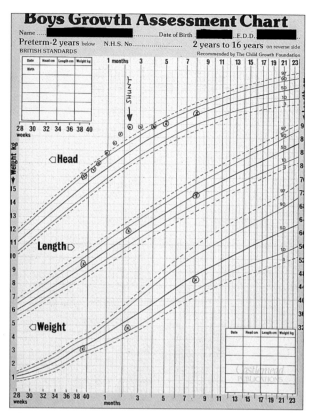

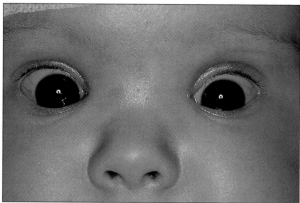

12.6 Paranaud's syndrome with failure of upgaze—'sun-setting'.

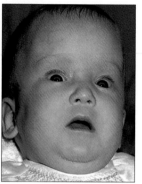

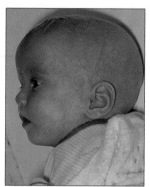

12.5 Chart to show head growth curves for children with third to 97 percentiles marked showing an example of a rapidly enlarging head crossing the centiles secondary to hydrocephalus.

12.7 and 12.8 Paranaud's syndrome in a child with hydrocephalus. Note prominent veins over forehead and lateral aspect of head.

cumference charts (**12.5**) provides early objective evidence of an excessive growth rate, where overt signs of raised intracranial pressure may be absent. In the first 12 months of life, a child's head should gain approximately 12 cms, the majority of this growth occurring within the first 6 months of life. It must be remembered that abnormally shaped heads, as seen in scaphocephaly, will have larger circumferences than normal but no underlying ventriculomegaly or hydrocephalus. The presence of a palpable anterior fontanelle is helpful in determining whether there is raised intracranial pressure. Changing the position of the head from a recumbent to a vertical posture should produce a flattening or dipping of the fontanelle, which is more overtly pulsatile in the normal child. A quantitive measurement can then be made by assessing the vertical distance from the ear to the clavicle when the fontanelle becomes flattened, giving an indication of intracranial pressure.

In hydrocephalus, the splaying of the sutures can be palpated and head percussion produces the so-called 'cracked pot' note. The raised intracranial pressure associated with hydrocephalus produces distension of the scalp veins which are particularly prominent in the fronto-temporal regions. In extreme cases of raised intracranial pressure, the distortion of the peri-aqueductal tissues

caused by the progressive ventricular enlargement leads to the development of 'sun-setting' (**12.6–12.8**). The child's eyes are fixed in a permanent downward gaze relative to the horizontal, with covering of the lower iris and exposure of the upper sclera. Fundoscopy may reveal papilloedema, but this is not common in infants. The presence of haemorrhages in the retina are more suggestive of subdural haematoma secondary to accidental or non-accidental head injury.

In young and premature babies, bradycardia and apneoa are signs of raised intracranial pressure, although not diagnostic. In older children, an exaggerated sinus arrythmia may be seen. When a large head is seen in association with delayed development, hydrocephalus should be excluded. It must be remembered that the commonest cause of a large head is to have a parent with a large head, and that some children with familial macroencephaly show dissociated motor development. In these children, all intracranial CSF spaces may be increased in size on the CT scan, at least for the first two or three years of life.

In the older child, the symptoms of hydrocephalus are related to how rapidly it develops. In the slowly progressive type, the clinical features are those of headache typically worse in the morning and often associated with nausea or vomiting, or a deterioration in school performance over a period of time and an alteration in gait and fine motor control often described by teachers, family and friends as increasing clumsiness. Fundoscopy may reveal pale discs secondary to optic atrophy, a long-term pressure effect, or frank papilloedema, depending on the underlying pathological cause. Other associated lower cranial nerve palsies, cerebellar signs and long-tract signs may be seen.

In acute hydrocephalus, the symptoms are those of a rapid onset of severe headache associated with vomiting. There may be signs of a third or sixth cranial nerve palsy with an eye movement disorder, papilloedema with haemorrhages; confusion with a deteriorating level of consciousness is not unusual in severe cases.

Investigations

Head circumference measurements still provide the most readily available information on developing hydrocephalus in the young baby. Skull x-rays may demonstrate suture widening, as well as the 'copper-beaten' appearance of the effect of raised intracranial pressure on the skull vault (*see* **12.43**).

Role of imaging

1. To establish the diagnosis of hydrocephalus.
2. To evaluate the cause.
3. To monitor the response following treatment.
4. The detection of complications following treatment.

Currently, ultrasound examination in the infant provides accurate and easily repeatable information on ventricular size. Changes in size or configuration of the supratentorial ventricular system are easily seen, and in certain cases, lesions within the posterior fossa may be identified on transfontanelle ultrasonography.

CT scanning is useful in all age groups for determiningventricular size as well as the possible sites of CSF obstruction. It is the only tool suitable for investigating a child in whom the sutures and fontanelles have closed. Where used as a sequential investigation to observe changes in size of the ventricular system, a limited CT scan without orbital slices can be obtained, thereby reducing the dose of ionising radiation given to the lenses of the eyes. The use of intravenous contrast material provides further information on structural lesions within and around the brain parenchyma.

Magnetic resonance (MR) scanning provides a non-invasive means of assessing ventricular size and configuration. The use of different scanning sequences enables the clinician to distinguish between fluid-filled structures containing CSF and others containing fluid with a high protein content, which might not be so clearly distinguished on CT scanning. The MR scan is capable of using multiplanar imaging techiniques and thereby enables anatomical variations to be defined more clearly. It is particularly useful in imaging the craniocervical junction, where CT scans are limited in their usefulness.

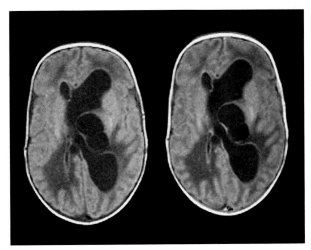

12.9 MR scan of intense ventriculitis secondary to infected shunt. Note the scan on the right is with Gadolinium DTPA enhancement but shows no increase in signal from the ependymal lining compared to the scan on the left. The ependymal lining is stripped away from the lateral wall of the left lateral ventricle, and can be mistaken for a tumour.

Furthermore, the presence of signal voids where flow is occurring enables the MR scan to be used for measurement of CSF flow, although this is not a practical clinical tool at present.

In certain cases, the use of intraventricular iodine-containing contrast medium can provide information on the communication of cystic lesions with the ventricular system. This means of invesigation is less widely used since other non-invasive techniques became available. Pneumoencephalography is almost never used. Angiography is used to investigate children with structural lesions such as tumours which may be causing an obstructive hydrocephalus, but this use is being largely superseded by MR scanning (**12.9**). The use of MR scanning with three-dimensional reconstruction may possibly replace invasive cerebral angiography even in the management of arteriovenous malformations.

Hydrodynamic investigations of CSF production require the placement of a catheter within the CSF space either within the ventricle itself, usually through a frontal burr hole (**12.10 and 12.11**), or in the subarachnoid space, usually via a lumbar puncture. In this way, the chemical composition of the CSF can be determined, the absolute pressure measured on a continuous or intermittent basis, and where continuous monitoring is carried out, the presence ofabnormal pressure waves can be clearly documented (**12.12 and 12.13**). The injection of isotope within the CSF space and its rate of clearance is still used from time to time to monitor cases where the diagnosis of hydrocephalus is in doubt.

CT findings in hydrocephalus

1. Early dilatation and rounding of the temporal horns is

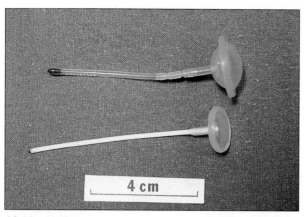

12.10 An Ommaya reservoir (top) and Rickman reservoir.

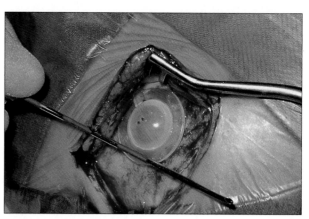

12.11 Insertion in right frontal region of CSF reservoir through a curivlinear incision.

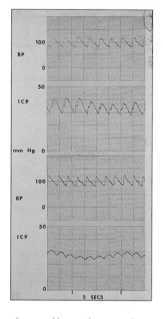

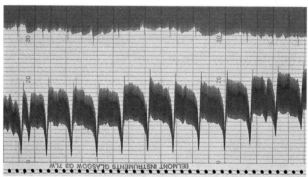

12.12 (left) Chart recording to demonstrate intracranial pressure and blood pressure measurement.

12.13 (right) 'A' waves demonstrated on ICP recording with pressure rises of greater than 50 mm of mercury for more than 5 minutes (see Chapter 7).

the earliest sign, and may be seen before obvious enlargement of the bodies of the lateral ventricles. The early dilatation of the temporal horns in hydrocephalus is readily differentiated from temporal horn dilatation occurring as a manifestation of temporal lobe atrophy, in which condition it is invariably associated with enlargement of the Sylvian fissures and other signs of temporal lobe atrophy.

2. Rounding and enlargement of the frontal horns with an acute angle formed by the medial walls of the dilated frontal horns, the septal angle. In atrophy, the frontal horns are enlarged but not ballooned and the angle is typically obtuse.

3. Enlargement and ballooning of the third ventricle.

4. Dilatation of the bodies of the lateral ventricles tends tobe greater than that occurring secondary to atrophy.

5. Enlargement of the fourth ventricle suggests extraventricular obstructive hydrocephalus.

6. Preservation or accentuation of grey/white matter differentiation.

7. Sulcal effacement, when present, is a diagnostic sign of hydrocephalus. It should be remembered, however, that the sulci may dilate when obstruction is at the level of the arachnoid granulations.

8. Periventricular oedema occurs mainly in the periventricular matter of the frontal horns in the acute and subacute phases of hydrocephalus. The presence of periventricular low densities on CT scanning is suggestive if not indicative of raised intracranial pressure: the transluminal spread of CSF through the ventricular ependymal lining indicates a reversal of CSF flow through the white matter to reach the CSF subarachnoid spaces as a potential route of absorption.

Neuroradiology and intraventricular obstructive hydrocephalus (IVOH)

Accurate classification of IVOH is possible, because the ventricles dilate proximally to but not distally to the obstruction (*see* **Table 12.1**).

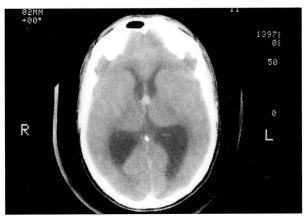

12.14 CT scan of colloid cyst.

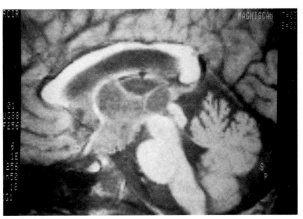

12.15 MR scan of posterior third ventricular tumour with occlusion of the origin of the aqueduct of Sylvius.

Obstruction can occur at a number of sites:

Lateral ventricles Congenital coarctation is a rare form of obstruction, occurring usually at the trigone or within the temporal horn. The narrowing may be a congenital maldevelopment or a consequence of intra-uterine ventriculitis with adhesion formation. Obstruction of the

TABLE 12.1 Hydrocephalus: Communicating, Non-Communicating

Clinical signs in infants

> Increased head size
> Bulging fontanelle
> Sun-setting
> Prominent scalp veins
> Apneoa\bradycardia

Clinical signs in older children

> Headaches
> Nausea\vomiting
> Papilloedema
> Occular motor signs
> Gait disturbance
> School performance deterioration
> Lower cranial nerve palsies

Investigations

> Skull x-ray
> Ultrasound
> CT scan
> MR scan

atrium by an intraventricular tumour produces enlargement of the temporal horn.

Foramen of Monro Obstruction of the foramen of Monro is rare (**12.14**). Obstruction of CSF flow between the lateral and third ventricles causes lateral ventricular enlargement and usually third and fourth ventricular contraction on CT. The foramen of Monro may be obstructed by an ependymoma, teratoma, adjacent glioma, a tuber, papilloma or meningioma. The foramen of Monro may be partially obstructed by extra-axial suprasellar masses and arachnoid cysts of the suprasellar cistern. Other causes are intraventricular haemorrhage and infection. Obstruction of one intraventricular foramen, where one ventricle enlarges to displace the midline structures to the opposite side, may be seen in some cases of tumour.

Third ventricle The commonest obstructive lesions are extrinsic to the third ventricle (**12.15**). These include craniopharyngioma and paraventricular glioma (thalamus, optic chiasma, hypothalamus), and mass lesions related to the posterior third ventricle (gliomas of the posterior hypothalamus and thalamus), tumours of the pineal region, arteriovenous malformations, aneurysms of the basilar artery and of the vein of Galen.

Aqueduct When CSF flow is obstructed at the aqueduct, the third and lateral ventricles enlarge, whereas the fourth usually shrinks. Aqueduct stenosis is the commonest cause of IVOH. The causes of obstruction are a congenital web or atresia, often in association with an Arnold–Chiari malformation or a tumour of the mesencephalon or pineal gland.

Congenital aqueduct stenosis more commonly occurs with the Chiari II malformation. Four main types of anomaly have been described:

1. Stenosis.
2. Forking—two main channels of greatly reduced dimension found side by side.

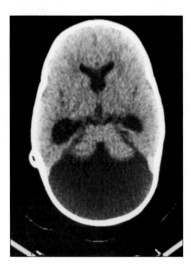

12.16 Dandy–Walker cyst with absence of the vermis. Note enlargement of the supra-tentorial ventricular system.

3. Septum formation.
4. Gliosis.

If the Arnold–Chiari type II malformation is present, the CT appearances of the malformation will be seen on the lower sections.

Once aqueductal stenosis is detected, benign congenital obstruction must be distinguished from that due to tumour. In these patients, magnetic resonance imaging, positive CT cisternography or possibly ventriculography combined with CT may be necessary to demonstrate the obstructing lesion.

MRI is also of value in assessing aqueductal patency, since it is able to identify flowing CSF (*see* above).

Fourth ventricle　Obstruction at the fourth ventricular level may be congenital (e.g. Dandy–Walker cyst) or acquired (**12.16**). Inflammation and scarring in the ependyma from haemorrhage or infection can cause acquired obstruction of the fourth ventriclar outlets. CT then shows the enlarged fourth, third and lateral ventricles, but without hypoplasia of the cerebellum. This condition may be difficult to differentiate on CT from extraventricular obstructive hydrocephalus, since the pattern of ventricular enlargement is the same in the two conditions. Many mass lesions can cause fourth ventricular obstruction, including extraventricular intra-axial neoplasms (astrocytoma, medulloblastoma, brainstem glioma), abscess, cerebellar oedema, and extra-axial masses such as arachnoid cysts, chordoma and subdural haematoma.

If both the aqueduct and fourth ventricular outlets areobstructed, as a complication of ventriculitis orintraventricular haemorrhage, the fourth ventricle may enlargeeven after the lateral ventricles are successfully shunted. This is referred to as an isolated or 'trapped' fourth ventricle.

Neuroradiology in extraventricular obstructive hydrocephalus (EVOH)

In EVOH, the block to CSF flow is distal to the ventricular system and occurs either at the skull base or at the arachnoid granulations. Formerly, the hydrocephalus was described as communicating hydrocephalus, that is, the ventricular system communicates with the extraventricular subarachnoid spaces. EVOH is a more accurate term. The aetiology is usually obliteration of the subarachnoid space or alteration of the arachnoid villi. In most cases, the CT diagnosis of EVOH is not difficult. CT shows symmetrical enlargement of the lateral, third and often fourth ventricles and effacement of the cortical sulci. There is, however, one area of potential diagnostic difficulty in children with bilateral subdural fluid collections who show enlarged cortical subarachnoid spaces and ventricles. With this exception, the demonstration of enlarged sulci and ventricles usually excludesthe diagnosis of hydrocephalus. The differentiation of cerebral atrophy from hydrocephalus and bilateral hygromas in children requires clinical information. A small head and a low-tension fontanelle support the diagnosis of atrophy, whilst an enlarging head and bulging fontanelle will suggest the diagnosis of a subdural haematoma.

Causes of EVOH　The CT scan may show evidence of meningeal enhancement in meningitis or carcinomatosis, subarachnoid haemorrhage, evidence of trauma, or the classical defect in the enhanced straight or sagittal sinus in cases of sagittal sinus thrombosis. The deformed cranial vault in craniosynostosis, Hurler's syndrome or achondroplasia is readily detected. However, in the majority of patients with hydrocepalus, CT provides no specific clues to the diagnosis.

Neuroradiology and the Dandy–Walker syndrome and Chiari malformation

The Dandy–Walker syndrome is characterised by a cystic dilatation of the fourth ventricle, hypoplastic cerebellar hemispheres and absent vermis. Hydrocephalus is frequently associated with these features, and other associated malformations which may be present include agenesis of the corpus callosum, gyral anomalies and heterotopias, holoprosencephaly and encephalocoeles. The main imaging characteristic of a Dandy–Walker cyst is a large CSF-containing cyst occupying most of the posterior fossa. The fourth ventricle is not visualised. Tentorial malposition is present, recognised by the inverted malpositioned tentorial bands which bulge outwards and straightening of the normally concave tentorial borders. This appearance suggests the presence of the Dandy –Walker syndrome even when there is no ventricular dilatation. The differential diagnosis of the Dandy –Walker syndrome imaging includes:

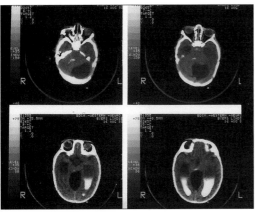

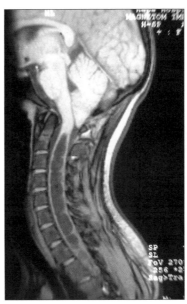

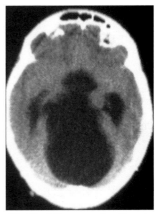

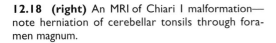

12.17 (above) Arachnoid cyst of supra-cerebellar region. Intrathecal contrast has collected in posterior aspect of third–fourth ventricles.

12.18 (right) An MRI of Chiari I malformation—note herniation of cerebellar tonsils through foramen magnum.

12.19 CT scan of a Dandy–Walker cyst

1. Mega cisterna magna.

2. Trapped fourth ventricule due to occlusion of the aqueduct of Sylvius and the foramena of Luschka and Magendie.

3. A retrocerebellar arachnoid cyst (**12.17**).

The Chiari I malformation consists of inferior displacement of the cerebellar tonsils and cerebellum without a displacement of the fourth ventricle or medulla. This is readily visualised in the sagittal plane on MR or on CT myelography (**12.18 and 12.19**). The Chiari II malformation (Arnold–Chiari malformation) is the commonest type seen in neonates and infants. It consists of a protrusion of the lower part of the cerebellum which is accompanied by elongation of the fourth venticle, extending into the spinal canal. There is an associated meningomyelocoele. The CT appearance of this malformation may be divided into three groups:

1. Abnormalities of the bone and dura. The skeletal anomalies are due to dysplasia of the membranous skull bones and include craniolacunae, scolloping of the petrous bone and clivus, enlargement of the foramen magnum (best seen on coronal and sagittal sections), partial absence and/or fenestration of the falx and hypoplasia of the tentorium. Hypoplasia of the falx and tentorium are best visualised on contrast-enhanced axial and coronal CT scans respectively.

2. Abnormalities of mid-brain and cerebellum including elevation of the cerebellum superiorally through the wide incisura resulting in the formation of a heart-shaped mass referred to as a cerebellar pseudo-tumour.

3. Abnormalities of the ventricles and cisterns include elongation of the fourth ventricle which on sagittal MR is shown to be flattened and extending into the cervial canal. The third ventricle is usually mildly dilated in the Chiari II malformation. The massa inter-media is unusually large, with the third ventricle thereby appearing small in comparison with the lateral ventricle. The lateral ventricles are dilated in most cases of Chiari II malformations. Thinning of the cortical mantle over the occipital lobes and vertex is readily recognised on imaging. In 40 % of cases, the septum pellucidum is absent and is best seen on axial and coronal sections. The subarachnoid basal cisterns are poorly visualised and the interhemispheric fissure may be either obliterated in cases of ventricular dilatation, or widely patent and increased in width in patients with large head circumference.

Neuroradiology in untreated hydrocephalus

The white matter is affected more than grey matter by the extent of hydrocephalus, as the latter is to some extent protected by its glial structure. The periventricular white matter becomes infiltrated with extracellular oedema fluid, which is most marked in the immediate periventricular region.

This extracellular periventricular oedema represents transependymal flow of CSF or ventricular CSF extravasation.

Periventricular oedema is recognised on CT as blurring or loss of the normally sharp ventricular margins where the ventricles lie against the white matter. The blurring is usually most severe near the superolateral angles of the frontal horns, but may also be seen along the other portions of the ventricles that are adjacent to the white matter. The ventricular margins adjacent to the grey matter of the caudate nucleus are relatively spared until very late. Clinically, periventricular oedema is associated with acute and subacute hydrocephalus with high intraventricular pressures and impaired levels of

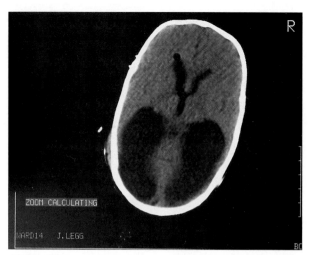

12.20 CT scan demonstrating preferential ventriculo-megally in a child with hydrocephalus affecting the occipital horns,. Note the normal-sized frontal horns.

consciousness, rather than with normal pressure hydrocephalus or chronic, relatively compensated hydrocephalus, as seen in aqueduct stenosis.

The ventricular dilatation is determined, in part, by the distensibility of the brain, dura, and calvarium that surround and support the ventricle.

The atria and occipital horns are often disproportionally dilated when compared to the frontal horns (**12.20**). This has been attributed to the varying effects of hydrocephalus on grey and white matter and the variable distensiblity of the vertex and skull base. The relative rigidity of the skull base restrains expansion of the frontal horns, whereas the vertex is distensible, which permits dilatation of the atria and occipital horns. Progressive thinning of the cerebral mantle occurs with increasing ventricular dilatation. This change is attributed to stretching of axon fibres and sheaths passing around the dilated ventricles.

Attenuation of the ependyma and cerebral mantle by hydrocephalus may lead to focal dehiscence of the ventricular wall with formation of unilateral or bilateral pulsion diverticula of the ventricular wall.

Neuroradiology in treated hydrocephalus

Successful intraventricular shunt therapy leads to a numberof changes on the brain parenchyma which can be recognised on CT.

1. Periventricular oedema regresses significantly or even disappears in the first few weeks after shunting.

2. The decrease in ventricular size after shunting is often assymetrical, the shunt-containing ventricle being smaller. Shunt-induced haemorrhage with fibrosis may contribute to the inequality in ventricular size and may not permit symmetrical ventricular enlargement with shunt malformation.

3. The reduction in size of the frontal horns is often greater than that of the atria and occipital horns, as the grey matter rapidly returns to normal compared with the more severely-damaged white matter. Shunting therefore often increases the disparity in size between the frontal horns and atria.

4. The cerebral mantle may increase in thickness after shunting in early hydrocephalus.

5. The thalami move superomedially. The corpus callosum folds downwards. These changes result in small ventricles with sharpened lateral angles and an acute callosal angle, which is the angle subtended by lines drawn along the roofs of the lateral ventricle in the coronal plane.

6. The lateral ventricles may become nearly invisible. In such instances, there is absence of cortical sulci and formation of a diamond-shaped CSF space at the apex of the incisura, composed of the dilated confluent superior vermian and velum interpositum cisterns. Patients with meningomyelocele and Chiari II malformation frequently exhibit upward transincisural growth of the so-called cerebellar pseudotumour.

7. Fissures and sulci may appear to be widened, with focal or diffuse invagination of the cortical surfaces. The interhemispheric fissures widen just above the corpus callosum.

Treatment

The rationale of treatment of hydrocephalus is based on the supposition that a cortical mantle of a certain minimum thickness is necessary to optimise the intellectual and physical development of a growing infant. Whilst sporadic cases of extreme ventriculo-megally in children with high IQs have been described, such anecdotes do not negate the rationale of treating repeated pressure fluctuations which necessarily lead to local ischaemic change.

Early treatment consisted of the application of tight-bandages around the head which led to raised intracranial pressure and abnormally shaped heads with vertical elongation. Currently, the management may be by surgical or medical means. There has been no good evaluation of the relative merits of different medical methods of treatment by controlled trials. Repeated lumbar puncture, and diuretic therapy using frusemide, acetazolamide (Diamox) or osmotic agents, have all been tried. Diuretics reduce CSF production and may prove successful in the management of children where overabsorption of CSF is only moderately outstripped by the production rates. They are, however, rarely effective as a sole method of treatment but can act as a temporising measure. Osmotic diuretics may have profound side effects in young children.

Choroid plexectomy was first used to treat hydrocephalus in 1918, though we now know the choroid plexus is responsible for only 50 % of CSF production and this procedure is no longer practised. The use of bypassing procedures, draining CSF from within the ventricle to a site distal to the obstruction has been well

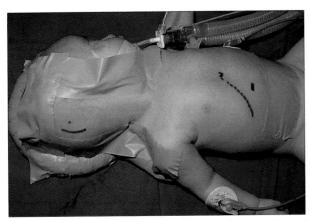

12.21 Operative slide to show technique for insertion of ventricular peritoneal shunt. Note positioning of patient with support under shoulder.

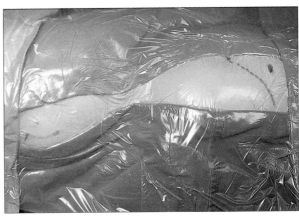

12.22 The patient is positioned and the skin prepared and draped.

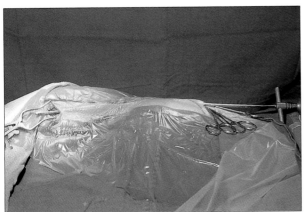

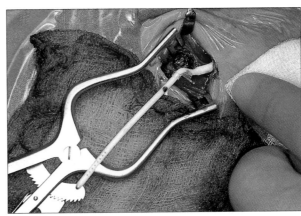

12.23 and 12.24 Incisions are made over the posterior parietal and right hypochondrial regions (**12.23, left**) and connected via a single subcutaneous passage without intervening skin incisions (**12.24, right**).

recognised since the time of Hippocrates. Various sites in the body have been used, but it was the development in the mid-50's of a non-returnable pressure-controlled valve which revolutionised the success rate of the diversionary procedures. The catheter within the ventricle is connected to a one-way flow pressure-controlled valve connected to a distal catheter. The distal catheter is usually sited in the peritoneal cavity or, where inappropriate, the right atrium (**12.21–12.24**). In rare cases, a ventriculo-pleural shunt can be used, but only as a temporising procedure. Flow-controlled and more sophisticated variable pressure-controlled valves are now available.

Complications

The major complications in the treatment of hydrocephalus with shunts inserted are infection, mechanical failure, wrong placement, overdrainage, seizures and other complications peculiar to each particular catheter (**12.25–12.30**). Infection is essentially a surgical techni-cal problem. The rate of infection varies from 0.14 % to 30 % in current published series, with an average rate of 5–7 % infection rate in most paediatric neurosurgical units. The typical infecting organism is *Staphylococcus epidermis*, and treatment of such infection requires removal of the infected shunt system and the administration of intravenous and intrathecal antibiotics, with the maintenance of external CSF drainage whilst the shunt system has been removed. Once the cell count within the CSF demonstrates resolution of the infection, a new internalised shunt system is inserted and the external CSF drainage discontinued.

A particular complication of ventricular atrial shunts is related to microemboli affecting the kidneys, causing a shunt nephritis. This produces changes within the renal structure which on removal of the infected shunt are usually reversible.

Mechanical failure is usually due to separation of the proximal catheter from the valve which is less common now that unitised systems are used, or by blockage of the

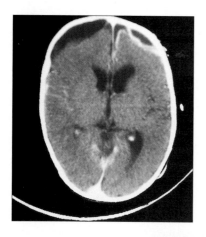

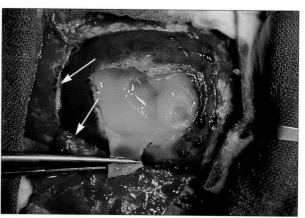

12.25 and 12.26 Complication with subdural drain placement with subdural empyaema. Note enhancing meninges (**12.25, left**). Operative photograph (**12.26, right**) to show thick pus lying enclosed in a membrane which is held between the forcep. The dural edge is marked with solid white arrows.

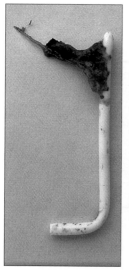

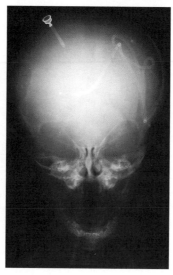

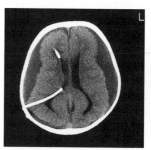

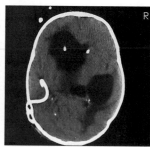

12.29 Subdural collections following VP shunt insertion; treated by exchange for higher pressure system.

12.30 Shunt complication withinsertion of ventricular catheter into left temporal lobe.

12.27 Shunt complications: mechanical obstruction due to blockage by choroid plexus.

12.28 Shunt complication with migration of entire VP shunt inside the ventricle.

ventricular catheter with choroid plexus. The placement of the ventricularcatheter may have some effect on the likelihood of mechanicalblockage. Although there is no general agreement on where tosite the ventricular catheter, traditionally it has been placed beyond the foramen of Monro. Malplacement of the ventricular catheter within a peripheral CSF space or the brain parenchyma itself is often seen to cause shunt malfunction. Peritoneal catheters may be malplaced within the lesser sac or the rectus sheath; perforation of a viscus by a reinforced peritoneal tube has been reported. In some cases, failure to fix the catheter system adequately has led to migration of the whole shunt eitherwithin the head, or within the peritoneal cavity.

Over-drainage remains a major problem, seen in pressure-controlled valve systems occurring in approximately 2 % of cases. It is typically seen in older ambulant children who have adopted a vertical position and is thought to be due to a syphoning effect. This can be overcome by the insertion of an antisyphon device or by the use of more modern flow-control valve systems.

Neuroradiology and intracranial complications of shunts

The shunt system consists of a proximal ventricular catheter that extends from the lateral ventricle through a burr hole and a distal portion that continues into the superior vena cava, pleural or peritoneal cavities. As children with hydrocephalus frequently have a fenestrated or absent septum pellucidum, it isnot unusual to see the shunt catheter across the midline into the opposite lateral ventricle. Multiple intraventricular shunts may lead to ventricular loculation.

Shunt malformation is not infrequent and is recognised by:

1. Renewed separation and bulging of sutures and fontanelles in children.
2. Renewed periventricular oedema.
3. Fullness of ventricular contours.
4. Increasing size of the ventricular system.

Spina bifida

Spina bifida results from failure of closure of the neural tube or overlying mesodermal tissue or skin (*see*

12.31 (left) Spina bifida opperta at the lumbar-sacral level.

12.32 (right) Spina bifida occulta with hairy patch.

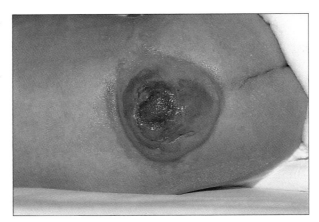

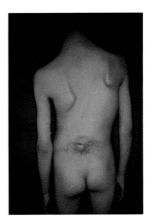

Chapter 10). It may be either open or closed, and is referred to as either spina bifida opperta or spina bifida occulta (**12.31 and 12.32**).

At about day 16 of embryonic life, a cord of cells develops: the neural plate, called the notochordal process. Initially solid, the extension of the primitive pit at Henson's node burrows into the solid notochordal process, forming a cylinder of cells surrounding the notochordal canal. This cord of cells fuses with the endoderm ventrally, and this fusion allows the notochordal plate to open into the yoke sac (see **11.2**, Chapter 11). This process is called intercalation of the notochord into the endoderm, but subsequently from the cranial end of the embryo the notochordal plate reforms a canal separating again the notochord from the endoderm. This process is called excalation of the notochord.

At this stage, the notochord induces the overlying ectoderm to form a neural plate from which the CNS develops. At day 22, of embryonic life, the neural groove deepens in the neural plate and this plate of cells folds over to meet in the midline and form aneural tube. This first fuses from the optic plate to the level of the 12th somite and subsequently continues to fuse cranially and caudally in pace with the developing embryo. This process is completed cranially at the anterior neuropore which is at thel evel of the future lamina terminalis, the anterior aspect of the third ventricle. Caudally, the neural tube closes at the level of the posterior neuropore which is approximately at the L1/2 level. Distal cord and cauda equina development occurs by a process called canalisation of the tail bud by connection of vacuoles in the caudal cell mass, coalescing and joining with the neural tube. The closure of the neural tube draws in cutaneous ectoderm on either side to form the overlying skin structures to the spinal canal. Coalescence of masses of mesoderm forms the bony elements and lateral spinal masses. The failure of intercalation and excalation of the notochord is the probable explanation for occult spina bifida, diastematomyelia, neurenteric cysts and combined anterior and posterior spina bifida, whilst mal development of the neural tube gives rise to the more severe forms of open spinal disraphism.

The failure of closure of the neural tube leads to fail-

ure of closure of the overlying ectodermal structure, and in this respect, the baby presents with an open lesion where the underlying neural placode is exposed to the exterior, with CSF draining through the central canal. The dura is deficient and fuses laterally to the paraspinal muscle fascia and the skin at the margins of the defect. The pedicles of the vertebral bodies are splayed open and the laminae are hypoplastic. The neurological deficit depends on the level of spinal canal affected. The various subgroups of spina bifida opperta include:

1. Myeloschisis where the neural tube is totally open.

2. Myelomeningocele where the central canal has been partially formed and opens onto the neural placode.

3. Meningocele where the neural structures have developed normally and there is merely an outpouching of the meninges.

Associated features of spina bifida opperta include the Arnold Chiari malformation which occurs in 90 % of all children with spina bifida opperta. In this anomaly, the cerebellar vermis and tonsils together with the fourth ventricle are displaced caudally together with the cervico-medullary junction. The normal ponto-medullary angle is kinked, and there may be developments of hydrocephalus and hydromyelia with or without a syrinx.

Spina bifida opperta occurs in approximately 1/1000 live births, but this incidence varies from country to country and is as high as 4 to 5/1000 live births in some parts of Ireland. Notwithstanding the effect of antenatal diagnosis and termination of pregnancy, the true incidence of spina bifida opperta appears to be declining in most areas, other than in third world countries. This decline in incidence may well reflect a general improvement in standards of nutrition. The Medical Research Council intervention study showed that supplementary folic acid can significantly reduce the risk of recurrence of a neural tube defect in women with a previously affected baby.

The recommendations of the Department of Health's Expert Advisory Group is that a first occurrence of a neural tube defect might be prevented by all women taking extra folate prior to conception and for the first 12 weeks of pregnancy as a daily medicinal or food supple-

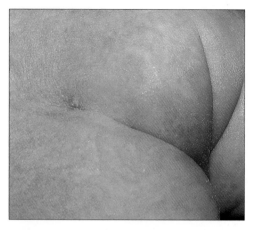

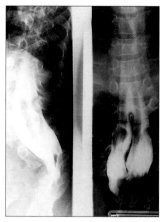

12. 33 (left) Dermal sinus.

12.34–12.36 (right and below, left and right) Diastematomyelia with diplomyelia. Note bony centre of dural sac on operative slide.

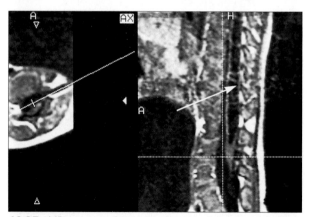

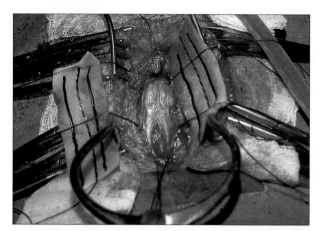

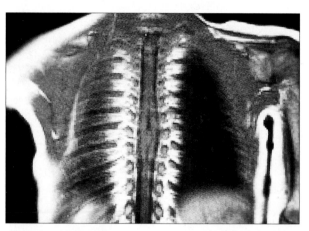

12.37 MR scan to show anterior sacral meningocele with communication through the left lateral aspect of the spinal column (see dotted line aand reconstructed image). NB: there is an associated extensive syrinx of the cord (see arrow).

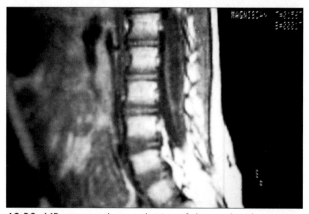

12.38 MR scan to show tethering of the cord with associated lipoma.

ment. To prevent a recurrence, 5 mg of folic acid should be taken for the same period. A number of departments of clinical genetics have now set up a register and counselling service for families who already have an affected child. This is of value not only in reducing recurrence risk but also in addressing the attendant health education and psychological issues.

Spina bifida occulta

Maldevelopment of the notochord is the origin of spina bifida occulta. Manifestations include congenital dermal sinus, diastematomyelia, neuroenteric cysts, tethered cord, lumbosacrallipoma and lipomyelomeningocele, and combined anterior and posterior spina bifida (**12.33–12.38**).

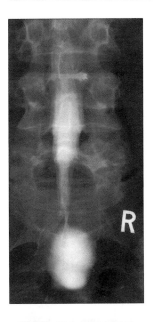

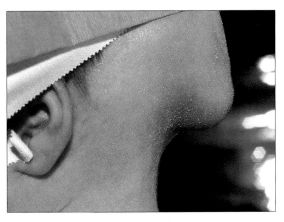

12. 39 (left) X-ray to show intrasacral meningocele.

12.40–12.42 (above, right and below, left) Occipital encephalocele showing intraoperative findings.

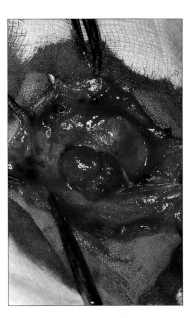

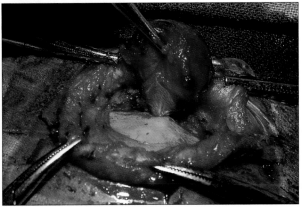

12.40 Occipital encephalocoele showing intraoperative findings.

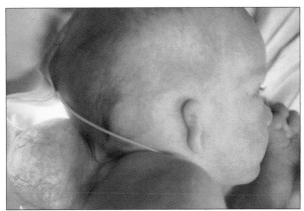

12.43 Occipital encephalocele containing no solid matter.

Clinical features

In spina bifida opperta, the lesion is obvious and the extent of the neurological deficit depends upon the level of the spine involved and the degree of maldevelopment that has occurred. Clearly in the case of a meningocele, neurological function is intact, and surgical repair is directed at restoring full coverage of the neural structures together with a water-tight enclosure of the CNS (**12.39–12.42**). Replacement of skin cover can usually be achieved by undermining laterally the intact skin margins and attempting a primary closure. With the more severe myelomeningoceles, resection of the neural placode together with attempts at reformation of a neural tube with a central canal by involution of the neural placode has been tried. The attempt to reform a normal appearance from abnormally developed structures may result in worsening of the neurological deficit (**12.43**).

The aim remains to achieve a water-tight closure of the central canal with skin cover of the defect without worsening of the neurological deficit. Once a water-tight closure has been achieved, the development of hydrocephalus is found in approximately 75 % of cases of myelomeningocele, while spina bifida occulta occurs in up to 30 % of the population *in some series* (**12.44 and 12.45**).

Typically, over 75 % of myelomeningocele andmeningocoeles will be found at the thoraco-lumbar and sacral region, with only 10 % in the thoracic area and 5 % at the cervical region. The clinical features will depend to a large extent upon the neurological deficit. In addition to the Arnold–Chiari malformation and hydrocephalus, the loss of neurological function in the limb girdle and lower limb muscles will lead to the development of kyphoscoliosis, dislocation of the hips, and club feet. Furthermore, the involvement of the sacral roots gives rise to bladder

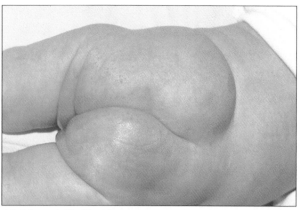

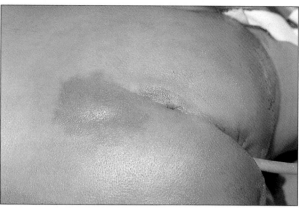

12.44 and 12.45 Myelocystocele.: first example (**12.44, left**) showing severe distortion of natal cleft and asymmetric folds in the left thigh and buttocks; the second example (**12.45, right**) shows a myelocystocele associated with a dermal sinus.

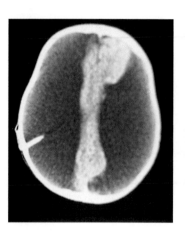

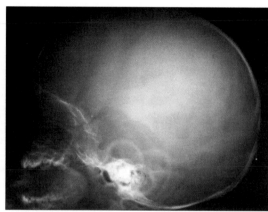

12.46 (left) Holoprosencephaly with shunt placement for cosmetic care (*see* Chapter 11).

12.47 (right) Lateral skull x-ray to show widening of the sutures associated with raised intracranial pressure.

dysfunction, which in the past was a major cause of morbidity and mortality, as ascending urinary tract infections led to renal failure.

Neuroradiology and spinal dysraphism

Imaging techniques Plain radiography is highly sensitive and demonstrates the osseous defects, scoliosis and bony spurs which accompany dysraphism. Normal radiographs do not exclude a significant dysraphic cord abnormality. CT myelography has been replaced by MRI, which has greater sensitivity for demonstrating neural tissue. The multiplanar capability allows complete delineation of the dysraphic abnormality. Both CT and MRI have the capability of displaying the full extent of any extradural component. MRI has the additional advantage of detecting any intramedullary abnormality such as a cavity or myelomalacia.

Treatment

Initially, the aim is to restore cover to the overlying skin defect after repair of the central canal and attempted reformation of the neural tube. A full pre-operative neurological examination will give an indication of the likely level of function to be expected from the child, but worsening of neurological function immediately post-operatively is not unusual. The presence of a defect involving D12 and L1 has a major impact because of the embryology of the developing nervous system on cauda equina function and hence the likely outcome in terms of neuronal function within the lower limb.

After closure of the defect, the management involves a multidisciplinary team: a urologist for the assessment of renal and bladder function, an orthopaedic surgeon, and physio- and occupational therapists for the treatment of the limb and muscle complications secondary to neural damage. The need for shunting becomes apparent with increasing head size, and signs and symptoms of raised intracranial pressure. Shunting is usually carried out within a week of closure of the defect in those children who will develop hydrocephalus (**12.44–12.47**).

The treatment of spina bifida occulta will depend upon the defect noted. Clearly, the presence of a pit in the midline low down over the sacrum may be a manifestation of spina bifida occulta. The investigations carried out here would usually include plain x-rays, and/or ultrasound examination of the underlying spine, but in the absence of neurological deficit would not require any further management. The controversies currently surrounding the management of the tethered cord have still to be resolved. Many authors suggest early intervention for the release of the tethered cord even in the absence of a neurological deficit, on the basis of prevention is better than cure. The long-term results of this intervention have yet to be evaluated. Clearly, there is a good argument for non-intervention in the absence of either pain or progressive neurological deficit. Where a punctum exists or where a subcutaneous fatty lump is present in the presence of a midline pit, then investigation including MR scanning or CT myelography is mandatory to determine whether there is connection between the skin and the spinal canal, and in such circumstances whether a dermoid cyst is present. The discharge of matter from a punctum or leakage of clear fluid is a mandatory indication for urgent investigation.

Chapter 13: Inborn Errors of Metabolism

Ed Wraith

Introduction

The inborn errors of metabolism are a family of genetic disorders in which an enzyme deficiency usually results in the accumulation of a 'toxic' intermediary compound. In addition, for certain disorders, an essential end product is not produced in adequate amounts (**13.1**). Any one or multiple organs may be compromised in an affected individual, but the brain and nervous system seem particularly vulnerable to metabolic insult. Rapid diagnosis depends on sending the appropriate samples to a laboratory experienced in the interpretation of metabolic investigations. For most disorders, prenatal diagnosis is possible, emphasising the importance of establishing an accurate diagnosis in affected infants.

This chapter concentrates on disorders which have the potential to cause profound neurological damage in the untreated child.

Disorders of amino acid metabolism

Phenylketonuria

Classical phenylketonuria due to phenylalaninine hydroxylase deficiency is the most common amino acid disorder in Caucasians, with an incidence of 1:10,000 in the UK (**13.2**). The excellent response to a low phenylalanine diet has led to the introduction of successful neonatal screening programmes in most developed countries (**13.3**).

The enzyme deficiency leads to persistent hyperphenylalaninaemia (plasma levels: >1200 μmol/l; normal 60–90 μmol/l) as well as disturbances of tyrosine and tryptophan metabolism and impairment of catecholamine, melanin and serotonin production. If untreated, the disorder leads to severe learning difficulties (IQ <50) and epilepsy in most patients. The exact cause of these abnormalties is unknown, but it is likely that the amino acid imbalance leads to a disturbance in myelin and neurotransmitter production (**13.4 and 13.5**). In addition, hair and eye pigmentation is abnormally pale, and the skin is prone to eczematous change.

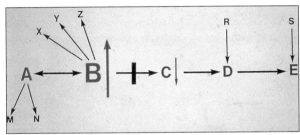

13.1 Inborn errors of metabolism; principles simplified. An enzyme block prevents substrates A and B from being converted to products C and D. The substrate which may be toxic accumulates, an essential end product may be deficient. The metabolic block may be limited to a subcellular organelle, for example, abnormal storage in lysosomes. Alternative pathways (X and Y) may be utilised; the metabolites may be useful in diagnosis.

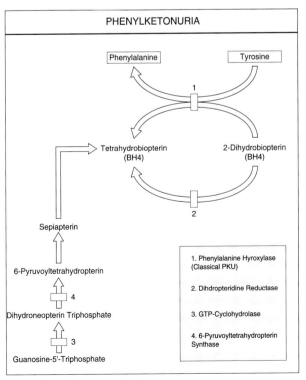

13.2 Phenylalanine metabolism.

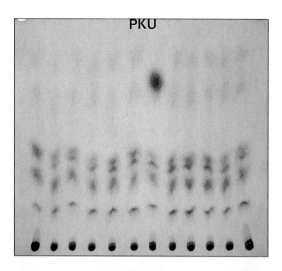

PKU

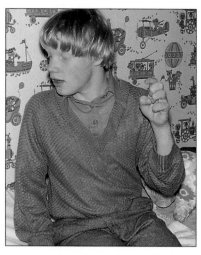

13.3 (left) A dense spot of phenylalanine in a newborn screening sample.

13.4 (right) Phenylketonuria: an untreated child with microcephaly, behaviour disorder and epilepsy. Note fair hair and blue eyes.

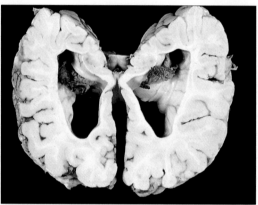

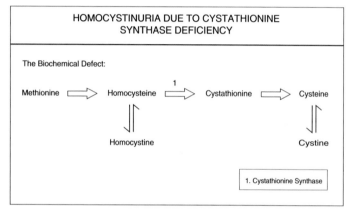

13.5 The brain in untreated phenylketonuria: cerebral atrophy with abnormal myelin.

13.6 Homocystinuria: methionine metabolism.

A strict, low-phenylalanine diet, started early in life, prevents these complications. The length of dietary treatment is controversial, but the recent reports suggesting that outcome is not ideal, plus the occurrence of neurological abnormalities in adult patients no longer subject to dietary treatment, have led to a positive move towards a 'diet for life' policy in many clinics. The success of dietary treatment has led to many healthy females with phenylketonuria reaching chid-bearing age. High levels of phenylalanine are teratogenic and lead to microcephaly, learning disability, congenital heart disease and other malformations. To avoid these complications, females with phenylketonuria considering pregnancy should return to strict dietary control before conception and maintain tight control of phenylalanine levels throughout the period of gestation.

In addition to classical phenylketonuria, there are a number of variants resulting from an abnormality in the synthesis or regeneration of biopterin cofactors. These cofactors are essential not only in the metabolism of phenylalanine, but also in the synthesis of neurotransmitters. These disorders have been labelled 'malignant' phenylketonuria as mental deterioration is not prevented by a low-phenylalanine diet alone and treatment must

include neurotransmitter precursor therapy if severe neurological handicap is to be avoided.

Homocystinuria

This disorder is due to an abnormality of methionine metabolism secondary to a deficiency of the enzyme cystathionine synthase (**13.6**). It has an incidence of approximately 1:100,000 in the UK, although it is more common in Ireland (1:50,000). The resulting accumulation of homocystine interferes with cross-linkage in both collagen and elastic fibres, impairing their natural strength. The clinical disorder is very similar to that of Marfan's syndrome, but the brain is also affected, leading to severe learning disabilities and seizures. Patients are tall with arachnodactyly and develop lens dislocation (**13.7 and 13.8**). In addition, osteoporosis leads to kyphoscoliosis and genu valgum. The cardiovascular system is also involved, with premature arterio-venous thrombosis leading to early death from myocardial disease (**13.9**). In 50 % of the patients, large doses of vitamin B6 (pyridoxine), a cofactor for normal cystathionine synthase activity, produces a marked biochemical improvement. These patients are termed 'pyridoxine-responsive' and require no additional therapy. Patients

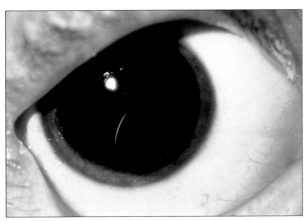

13.7 Homocystinuria: lens dislocation.

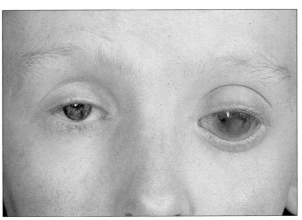

13.8 Homocystinuria: lens dislocation leading to acute glaucoma.

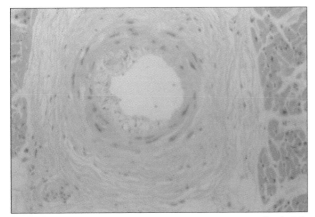

13.9 Homocystinuria: coronary artery narrowing; death followed, age 21, with pulmonary embolism.

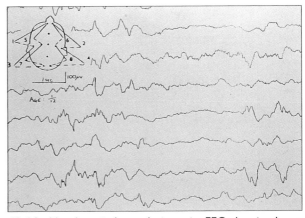

13.10 Non-ketotic hyperglycinaemia: EEG showing burst suppression.

who fail to respond to pyridoxine require a life-long low-methionine diet.

Early detection and treatment produce excellent results if compliance is maintained. Treatment of patients already affected is less rewarding, though there is some evidence that dietary treatment at this stage prevents further deterioration of the ocular and possibly thromboembolic complications.

Non-ketotic hyperglycinaemia

Although this disorder is very rare, it deserves mention as it produces a characteristic, devastating neurological illness in the newborn period. In affected patients, the molecular defect is in the glycine cleavage system which results in a massive accumulation of glycine in body fluids, particularly the CSF. Clinically, the infants present very soon after birth (often in the first hour or so of life) with a life-threatening illness which rapidly leads to apnoea and coma. The infant appears unresponsive and flaccid, and, unless supported by mechanical ventilation, death follows promptly. Most infants die during this acute presentation. Survivors develop intractable myoclonic seizures and hiccups, and make no intellectu-

al progress. The EEG characteristically reveals a burst suppression pattern (**13.10**), although hypsarrhythmia has also been reported. Neuroradiology often reveals agenesis of the corpus callosum and other anatomical defects, highlighting the potential for biochemical abnormalities to cause errors in brain development (**13.11**).

Diagnosis is established by finding a grossly elevated CSF glycine. There is no effective treatment.

Other amino acid disorders

There are a number of other rare abnormalities of amino acid metabolism in which learning disabilities may be a presenting feature. These disorders are too rare to consider in detail, but highlight the importance of requesting urine and plasma amino acid analysis in all children with unexplained learning disabilities.

Organic acidaemias

These disorders (**13.12**) are characterised by the accumulation in the plasma and excretion in the urine of low molecular weight, water soluble, carboxylic acid metabolites of amino acids, carbohydrates or fats.

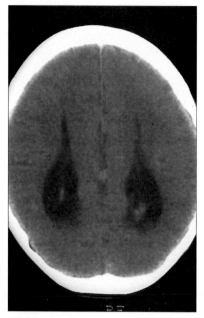

13.11 Non-ketotic hyperglycinaemia: agenesis of the corpus callosum with widely spaced ventricles and dilated posterior horns.

THE BIOCHEMICAL DEFECTS LEADING TO
A NUMBER OF ORGANIC ACIDYRIAS

Branched Chain Amino Acids

1-leucine	Isoleucine	Valine
2-Oxo-Isocaproate	2-Oxo-3-methyl-n-valerate	2-Oxoisovalerate
Isovaleryl-CoA	2-methylbutyryl-CoA	Isobutyryl-CoA
Isovaleric acidaemia		
3-methylcrotonyl-CoA	Tiglyl-CoA	Methylacrylyl-CoA
3-methylcrotonyl CoA carbox. def.		
3-methylglutaconyl-CoA	2-methyl-3-(OH)butyryl-CoA	3-(OH)isobutyryl-CoA
3-methylglutaconyl acidaemia		
3-(OH)-3-methylglutaryl-CoA	2-methylacetoacetyl-CoA	3-(OH)isobutyrate
HMG CoA lyase def.	*b-ketothiolase def.*	
Acetacetic acid	Acetyl-CoA	Methylmalonyl semialdehye

Propionyl-CoA

Propionic acidaemia

Methylmalonyl-CoA

Methylmalonic acidaemia

Succinyl-CoA

13.12 The biochemistry of the common organic acid disorders.

Increasing diagnostic sophistication has led to the recognition of many new conditions in recent years. Clinical presentation can be very variable. In the neonatal period, the infant may present with an encephalopathic illness with associated metabolic acidosis and ketosis. Other infants who avoid or survive the acute neonatal presentation may present with unexplained learning disability often associated with feeding difficulties, recurrent vomiting and failure to thrive. Occasionally, such infants will present with encephalopathy after a minor catabolic stress such as intercurrent infection (which may be trivial), fasting or surgery. Examples of conditions presenting either in the newborn period or later with encephalopathy include methylmalonic acidaemia, propionic acidaemia, maple syrup urine disease or isovaleric acidaemia. The key to the diagnosis of affected infants is a high index of suspicion on the part of the clinician. Formal clinical examination rarely leads to a diagnosis as the clinical signs are mimicked by a large number of

commoner childhood illnesses. Important clues in the history include parental consanguinity or previous stillbirth or neonatal death. 'Spot' testing of the urine for ketones (strongly positive in cases of organic acidaemia) can be helpful. Infants with propionic acidaemia can present with profound neutropenia as well as acidosis, leading to a mistaken diagnosis of sepsis by those unaware of this association. The most important step in treatment is to achieve an anabolic state in the affected infant. A combination of glucose, lipid emulsions, insulin and the early introduction of protein to the diet is the most effective early treatment. The removal of toxic metabolites, by either peritoneal dialysis or arteriovenous haemoperfusion is of secondary importance. For some disorders a vitamin cofactor, such as vitamin B12 in some cases of methylmalonic acidaemia, can lead to a correction of the biochemical defect. In vitamin-unresponsive conditions, some limitation to daily protein intake is necessary.

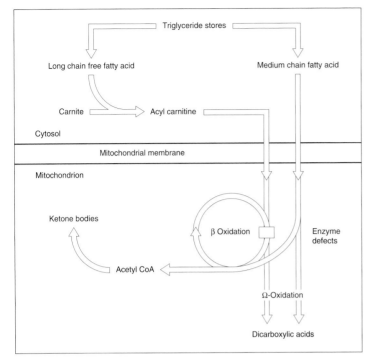

13.13 Fatty acid metabolism simplified, with a block in normal Beta-oxidation leading to the production of dicarboxylic acids typical of fatty acid oxidation defects.

13.14 Urea cycle enzymes; blockage leads to hyperammonaemia.

Fatty acid oxidation defects

A defect in the beta-oxidation pathway can have a profound effect on normal cellular metabolism (**13.13**). This is manifested biochemically by the production of abnormal metabolites: dicarboxylic acids and a failure to produce normal ketone bodies. Hypoglycaemia is common. Clinically, the end result is encephalopathy and resembles Reye's syndrome with prominent fatty change in the viscera noted at postmortem. The disorder is one cause of sudden infant death.

The most commonly diagnosed defect—medium chain fatty acyl CoA dehydrogenase deficiency (MCAD) —usually presents within the first two years of life, often after an episode of intercurrent, mild infection. A common mutation in the MCAD gene is seen in 85 % of affected individuals, and can provide the basis for a very rapid, specific diagnosis of this disorder in infants with encephalopathy. Treatment of affected infants involves dietary manipulation to limit fat and increase carbohydrate intake, as well as the avoidance of fasting.

Urea cycle defects

The urea cycle provides the route for the elimination of toxic compounds produced as a result of protein catabolism (**13.14**). In addition, it provides the mechanism for the *de novo* synthesis of the amino acid arginine. The cycle consists of a series of five chemical reactions, and a defect in the normal activity of the enzymes of the urea cycle leads to hyperammonaemia of varying severity. In carbamoyl phosphate synthetase (CPS), ornithine carbamoyl transferase (OCT), arginosuccinic acid synthetase and argininosuccinase deficiencies, the clinical picture is dominated by severe neonatal hyperammonaemia. In arginase deficiency, progressive spasticity and learning disability are more common than acute encephalopathy.

OCT deficiency is X-linked, and symptoms are relatively common in manifesting female heterozygotes, particularly at times of catabolic stress such as pregnancy. The other disorders are recessively inherited. Mild variants are common and may present with behavioural disturbance often associated with a history of dietary protein intolerance.

Treatment requires protein restriction and the utilisation of alternative pathways of waste nitrogen excretion. Many children survive with significant learning difficulties.

Glycogen storage disease

The common disorders of glycogen catabolism can be divided into those which primarily affect the liver and those that cause prominent muscular dysfunction (see **Table 13.1**, overleaf). A third presentation is due to a deficiency of the lysosomal enzyme, acid glucosidase, leads to a generalised intracellular accumulation of glycogen and presents clinically with profound hypotonia and cardiac failure (GSD II: Pompe's disease). The very rare Type IV GSD causes progressive liver cirrho-

TABLE 13.1 Glycogen Storage Disease

Name	Enzyme deficiency	Comment
I *(Von Gierke)*		
a	Glucose-6-phosphatase	Hepatic, severe hypoglycaemia and acidosis. Dependent on exogenous glucose. Adenoma and hepatoma may be late complications.
b	Translocase T_1	
c	Translocase T_2	
II *(Pompe)*	Lysosomal acid–glucosidase	Generalised lyosomal defect. Death from cardiomyopathy. Adult form may affect skeletal muscle only.
III *(Debrancher)*	Amylo-1, 6-glucosidase	Hepatic, mild type I, chronic myopathy—may be late complication.
IV *(Brancher)*	Amylo-1, 4→ 1, 6-transglucosidase	Causes liver failure, death in early childhood.
V *(McArdles)*	Muscle phosphorylase	Weakness and cramping of muscles. No rise in blood lactate during ischaemic exercise, myoglobinuria.
VI	Liver phosphorylase	Hepatic, mild.
VII	Phosphofructokinase	Symptoms identical to V.
VIII	Liver phosphorylase kinase	Hepatic, usually no hypoglycaemia. ('Benign hepatomegaly'.)

sis and death from hepatic failure at an early age.

The hepatic glygogenoses (Types I, III and VI) cause hepatomegaly and a tendency to hypoglycaemia which can be profound in Type I patients and also in some patients with Type III (**13.15**). In addition, there is growth retardation and in Type I a tendency to hyperlipidaemia, lactic acidaemia and hyperuricaemia. Some patients with Type III have a more generalised enzyme deficiency and, in particular, skeletal and cardiac muscle may also be affected (**13.16–13.18**). In these patients a slowly progressive myopathy may occur in adult life, and some develop cardiomyopathy with left ventricular outflow obstruction. Patients with primary muscle disease (Type V: McArdles's disease and Type VII) present with cramps and contractures during exercise. In most cases, presentation is delayed until the second decade although there is a history of exercise intolerance in many patients dating back to childhood. Myoglobinuria

is a rare complication and may lead to acute renal failure.

Diagnosis of all the glycogenoses is by appropriate enzyme assay. A number of stimulation and provocative tests have been described for both the hepatic and muscular forms of the disease. The ischaemic exercise test often suggested in McArdles's disease can be hazardous, leading to muscle necrosis in affected patients, and should no longer be recommended as a routine procedure. Treatment of the hepatic glycogenoses is aimed at maintaining normoglycaemia (**13.19 and 13.20**), whilst some patients with muscular forms of the disease may improve on a high protein intake.

Mitochondrial disorders

Mitochondria are the cellular organelles responsible for energy production. They are unique in that they contain their own genetic material which is inherited exclusively

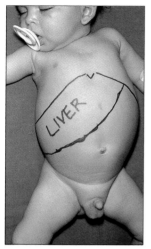
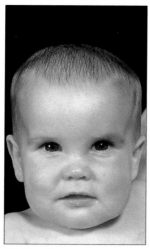
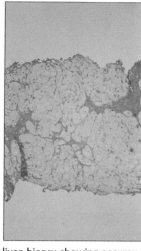

13.15 Glycogen storage disease type I: A baby with hypoglycaemia and hepatomegaly.

13.16 Glycogen storage disease III. 'Cherubic' facial appearance.

13.17 and 13.18 Same baby: liver biopsy showing accumulated glycogen.

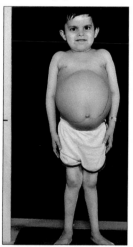
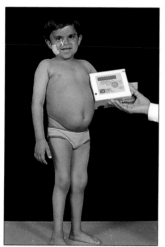
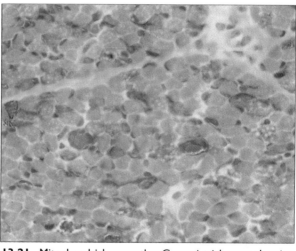

13.19 and 13.20 Glycogen storage disease I. A child seen before (**13.19, left**) and after (**13.20, right**) treatment with nocturnal glucose infusion via nasogastric tube.

13.21 Mitochondrial myopathy: Gomori trichrome showing characteristic ragged red fibres.

through the maternal line. Mitochondrial DNA (mt DNA) codes for proteins which form part of the mitochondrial respiratory transport and oxidative phosphorylation chain. It has become increasingly recognised that a number of encephalopathic, neuromuscular and multisystem disorders can result from specific disruption of the mitochondrial genome. The neurological disorders are characterised histologically by 'ragged red fibres' seen in muscle biopsy specimens (**13.21–13.23**). Clinical features may include encephalopathy, ophthalmoplegia, myopathy, seizures, strokes, ataxia, dementia or a multisystem presentation with hepatic involvement, deafness and cardiac abnormalities (**13.24**). The three main recognised syndromes are:

1. Kearns–Sayre syndrome (KSS): Onset before 20, ophthalmoplegia, pigmentary retinopathy, plus one of the following: heart block, cerebellar syndrome, CSF

protein above 100 mg/dl.

2. MELAS: Mitochondrial encephalomyelopathy, lactic acidosis and stroke-like episodes.

3. MERRF: Myoclonic epilepsy with 'ragged red fibres' which are seen on muscle biopsy.

Biochemically, the hallmark of mitochondrial dysfunction is the presence of lactic acidaemia which may be severe and resistant to treatment. Investigations of mitochondrial disorders include estimation of blood and CSF lactic acid, which are usually raised. Muscle biopsy abnormalities may consist of the presence of strongly reacting, more granular fibres with oxidative enzyme reactions (SDH and NADH stains) or the disrupted red staining 'ragged-red fibres' with Gomori trichrome stain. Electron microscopy may identify abnormal morphological changes of the mitochondria. Biochemical testing of the muscle biopsy will identify the specific abnormality.

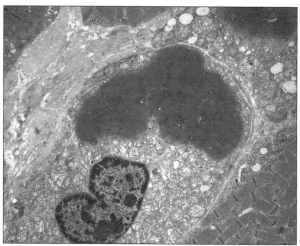

13.22 Electron micrograph (magnification x 3300) shows increase in size and number of mitochondria.

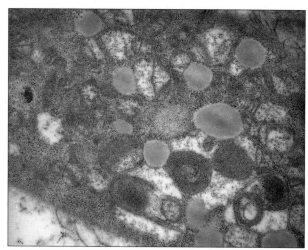

13.23 Electron micrograph (magnification x 12,800) of enlarged mitochondria, some of which have whorled membrane . This also shows increase in lipid.

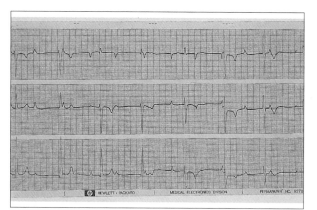

13.24 Mitochondrial cytopathy: Heart block.

Peroxisomal disorders

Peroxisomes are sub-cellular organelles responsible for, among other things, the biosynthesis of plasmalogens (a component of cell membranes), bile acid biosynthesis, peroxidase activity, pipecolic acid catabolism, β-oxidation of very long-chain fatty acids (VLCFA) and phytanic acid catabolism. A number of specific enzymes are housed within the peroxisome, and defects of peroxisomal biogenesis as well as specific enzyme deficiencies have been described.

Zellweger's syndrome

The prototype for this group of disorders is the cerebro-hepato-renal syndrome of Zellweger which is caused by a defective post-translational import of peroxisomal proteins to within the peroxisomal membrane. Histologically, this is characterised by an 'absence' of peroxisomes under electron microscopy, and functionally by a generalised deficiency of peroxisomal enzyme activity.

The clinical phenotype of classical Zellweger's syndrome is easily recognisable and consists of a dysmorphic facial appearance (high forehead, flat occiput, large fontanelles, low nasal bridge, epicanthus, micrognathia, abnormal ears) (**13.25**), cataracts, severe hypotonia, poor suck, seizures and severe psychomotor retardation. Affected infants rarely live more than a few months. Pathologically, in addition to the absent peroxisomes, examination of the CNS commonly reveals a striking disorder of neuronal migration. In addition to the classical patients described above, a number of infants with Zellweger phenotype, but with structurally intact peroxisomes, have been described. Most of these infants have specific peroxisomal enzyme deficiencies rather than the

A number of disorders are associated with specific deletions, duplications and point mutations in mtDNA: for example the Kearns–Sayre syndrome (heart block, ophthalmoplegia, retinitis pigmentosa and various CNS manifestations) is associated with large mtDNA deletions and occasional duplications, whilst Leber's optic neuropathy, MERFF (myoclonic epilepsy with ragged red fibres) and MELAS (mitochondrial encephalopathy with lactic acidosis and stroke-like episodes) are associated with point mutations in the mitochondrial genome.

Accurate diagnosis is required for genetic counselling in affected families. Inheritance of mitochondrial disorders will follow Mendelian lines if the mutation is of nuclear genes encoding mitochondrial proteins and will be maternally inherited if the mutation affects the mitochondrial gene, as mitchondrial DNA is derived exclusively from the oocyte.

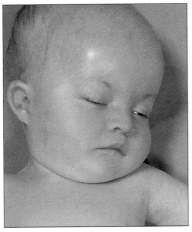

13.25 Zellweger's syndrome. Characteristic facial appearance: 'box-like' cranium.

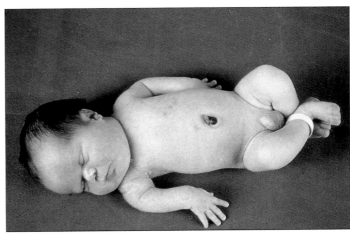

13.26 Rhizomelic chondrodysplasia puntata: mid-facial hypoplasia and short limbs.

13.27 Rhizomelic chondrodysplasia puntata: epiphysial stippling.

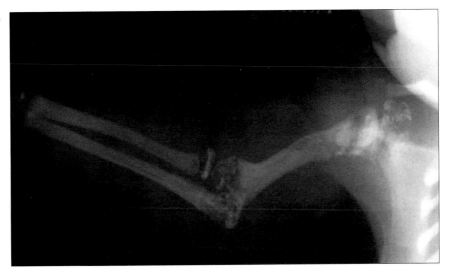

generalised dysfunction characteristic of Zellweger's syndrome.

Other peroxisomal disorders

Neonatal adrenoleucodystrophy (ALD) There is an apparent absence or deficiency of all peroxisomal β-oxidation enzymes. This must be differentiated sharply from X-linked ALD, where the defect is one of VLCFA activation (*see* below). Neonatal ALD is characterised by severe hypotonia and seizures, and the postmortem findings of atrophic adrenals.

Rhizomelic chondrodysplasia punctata (**13.26**) This also presents an easily recognisable phenotype (marked shortening of the proximal limbs, ichthyosis and cataracts). There is a profound disturbance of endochondrial bone formation with clefting of the vertebral bodies and striking chondrodysplasia punctata (**13.27**). Histologically, peroxisomes are present, but may be

abnormal in number and shape. Three characteristic biochemical defects have been demonstrated in affected patients.

X-linked ALD is characterised by a defect in the catabolism of VLCFA; peroxisomal structure appears normal. A number of differing phenotypes have been described. The childhood form of the disease is most common, and is characterised by the onset of dementia between the ages of four to ten years. Progressive neurological deficit leads rapidly to a vegetative state. Adrenal dysfunction is usually demonstrable by ACTH stimulation. Adrenomyeloneuropathy presents later (usually in young adult life) with a gait disturbance. Gradual paraparesis with sphincter disturbance precedes intellectual deterioration by many years. Clinical Addison's disease is usually apparent, and may precede the neurological deterioration. The course of the illness may be very protracted and may be mistaken for multiple sclerosis or other neurological syndromes.

Other less common phenotypes have been described, and a number of asymptomatic individuals with the biochemical defect have also been described. Diagnosis of ALD is based on the demonstration of high levels of VLCFA in plasma or skin fibroblasts.

Dietary treatment aimed at suppressing the synthesis of VLCFA as well as dietary restriction of these compounds can lower plasma levels in affected patients to within the normal range. Therapeutic trials are currently underway to see if this dietary modification can improve neurological outcome. Bone marrow transplantation as a means of enzyme replacement has been attempted on a small number of affected patients. Biochemical correction of the defect has been demonstrated, but it is too early to see whether this will influence the outcome.

Refsum's disease is a disorder of lipid metabolism caused by a failure to oxidise phytanic acid (a normal dietary constituent of dairy products and fats). An isolated defect in mitochondrial phytanic acid hydroxylase has been demonstrated in patients with classical Refsum's disease. (An infantile form of the disorder is associated with generalised peroxisomal dysfunction.) The clinical features include cerebellar ataxia, peripheral neuropathy, retinitis pigmentosa and sensori-neural deafness. CSF protein is often elevated. Treatment with a low phytanate diet can bring about significant improvement and, when combined with regular plasmapheresis, phytanic acid stores can be reduced to near-normal levels and arrest progress of the disease.

Neuroradiology and metabolic disorders

Mitochondrial disorders

Within the mitochondrial disorders, there is considerable overlap in radiological appearance. The MRI pattern of MELAS is not typical, but infarct-like lesions with an atypical distribution occurring at a young age suggests it. Also, extensive cortical laminar necrosis has been described, bordered by gliotic tissue. In MERRF, the MRI pattern is indistinct. A vacuolating myelinopathy may be seen in the central and cerebellar white matter, as well as in the cerebellar peduncles, together with degeneration of the dentate nucleus. In KSS, extensive calcifications are reported on CT, and severe involvement of the white matter on MRI. In Leigh's syndrome the lesions are located in the basal ganglia, brainstem tectum and tegmentum, periaqueductal grey matter, substantia nigra, thalamus, dentate nucleus and spinal cord.

Disorders of organic acid and amino acid metabolism

These disorders form a heterogeneous group. Many characteristic MRI patterns related to the nature and location of the enzymatic defect are recognised. First is a group with prevalent lesions in the arcuate fibres, which are confluent and generalised or patchy and irregular; this group can be with or without cerebellar involvement. Second, there are those with preference for the basal ganglia, in particular the caudate nucleus and the putamen, and combined with spongiform white matter degeneration (WMD). Third is a group with periventricular lesions. Fourth are those with WMD and calcifications. Finally, an unusual form with oedema having a typical pattern of spread. These manifestations may be accompanied by other abnormalities, such as pericerebral fluid collections, arachnoid cysts, cerebellar hypoplasia, and corpus callosum agenesis.

In phenylketonuria, the MRI changes in the white matter are mainly in the periventricular frontal and occipital white matter.

Maple syrup urine disease shows very specific CT and MRI patterns, initially with generalised diffuse oedema, in combination with localised, more severe oedema involving the deep cerebellar white matter, the dorsal part of the brainstem, the cerebral peduncles and the dorsal limb of the internal capsule. This oedema disappears during the second month of life, resulting in atrophy.

Peroxisomal disorders

A number of patterns have emerged, some of which can be considered either pathognomonic for a specific disorder as in X-linked adrenoleukodystrophy, or highly characteristic for a group of disorders, e.g. Refsum's disease.

Adrenoleukodystrophy is a hereditary, sex-linked disease of young males combining degenerative lesions of the CNS with adrenal insufficiency. Imaging has a major role in contributing to the clinical diagnosis. Typical lesions of WMD are noted in the posterior cerebral white matter extending asymmetrically into the frontal areas. Enhancement may occur anterior and adjacent to the WMD areas where there is an active demyelinating process. Typical findings include calcification. Mass effect is an unusual feature which may rarely be encountered in the active period of the disease. With progression of the disease, central and cortical atrophy ensues, indistinguishable from many other degenerative processes.

Chapter 14: Neurodegenerative Disease

Ed Wraith, Richard W. Newton, W. St. Clair Forbes

The neurodegenerative disorders are a group of conditions, often with an underlying biochemical basis that cause progressive and profound loss of neurological function over a variable time period. Many conditions demonstrate, in addition to CNS disease, disruption of other organ tissues and in some instances, as with the mucopolysaccharidoses, the disorders are associated with a dysmorphic physical appearance.

The most important aspect of investigation is a thorough history and clinical examination. The degenerative process may affect primarily the grey or white matter of the central nervous system and this may dictate the principal neurological findings. A combination of dementia, progressive deterioration of neurological function and seizures strongly suggests a neurodegenerative process, and the history should document clear regression of milestones.

Treatment of neurodegenerative disease is palliative only, but it is important to make every effort to establish an accurate diagnosis to allow the family to benefit from appropriate genetic counselling.

Table 14.1 details a classification of these disorders.

TABLE 14.1 Classification of Neurodegenerative Disease

1. Lysosomal storage disease:
    - i) Sphingolipidoses e.g. GM1-, GM2-gangliosidosis, Krabbe's disease, metachromic leucodystrophy etc.
    - ii) Glycoproteinoses e.g. mannosidosis, fucosidosis etc.
    - iii) Mucopolysaccharidoses.
    - iv) Mucolipidoses.

2. Peroxisomal disorders, e.g adrenoleucodystrophy (see earlier).

3. Organic acidurias, e.g. Canavan's disease.

4. Trace metal metabolism e.g Wilson's disease and Menke's syndrome.

5. Neuronal ceroid lipofuscinoses.

6. Spinocerebellar degeneration, e.g. Friedrich's ataxia, abetalipoproteinaemia, olivo-pontocerebellar atrophy, ataxia telangiectasia etc.

7. Basal ganglia degeneration, e.g. Hallervorden–Spatz disease and dystonia musculorum deformans.

8. 'Infections', e.g. subacute sclerosing panencephalitis, progressive multifocal leuco-encephalopathy, prion disease.

9. Miscellaneous, e.g. Pelizaeus–Merzbacher and Alexander's disease.

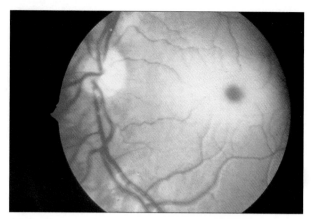

14.1 Cherry-red spot seen in GM1 gangliosidosis, Tay-Sachs and other neurodegenerative diseases.

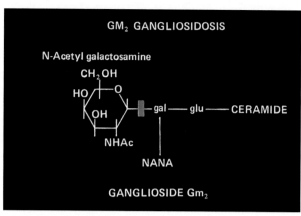

14.2 The biochemical defect in GM2 gangliosidosis.

From the list, it can be seen that whilst neurodegenerative disease may primarily be a problem of infancy, no age group is immune and many disorders present for the first time in early adult life. A number of the disorders will be considered in more detail.

Lysosomal storage disease

Sphingolipidoses

The sphingolipidoses are a family of disorders characterised by a failure to degrade lipids containing a sphingoid group. Sphingolipids are degraded sequentially by a series of exoglycosidases, a deficiency of which leads to the specific metabolic disorder. In GM1 gangliosidosis, a deficiency of β-galactosidase results in a storage disorder which can present at birth, early childhood or in adult life (infantile, juvenile and adult forms respectively). The affected child at birth has a mild Hurler (*see* below) phenotype with facial dysmorphism and skeletal dysplasia. In addition, there is a macular cherry-red spot (**14.1**), organomegaly, seizures, hypotonia and severe psychomotor retardation. Infants usually die before the age of two years from intercurrent respiratory infection. The adult form of the disease is characterised by a cerebellar ataxia with evidence of a superimposed upper motor neurone lesion. Intellectual impairment is mild, seizures are rare and vision is unaffected. The juvenile presentation produces a phenotype intermediate between these two extremes.

The GM2 gangliosidoses are caused by a deficiency of β-N-acetylhexosaminidase which exists as two isoenzymes, hexosaminidase A and B, which have a different subunit structure (**14.2**). A complete deficiency of hexosaminidase A causes classic Tay–Sach's disease, whilst a deficiency of both isoenzymes causes the clinically identical disorder Sandoff's disease.

Patients present in early infancy with weakness, hypotonia and feeding difficulties. A characteristic early symptom is an exaggerated startle response to sound. Psychomotor development reaches a plateau towards the end of the first year of life. Affected infants develop macrocephaly, hypotonia, blindness, deafness and ultimately decerebration. Seizures may be particularly difficult to control. A cherry-red spot is the classic macular hall-mark of the disease. Death usually occurs in early infancy. The high incidence of the carrier status for classical Tay– Sach's disease in the Ashkenazi Jewish population (1:20-25) makes heterozygote screening relevant to this population.

Krabbe's disease is due to a deficiency of galactocerebrosidase and causes a very aggressive neurodegenerative illness in affected infants. Presentation is often very soon after birth with feeding difficulties, severe spasticity, irritability, seizures and poor developmental progress followed by rapid regression. C.S.F. protein concentration is elevated. Death often occurs within the first year of life. Juvenile and adult forms of the disorder have been described.

A deficiency of arylsulphatase A causes metachromatic leucodystrophy (**14.3**). Clinical classification is again dependent on the age of onset of symptoms and is most conveniently divided into congenital (at birth), late infantile (1-2 years), juvenile (4–7 years) and adult (>16 years). The late infantile form of the disease is most common and presents with developmental delay, hypotonia and ataxia progressing to a severe spastic quadriplegia. Cranial nerve palsies and blindness occur late, and progressive neurodegeneration results in a vegetative state within three–four years of the onset of symptoms. The adult form is important as it may present with a psychosis many years before other features of neurological deterioration occur (**14.4**).

Both Gaucher's (B-glucocerebrosidase deficiency) and Niemann–Pick disease (sphingomyelinase deficiency) can present as non-neurological disorders. Indeed, in Gaucher's disease (Type I, non-neuronopathic or adult type) this is the most common mode of presentation. Affected patients develop massive hepatosplenomegaly with associated hypersplenism. Bone crises and other orthopaedic complications require attention, and a small number of patients develop compromised liver function.

14.3 (left) The biochemical defect in metachromatic leucodystrophy.

14.4 (right) Low attenuation in white matter: metachromatic leucodystrophy.

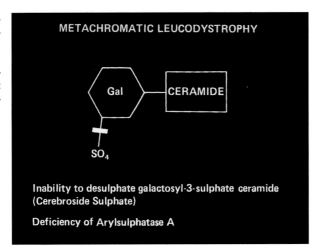

METACHROMATIC LEUCODYSTROPHY

Inability to desulphate galactosyl-3-sulphate ceramide (Cerebroside Sulphate)

Deficiency of Arylsulphatase A

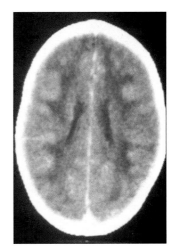

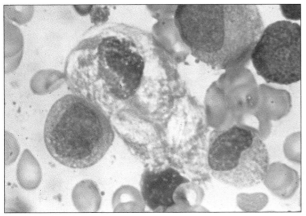

14.5 A Gaucher cell in bone marrow.

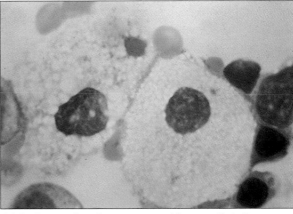

14.6 Foam cells in bone marrow: Niemann–Pick disease.

Patients with Gaucher's disease Type II (acute neuronopathic) present in the early months of life with a characteristic triad of squint (due to cranial nerve palsy), head retraction and feeding difficulties. Developmental delay and hepatosplenomegaly are usually present. Seizures are often a problem and the neurodegenerative process is usually aggressive, leading to death in the first two or three years of life. Type III (Norbottnian type) is very rare and presents with a phenotype in between that of I and II. In all cases the typical Gaucher cell can be found on bone marrow aspiration and can be an important clue to diagnosis (**14.5**).

A number of variants of Niemann–Pick disease have been described. Presentation with hepatosplenomegaly and no neurological involvement is common (Type IB). Other patients present with features of an aggressive neurodegenerative process in the first year of life (Type IA). In addition, hepatosplenomegaly and respiratory involvement are common. Death usually occurs before the age of three years. Patients with type C disease have a cellular defect in cholesterol handling and do not have a demonstrable deficiency of sphingomyelinase. Onset is usually in early childhood with psychomotor retardation, vertical supranuclear ophthalmoplegia, seizures, ataxia

and death between the ages of 5–15 years. A small subgroup of patients present with liver failure in the newborn period. The classification of this group is currently undergoing revision, but in all cases characteristic foam cells may be seen in the bone marrow, offering a clue to diagnosis (**14.6**).

Glycoproteinoses, mannosidosis and fucosidosis

The glycoproteinoses, mannosidosis and fucosidosis, produce many features in common with the mucopolysaccharidoses and are part of the differential diagnosis of the child with 'coarse' facies.

Mucopolysaccharidoses (MPS)

The mucopolysaccharidoses are a family of disorders caused by a defective catabolism of glycosaminoglycans (GAGs) (**14.7**). Presentation is generally in one of three ways:

1) With a dysmorphic syndrome, as in MPS I and II.

2) With severe behavioural disturbance in the absence of gross somatic features, as in MPS III.

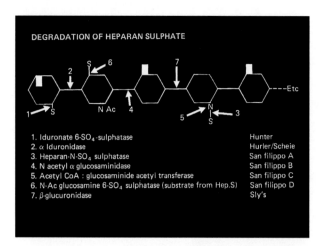

DEGRADATION OF HEPARAN SULPHATE

1. Iduronate 6-SO$_4$-sulphatase   Hunter
2. α Iduronidase   Hurler/Scheie
3. Heparan-N-SO$_4$ sulphatase   San filippo A
4. N acetyl α glucosaminidase   San filippo B
5. Acetyl CoA : glucosaminide acetyl transferase   San filippo C
6. N-Ac glucosamine 6-SO$_4$ sulphatase (substrate from Hep.S)   San filippo D
7. β-glucuronidase   Sly's

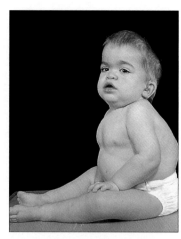

14.7 (left) The bio-chemical defect in some mucopolysaccharidoses.

14.8 (right) Hurler's syndrome: short neck and gibbus.

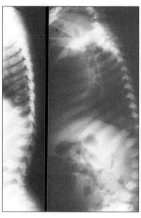 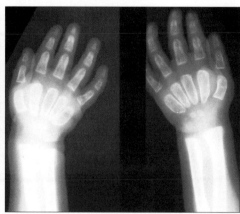 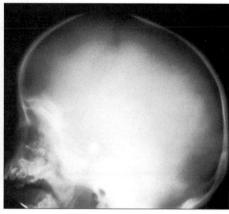

14.9 X-ray lateral spine in MPS IV (left) and MPS I (right). Universal platy-spondyly in MPS IV. Anterior beaking of lumbar vertebrae in MPS I.

14.10 MPS: metacarpals with proximal pointing.

14.11 MPS: lateral skull x-ray with expansion of the sella turcica.

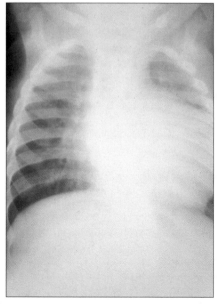

14.12 MPS IV: cardiac enlargement. Note anterior rib expansion.

3) As a skeletal dysplasia in a child of normal intelligence as in MPS IV.

Mild and severe variants are common in all MPS disorders. The prototype for this group of conditions is MPS IH (Hurler's syndrome) (**14.8**), a disorder which presents towards the end of the first year of life with developmental delay. In addition, affected children often have a large head, hepatosplenomegaly, and develop the characteristic 'coarse' facial appearance with corneal clouding typical of the MPS disorders. Recurrent herniae and ENT complications require surgical attention. A skeletal dysplasia (dysostosis multiplex) leads to short stature (**14.9–14.11**). Cardiac disease may be severe and is often a mixture of cardiomyopathy and valvular lesions (**14.12**). Death from a combination of neurodegeneration and heart failure is usual before the age of 10 years. MPS II (Hunter's syndrome) produces similar clinical findings: this disorder is X-linked.

In MPS III (Sanfilippo syndrome) somatic features are mild and the condition is dominated by severe

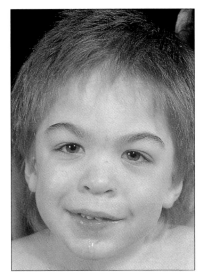

14.13 MPS III: only mild coarsening of facies.

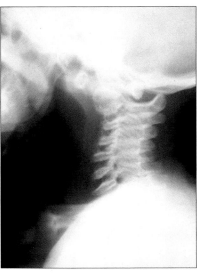

14.14 MPS IV: lateral cervical spine X-ray showing anterior atlanto-axial subluxation before surgery.

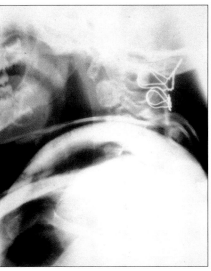

14.15 MPS IV: lateral cervical spine x-ray showing anterior atlanto-axial subluxation after surgery.

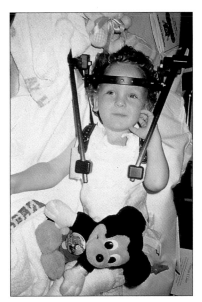

14.16 MPS IV: in halo post-operatively.

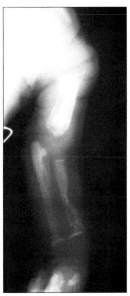

14.17 I-cell disease: periosteal cloaking of the humerus.

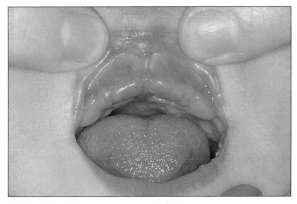

14.18 I-cell disease: hyperplasia of the gums.

behavioural disturbance and aggressive neurodegeneration (**14.13**). As appearance is often normal, diagnosis can be considerably delayed. Children with MPS IV (Morquio's syndrome) have a severe skeletal dysplasia which results in extreme short stature. Patients are of normal intelligence, but are at risk from cervical myelopathy secondary to atlanto-axial subluxation. Prophylactic cervical fusion is required to prevent this complication (**14.14–14.16**).

In all cases, diagnosis is made initially by examining the pattern of GAGs excreted in the patient's urine. Diagnosis is confirmed by specific enzyme assay.

Mucolipidoses

The mucolipidoses are a group of disorders due to defective post-translational modification of lysosomal enzymes. As a result, lysosomal enzymes are not targeted to lysosomes, and are lost from the cell. Functionally, this results in multiple lysosomal enzyme deficiencies. The most severe disorder is mucolipidosis II (I-cell disease) which presents with a severe Hurler-phenotype at or soon after birth. A severe skeletal dysplasia is present as well as a characteristic hypertrophy of the gums (**14.17–14.19**). Death occurs in early infancy.

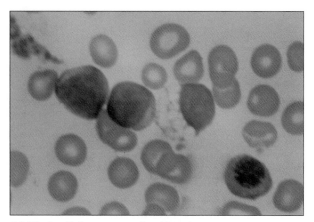

14.19 I-cell disease: vacuolated lymphocytes.

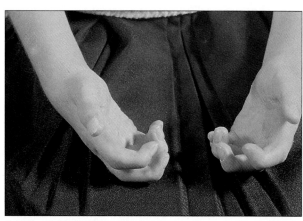

14.20 Mucolipidosis III: claw hand seen in other MPS-like disorders.

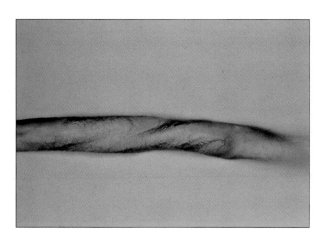

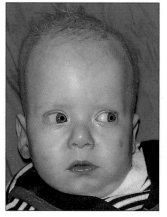

14.21 (left) Menke's disease: pili torti.

14.22 (right) Menke's disease: characteristic facial appearance.

Mucolipidosis III is a milder condition and children often present to rheumatology ororthopaedic clinics with joint stiffness. The disorder is compatible with low–normal intelligence and regression is usually not a feature of this disorder (**14.20**).

Canavan's disease

In this disorder, a spongy degeneration of the white matter leads to a clinical presentation dominated by macrocephaly, blindness, severe spasticity and developmental regression. Death usually occurs within the first two years of life. Recently the disorder has been shown to be associated with the excess excretion within the urine of N-acetylaspartic acid. The functional role of this compound within the CNS is not clear, but in patients with Canavan's disease the abnormal excretion hasbeen shown to be due to a deficiency of the enzyme aspartoacylase, thus allowing accurate biochemical diagnosis in suspected patients.

Menke's syndrome

This disorder is an X-linked recessive condition caused by an abnormal distribution of copper throughout the body associated with defective intestinal absorption. The clinical features include depigmented 'steely' or 'kinky' hair (**14.21 and 14.22**), characteristic facies, hypothermia, arterial degeneration (due to defective elastin synthesis), neurodegeneration, bladder diverticula and osteoporosis. Serum copper and ceruloplasmin levels are very low. Death commonly occurs before the age of two years.

Wilson's disease

This is caused by another defect in the handling of copper. In this instance biliary excretion of copper and incorporation into ceruloplasmin is severely impaired. The subsequent accumulation of copper causes a toxic effect on the liver and brain. The neurological effects are more common in adults and presentation with neurological symptoms is unusual before the age of 12 years. Dysarthria and poor coordination are the most frequent neurological symptoms. These are often accompanied by involuntary movements and dystonia. Pseudo bulbar palsy may occur early in the course of the disease, but deterioration in intellect is usually a late finding. The classic physical sign is the Kayser–Fleischer ring due to copper deposition on Descemet's membrane at the limbus of the corneum (**14.23**).

It is important to remember that this may only be visible by slit-lamp examination in the early stages of the disease. Biochemical findings include reduced serum ceruloplasmin and an increase in non-ceruloplasmin bound copper giving a net reduction in serum copper. Urinary copper is increased and this can be augmented by penicillamine therapy.

The condition can be treated successfully with D-Penicillamine, but side effects occur in up to 10 % of patients. The outcome of treatment depends upon the amount of damage that has occurred before treatment is started. Many of the neurological effects are reversible.

Batten's disease (neuronal ceroid lipofuscinosis)

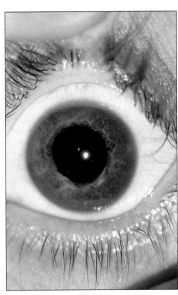

14.23 Wilson's disease: Kayser–Fleischer ring.

This is a neuronal storage disorder in which abnormal lipopigment accumulates in neurones. It is probably derived from the oxidation of polyunsaturated fatty acids. The stored substance is probably a proteolipid with the same aminio acid sequence and properties of subunit c of ATP synthase in childhood. Three clinical and genetically distinct entities all of autosomal-recessive inheritance are seen.

Late infantile form

This usually presents towards the end of the second year of life following a period of normal development. As in most of the neurodegenerative disorders development at first slows and then skills are lost. At about the age of three, seizures will ensue, they are usually primarily generalised, tonic or myoclonic.

A course truncal ataxia is a predominant feature with myoclonic jerks often superimposed. Optic atrophy and pigmentary retinal change are seen with the progressive emergence of pyramidal tract signs.

Progressive deterioration ensues, with death usually occurring by the age of six or seven years.

Juvenile form

This presents with progressive visual failure, usually between the age of five and seven years, and it may be three or four years before seizures develop. Dementia occurs at a late stage, with increasing short-term memory loss a common early feature. Lack of school performance may at first be attributed to psychological disturbance attendant on the progressive visual failure. Formal assessment may be very useful in resolving this issue.

Young people may remain mobile for many years but a coarse truncal ataxia then appears, followed by a progressive evolution of pyramidal, extrapyramidal and cerebellar signs. The rate of progression of the disease is variable, but death usually occurs between the ages of 13 and 20 years.

Infantile form

The early onset of this condition distinguishes it from the late infantile form. It is particularly common in Finland; the onset is between eight and 18 months. and the cardinal features are a progressive deterioration of intellectual function, ataxia, visual failure and myoclonic epilepsy. Rapid deterioration ensues for two years or so, following which children are reduced to a chronic vegetative state with a spastic quadraparesis following a period of hypotonia. Children may well stay in this state for some years, dying only towards the end of the second quinquennium.

Early juvenile form

These children resemble those with the late infantile form, showing ataxia as a presenting symptom followed by the early onset of seizures and a rapidly deteriorating course. Visual failure is a later feature but the biopsy findings (*see* below) resemble those seen in the juvenile form.

Diagnosis

Neuroradiology reveals cerebral atrophy, and standard metabolic tests are normal.

EEG The cardinal features of the late infantile type is polyspike wave activity of high amplitude evoked by slow flicker photosimulation (**14.24**). Runs of less well-defined spike wave complexes are seen in juvenile cases, whereas in the infantile form, the EEG is rather flat and featureless.

Evoked potentials ERG is usually absent or reduced in all forms (**14.25 and 14.26**). In the late infantile form, a grossly enlarged visually evoked response is seen in

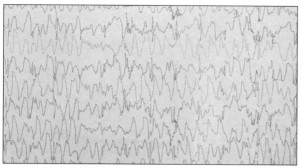

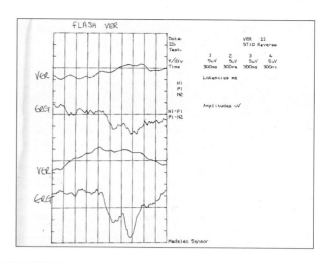

14.24 Typical EEG in Batten's disease: showing exaggerated following response to slow flicker.

14.25 (right) Absent ERG in Batten's disease, with control **(14.26, below left)**.

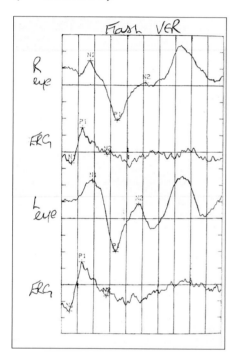

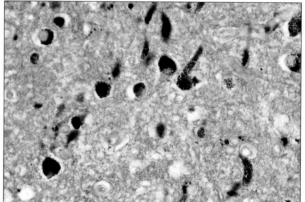

14.27 Batten's disease. Sudan black staining of frontal cortex showing positive staining (black) in neurons.

response to slow flicker photostimulation, but this is not seen in the Finnish infantile form.

Tissue biopsy Characteristic sudanophilic material **(14.27)** is seen on brain biopsy but less invasive methods of diagnosis are now usually pursued. Suction biopsy of the rectal mucosa offers a good alternative, showing intraneuronal inclusions which are curvilinear **(14.28)**. Similar deposits are seen in vascular endothelium and smooth muscles cells, autofluorescence in unfixed sections of PAS positive material is also characteristic **(14.29)**.

Skin biopsy is even less invasive and conveniently may show the characteristic curvi-linear bodies in sweat gland epithelium, vessel endothelium and smooth muscle cells. FIbroblasts are spared. EM for skin biopsy may not be as reliable in the juvenile form as in the late infantile form. Vacuolated lymphocytes are present in

about 25 % of the children with the juvenile form.

In the Finnish infantile form, brain biopsies reveal marked gliosis with neuronal and astrocytic deposition of a PAS-positive sudanophilic autofluorescent substance. This and skin biopsies may show granular osmiophilic deposits (Finnish snowballs!).

Alper's disease

This is a progressive neuronal degeneration of childhood with liver disease, a clinico-pathological entity more recently redefined by Huttenlocher, which leads to progressive degeneration of the cerebral cortex, with the emergence of hepatic disease as a terminal event. Children sometimes present with developmental delay followed by the emergence of intractable epilepsy. Death usually occurs within 10 months.

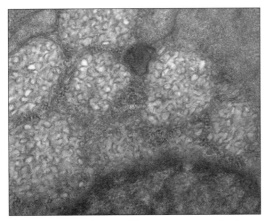

14.28 Batten's disease. Electron micrograph showing membrane-bound curvilinear bodies in fibro-blast (skin biopsy).

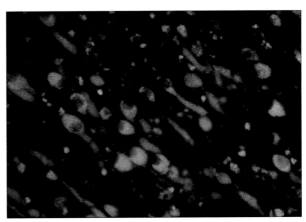

14.29 Apple-green autofluorescence as seen in neurons in a case of neuronal ceroid lipofuscinosis (section from frontal lobe).

The age of onset seems to be variable from the first weeks of life to the end of the second year of life. Failure to thrive may be a feature in early infancy.

Neuroradiology reveals cerebral atrophy with degeneration of both grey and white matter, particularly in occipital and posterior temporal lobes. The EEG tends to show multifocal discharges with sharp waves appearing on top of irregular slow-wave activity. At times these localise and may lead to continuous partial epilepsy.

The condition is probably due to a number of aetiologies with mitochondrial disease implicated in some. Liver biopsy at postmortem usually shows the sclerosis of a subacute hepatitis with fatty infiltration of hepatocytes.

The spinocerebellar degenerations: Friedreich's ataxia

Friedreich's ataxia is the commonest of the primary neuronal degenerations, with an incidence of about 1 in 10,000. It is autosomal recessive in inheritance. The gene is localised to chromosome 9. In the early stages, presentation is usually with progressive clumsiness. It should always be borne in mind when a girl of school age presents with clumsiness. Ataxia of the limbs and trunk with absent tendon reflexes and extensor plantars, dysarthria and loss of joint position sense usually appear within five years of presentation.

Less commonly, pes cavus with distal amyotrophy may appear as an early sign, leading to some difficulty in differentiating Friedreich's ataxia from some cases of hereditary sensory motor neuropathy. Choreo-athetosis, optic atrophy, nystagmus, deafness, scoliosis and cardiomyopathy are also recognised features.

The rate of progression varies but the picture is usually one of progressive dysarthria and gait deterioration, and most young people with the disorder are chairbound between the ages of 25 and 40. Further deterioration in the neurological disease may be very slow and the commonest cause of early death is the onset of a cardiomyopathy. Diabetes is also present in one in ten people with the condition. Most people with the condition will live into their 40's or 50's, many in particular the women, will marry, have children and live largely independent existences.

Where the condition is being considered, investigations should include chest x-ray, echocardiography and ECG to rule ou a cardiomyopathy, and a CT scan may occasionally show cerebellar atrophy and spinal x-rays in search of scoliosis.

Motor nerve conduction studies often give normal or slightly slow conduction velocity results. Sensory action potentials are often significantly reduced. There is no definite diagnostic test, the diagnosis being predominantly made on clinical findings. Localisation of the gene offers the best chance for confirmatory findings and appropriate antenatal diagnosis.

The hereditary spastic paraplegias (HSP)

There is often a history of normal motor development in early childhood followed by the emergence of symmetrical pyramidal signs which are mild but slowly progressive. The severity of the condition and its rate of progression vary greatly between families.

The commonest type is dominant in inheritance but parents may carry very few signs of the disorder. Brisk reflexes and a degree of pes cavus may be all that there is to see in the face of quite a fluent gait. More rare recessive but more rapidly progressive HSPs may also be found.

Full investigation is required, including neuroradiological imaging of the spinal cord. Congenital abnormalities of the cord are known at times to give a progressive picture of deterioration along with compression from tumours.

Even more rarely, HSP may be seen in association with progressive deterioration of cerebellar function, peripheral neuropathy in association with agenesis of the corpus collosum and optic atrophy (Charlevoix County disease); significant learning difficulties and ichthyosis; chronic GM2 gangliosidosis has also been known to present in this way.

The olivo-ponto-cerebellar atrophies may present in childhood with a chronic progressive ataxia although they usually present in middle age. Myoclonic seizures are the rule.

Chronic viral diseases

Subacute sclerosing panencephalitis (SSPE) is due to an altered host response to infection with measles virus. The onset is most often between the age of five and 15 years of age, and most children with the disorder have had measles at a mean age of three. A significant decline in the incidence of the disorder has been seen in the United States since the introduction of measles vaccination though the disorder itself may follow vaccination.

Initial presentation is often with a subtle deterioration in schoolwork. This is often seen in association with periodic episodes of unsteadiness. Intellectual deterioration then becomes more rapid and high amplitude myoclonic jerks become a dominant feature. They may be provoked by excitement or noise and are often repetitive showing characteristic periodicity with associated EEG seizure activity (burst supression).

Visual deterioration may ensue with cortical blindness and focal choroidoretinitis. Progressive gait disturbance ensues with the emergence of extrapyramidal and pyramidal dysfunction. Dementia then becomes severe, leading to decerebrate rigidity and a vegetative state. Death usually ensues within two or three years, with more rapid progression of the disorder being seen in older children. Exceptional cases of 'arrest' have been seen in the earlier stages of the condition.

Diagnosis is made from the very typical presentation, the picture of burst suppression on the EEG and the finding of intrathecal synthesis of measles-specific IgG.

Therapy has been tried with a number of agents includinginterferon transfer factor and antiviral agents but none have been shown to have proven value.

Progressive rubella panencephalitis

This disorder is usually seen towards the end of the second quinquennium. It too shows a progressive dementia with the evolution of pyramidal and extrapyramidal signs, myoclonic seizures and choreiform movement. A diagnosis is made from virological study.

Progressive multifocal leuco-encephalopathy

The disorder presents with focal generalised limb weakness, visual field defects, ataxia and dementia. The disorder is due to a papova virus which may be isolated at brain biopsy and is usually seen in immunosuppressed children.

Prion disease

These are the transmissible spongiform encephalopathies and include Kuru and Creutzfeldt–Jakob disease. Kuru seems to be confined to the New Guinea Highlander tribesman but Creutzfeldt–Jacob disease has been seen in the Western world in children receiving human growth hormone prepared from the human pituitary gland; transmission has also occurred following corneal transplantation. It presents as a progressive dementing illness with occasional cerebellar and visual dysfunction.

Retroviral infections and AIDS

Human T-lymphocytotrophic virus and human immunodeficiency virus (HTLV & HIV) are retroviruses which may both lead to human disease through the action of the enzyme reverse transcriptase. Children usually acquire HIV infection either perinatally from their infected mother or by transmission from blood products. Most children present with very non-specific symptoms including failure to thrive, lymphadenopathy and hepatosplenomegaly. Repeated infection with fungi or pneumocystis carinii is common. Neurological involvement in childhood is either due to opportunistic infection of the central nervous system or direct invasion of the brain by virus. Manifestations of the disorder therefore include demyelinating symptoms, opportunistic infection with toxoplasmosis or cryptococcus, infarction and haemorrhage.

Diagnosis is made on clinical grounds and appropriate biological and viral laboratory investigations.

Leucodystrophies

Metabolic basis unknown.

Pelizaeus–Merzbacher disorder

This disorder seems to be due to defective biosynthesis of proteolipid protein. There is a conatal form with onset in the first few weeks or months of life with rapid progression leading to death in the first 2 years of life (Type II). Type I has onset in the first year of life with slow progression leading todeath in the second or third decade.

The characteristic neurological features include striking nystagmoid eye movement which may be associated with oscillatory movement of the head, laryngeal stridor, pyramidal cerebellar and at times dystonic features. Optic atrophy with eventual visual failure is common.

Alexander's disease

The onset of this disorder may be very insidious, and the features are progressive. White matter degeneration leading to dementia, seizures and spasticity are seen. Enlargement of the brain and skull are common and megalencephaly is a striking feature.

Neuroradiology and the degenerative disorders

The role of imaging

1. In some disorders the appearance may be diagnostic, precluding the necessity for brain biopsy.

2. Specific disease processes, such as infarction or tumour, which may initially produce similar clinical symptoms, can be excluded. CT may distinguish diseased grey and white matter from normal brain tissue. Almost all degenerative disease will eventually demonstrate ventricular enlargement.

White matter disorders (WMD)

In WMD, MRI is the imaging modality of choice as it provides more detailed information about the structures involved which may lead to the correct diagnosis. In most cases of WMD, clinical and laboratory data are necessary to ensure correct diagnosis, but MRI may guide the diagnostic pathway in the correct direction. MRI however cannot differentiate between a selectiveWMD and selective myelin disorders. WMD therefore can be subdivided into acquired and hereditary disorders.

Patterns of white matter degeneration

Degenerative disease of white matter may be detected on CT and MR by changes in the frontal lobes, occipital lobes, the centrum semi-ovale and the internal capsule. Three patterns of CT and MR abnormality in disease of the white matter have been described: demyelination, dysmyelination and a combination of the two.

In demyelinating disorders (multiple sclerosis, anoxia, under-nutrition, progressive multifocal leukoencephalopathy) there is formation of the normal myelin, which is subsequently destroyed. The increased water content of the white matter results in an increased signal on MR and low density on CT. There may be enhancement following contrast in active disease.

In dysmyelinating disease (e.g. metachromatic leukodystrophy and Alexander's disease) there is abnormal formation and maintenance of myelin as a result of enzymatic disturbance. Dysmyelinating diseases are less likely to demonstrate mass effect or abnormal contract enhancement. Adrenoleukodystrophy shows large areas of low attenuation with peripheral advancing zones of gliosis that may show enhancement. The patterns of white matter degeneration which may be recognised on CT and MR are listed in **Table 14.2** (overleaf).

Lysosomal storage disorders

Among the spingolipidoses, the MRI patterns of T2-weighted sequences are of symmetrical, confluent, periventricular hypointense lesions, spreading centrifugally.

In the storage disorders, mucopolysaccharidoses (MPS), CT and MR demonstrate symmetrical areas of WMD, particularly in the parietal region, that may correlate with cavitation and with dilatation of the perivascular spaces. Follow-up scans may detect progressive hydrocephalus which is a relatively common complication in MPS I,II,III and VII. Spinal cord compression may result from atlanto-axial subluxation in Type IV (Morquio) Type IH (Hurler) and Type VI (Maroteaux-Lamy disease) (*see also* Chapter 17). CT of the upper cervical spine and skull base is indicated.

In Canavan's disease, the white matter takes on an oedematous, swollen appearance and the lateral ventricles are small and appear compressed. Later, the lateral ventricles become progressively enlarged and the decrease in density on CT of the white matter continues with the appearance of small cavities of CSF density.

Disorders with unknown enzymatic defects

In Alexander's disease, the MRI features correlate well withthe underlying vacuolating myelinopathy. There is swelling of the white matter with preferential involvement of the frontal lobes where the lesions are extensive and may be associated with compression of the frontal horns of the lateral ventricle. Contrast enhancement on CT is variable, being absent in some children, whilst in others there is a striking symmetrical enhancement with the caudate nuclei and anterior periventricular brain substance.

Acquired WMD

Non-infectious inflammatory disorders

In demyelinating condtions, MRI has a much more specific role than CT in demonstrating the plaques of demyelination. T2-weighted images demonstrate these plaques as areas of increased signal in the periventricular white matter and in the white matter of the cerebellar hemispheres. Enhancement with Gadolinium DTPA may enable active lesions to be identified. On CT, the plaques are less reliably identified as areas of low attenuation. In the acute phase, a significant mass effect may occur with focal areas of contrast enhancement which are usually small, round or ovoid and homogeneous, although thick-walled ring-like lesions may occur. These enhancing foci are located in the same general areas as the hypodense lesions.

Hypoxic-ischaemic lesions

In infants and children, MRI has been shown to be the imaging modality of choice for the follow-up of post hypoxic-ischaemic damage. There is a good correlation between the severity of the abnormalities and the extent of the lesions (*see also* Chapter 15).

Toxic-metabolic encephalopathies

Wilson's disease demonstrates extensive white matter involvement on MR. Focal abnormalities are found in the lenticular, thalamic and caudate nuclei, as well as in the brainstem. With the use of high field (1.5T) the potential for preferential T2 paramagnetic shortening exists. MR is generally more sensitive than CT in this disease. Grey matter lesions show characteristic bilateral symmetry, whereas white matter involvement, if present, is typically asymmetrical and is most frequent in the frontal lobes.

TABLE 14.2   Patterns of White Matter Degeneration

Focal symmetrical degeneration of white matter
      e.g.   adrenoleucodystrophy
              disseminated necrotising leucoencephalopathy

Focal asymmetrical degeneration of white matter
      e.g.   progressive multifocal leucoencephalopathy

Periventricular degeneration of white matter
      e.g.   multiple sclerosis

Centrum semi-ovale pattern of white matter degeneration
      e.g.   chronic subcortical ischaemic encephalopathy

Generalised white matter degeneration
      e.g.   Alexander's disease
              anoxic encephalopathy

Basal ganglial degeneration
      e.g.   Wilson's disease
              Huntingdon's disease
              Parkinson's disease
              Leigh's disease

Central pontine myelinolysis

Chapter 15: The Static Encephalopathies

Pamela I. Tomlin, W. St. Clair Forbes

Cerebral palsy

Cerebral palsy is a disorder of movement or posture due to a non-progressive brain abnormality. The term 'static encephalopathy' refers to the non-progressive nature of the underlying cause, which may be of pre- or perinatal origin or be acquired postnatally up to two years. The complex mechanisms of cell multiplication, migration and organisation make it easy to understand why it is that the effects of the original cause rarely remain static. Clinically, cerebral palsy is an evolving condition whose presence is often difficult to ascertain in the first six months of life. The manifestations of cerebral palsy depend on the developmental stage. Growth itself can worsen the contractures of spastic cerebral palsy (Dwyer *et al.*, 1989). Spastic muscles do not grow at the same rate as bone so that growth spurts, especially at puberty, can worsen the handicap.

Aetiology

It is now becoming clearer that the contribution of birth asphyxia to the origin of cerebral palsy is limited, and confined to perhaps 10–14 % of cases. Congenital and prenatal factors operate in more than 50 % of cases (Nayeye *et al.*, 1989; Torfs *et al.*, 1990).

Clear disproportion between head size and length at birth should be investigated for a congenital intrauterine viral infection, especially in a neurologically abnormal baby. Neonatal identification of viral excretion is essential as subsequently an acquired disorder cannot be ruled out (**15.1**). Cytomegalovirus is the commonest finding. Metabolic screening is best carried out when feeding is established (*see* Chapter 13). The neuro-radiological investigation is described below.

In some circumstances, as following placental abruption, birth asphyxia is clearly the cause of the cerebral palsy; these circumstances are rare. No one factor of foetal or cord pH, meconium staining, Apgar score, or the time of onset of spontaneous respiration is proof of birth asphyxia. However, when these factors are seen in the context of a neonatal illness involving irritability, hypertonia, or, more worryingly, flaccidity, hypogly-

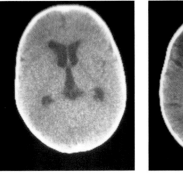

15.1 Intracranial calcification on CT scan in congenital cytomegalovirus infection.

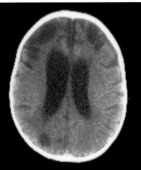

15.2 and 15.3 Multiple cysts in the frontal and parietal cortex with changes of cerebral atrophy following hypoxic-ischaemic change.

caemia, disseminated intravascular coagulation and renal failure, then hypoxic-ischaemic encephalopathy is the most likely diagnosis (Freeman and Nelson, 1988) (**15.2 and 15.3**). Seizures worsen the prognosis, as does a low-voltage or discontinuous EEG, ultrasound evidence of subcortical cystic change, and abnormal somatosensory potentials (**15.4–15.13**). To attribute the

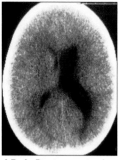

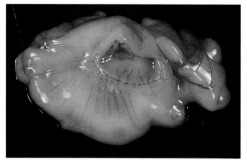

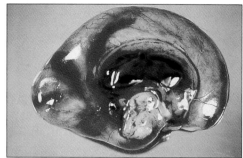

15.4 Periventricular leukomalacia. Axial CT: large right lateral ventricle.

15.5 Periventricular leukomalacia: early dilatation of ventricle.

15.6 Grade IV intraventricular haemorrhage IVH in premature infant.

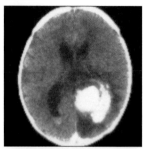

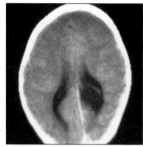

15.7 and 15.8 Intraventricular haemorrhage (IVH): CT scan. Axial sections show (**15.7, left**) a recent haematoma as an area of increased density with the right lateral ventricle extending into the adjacent parenchyma. (**15.8, right**) Late scan showing low-density area (porencephalic cyst) at the site of the bleed.

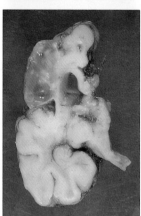

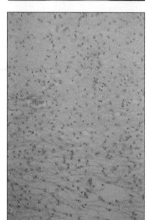

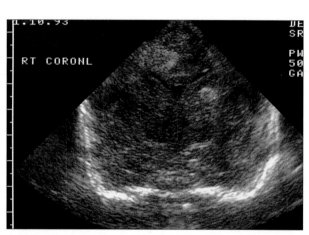

15.9 Periventricular leukomalacia (PVL). Late—surrounding cystic change.

15.10 PVL. Histological change—lower half—reactive gliosis and spongy degeneration of white matter.

15.11 Periventricular leukomalacia on ultrasound scanning.

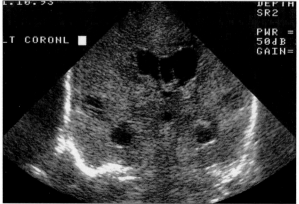

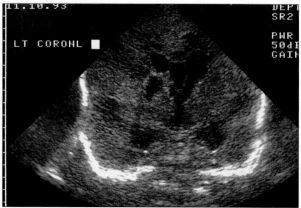

15.12 and 15.13 Subcortical cystic change on ultrasound scanning.

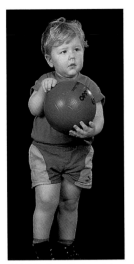

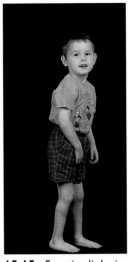

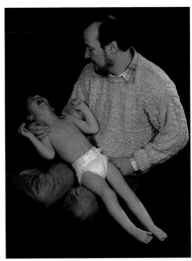

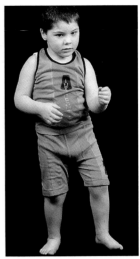

15.14 Spastic hemiplegia—right sided. Hyperpronated arm.

15.15 Spastic diplegia. Both legs show internal rotation and adduction at hip and pes planus.

15.16 Four-limb spastic cerebral palsy.

15.17 Ataxic 3-year-old child showing broad-based gait and elevated arms.

cause of cerebral palsy to birth asphyxia, there must be a clear story of hypoxic-ischaemic encephalopathy.

Spastic cerebral palsy

Spastic cerebral palsy is due to dysfunction in the cortico-spinal tracts, leading to increased muscle tone, hyperreflexia, and a tendency for joint contractures to develop, especially at the ankle, hip, knee, wrist and elbow. Initially, axial tone tends to be low; the increased tone of true spasticity tends to evolve as the first year of life progresses. There is often persistence of the primitive reflexes (*see* Chapter 2).

In hemiplegia, one side of the body is involved, the arm being affected more than the leg (**15.14**). Diplegia refers to bilateral involvement, the legs being affected more than the arms (**15.15**). Tetra- or quadriplegia is the most severe form, not confined to all four limbs, but affecting trunk and head control too (**15.16**). Monoplegias and triplegias are more rarely seen. Where there is a clear asymmetry in signs, it is most likely that an underlying cause will be found; diplegia may be traced to adverse perinatal factors. A genetic cause and higher risk of recurrence are more likely in symmetrical forms.

Poor foetal cerebral perfusion may lead to stroke-like episodes, at times perceived by the mother as a sudden fall off in foetal movements. Subsequently, a porencephalic cyst may develop in the affected area (*see* Chapter 11). A spastic hemiplegia on the contralateral side is the usual clinical manifestation. Similarly, focal infarction can occur after birth in the course of meningoencephalitic illness, hypotensive episodes, emboli or trauma. Pre-term infants may experience haemorrhagic or hypotensive ischaemia with subsequent periventricular leukomalacia (Sinha *et al.*, 1990). Diplegia is a common consequence, and later CT scanning may reveal ventricular dilatation.

Spastic quadriplegia is commonly associated with special sensory defects, epilepsy and mental handicap. Where there is a discernible cause, the insult is diffuse. There may be a gross underlying dysgenesis of the brain or evidence of intra-uterine infection with intracranial calcification. An acute infantile presentation of diffuse scattered contusions with fronto-temporal predominance and posterior subdural collections on CT scanning is pathognomonic of the shaken baby syndrome (*see* Chapter 9); full recovery is possible but spastic tetrapelgia can be the outcome, with associated cortical blindness, mental handicap and epilepsy. Arterio-venous malformations can rupture perinatally as well as in infancy or later childhood. The acute presentation may be indistinguishable from the shaken baby syndrome, but the CT scan shows much more obviously focal parenchymal haemorrhage.

Recessively inherited forms of quadriplegia also exist although the underlying metabolic cause has not been identified. This emphasises the need for all families of chidren with disability to receive adequate genetic counselling (*see* below and Chapter 18).

Ataxic cerebral palsy

The origin of ataxic cerebral palsy is in the cerebellum and its connections. Affected infants are slow to develop equilibrium reactions and are obviously delayed in all their motor milestones (**15.17**). Affected children are usually hypotonic, but increased tone is evident in the ataxic-diplegia syndrome. The children have poor coordination, are unsteady and often have associated learning difficulties. In the ataxic-diplegic form, the causes are similar to those of spastic diplegia. In the pure ataxic presentation, cerebellar hypoplasia may be evident on CT scanning. Sometimes the ataxia is a component of a genetic syndrome, like Joubert's, with vermis hypopla-

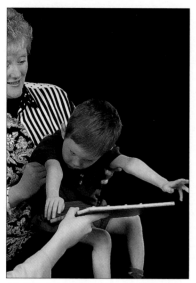

15.18 A child with dyskinetic cerebral palsy, showing uncontrolled patterns of arm movements and flaccid trunk, whilst attempting to reach out.

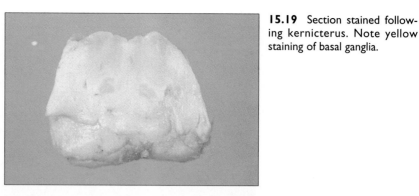

15.19 Section staining following kernicterus. Note yellow staining of basal ganglia.

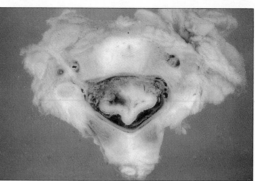

15.20 Cervical cord birth trauma—potentially avoidable.

sia. Hydrocephalus with or without a Dandy–Walker syndrome may underly the presentation. Screening of amino acids and organic acids may reveal an underlying metabolic cause.

Dyskinetic cerebral palsy

This form of cerebral palsy involves the basal ganglia and extra-pyramidal pathways. It may be seen in a pure form or in a mixed form with spasticity. Pure forms and all symmetrical presentations may have genetic implications. Where there is asymmetry, the aetiologies parallel those of spastic cerebral palsy. Dyskinetic cerebral palsy manifests as involuntary athetoid movements of the limbs, or as more sustained dystonic posturing of the trunk and limbs (**15.18**). Global ischaemic insults in the perinatal history may show as bilateral basal ganglia calcification on CT scanning. The association of athetosis and deafness with kernicterus is now rarely seen but can occur with ischaemic insults (**15.19**). Herpes simplex virus has a predilection for temporal and occipital lobes and can affect the extrapyramidal system. Hemichorea can occur as the result of a head injury. Contusions and axonal disruption occur because of the shearing effect between the different densities of the cortex and brain stem structures.

Prevention

There was an overall decline in the incidence of cerebral palsy from the mid 1950's to 1970, associated with improved obstetric and perinatal care (**15.20**). This is exemplified by the preventative work in Rhesus negative mothers with the advent of the postnatal administration of anti-D antibody and the early exchange transfusion of affected neonates. Since 1970, the incidence of cerebral palsy has remained relatively stable and there is evidence that it is rising in the low and very low birth-weight babies (Pharoah *et al.*, 1990). The evidence is that babies with impairment are surviving because of improved neonatal care. Further research into the aetiology of cerebral palsy, including the use of magnetic scanning and magnetic-resonance spectroscopy promises to be informative, particularly in relation to the neuronal migration problems (*see* Chapter 11).

The need to avoid alcohol and smoking in pregnancy is well advertised, though the consequences are still seen. The small for dates baby, especially if pre-term, is at higher risk for cerebral palsy than the appropriately grown infant. Regular antenatal care is not always taken up by the socially disadvantaged or pregnant teenager so that the foetus who is not thriving *in utero* may be detected late. There is a place for health education in the senior school years for both sexes (**15.21 and 15.22**).

There are genetic syndromes in which cerebral palsy is a component. Characterisation in the index case may be sufficient to allow genetic diagnosis early in subsequent pregnancies, as in Angelman's syndrome (Pembrey *et al.*, 1989) and the Miller–Dieker syndrome (Sharief *et al.*, 1990). However, these are very infrequent, and the majority of children with cerebral palsy show no genetic markers. Improved recognition and data-basing of cerebral palsy will facilitate this area of research.

The immunisation programme for rubella and the antenatal screening of mothers for infections and meta-

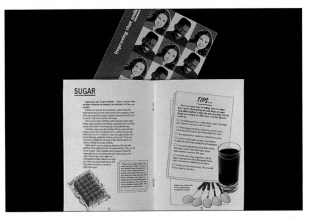

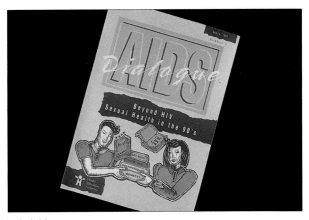

15.21 (left) and 15.22 (right) Health education poster for school children.

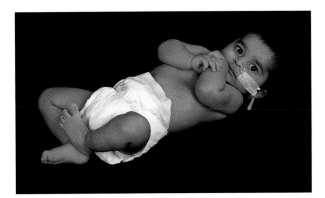

15.23 Central hypotonia—preserved active movements.

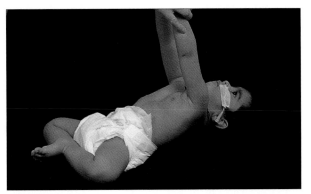

15.24 Central hypotonia—complete head lag and lack of limb tone.

15.25 Central hypotonia—rounded sitting.

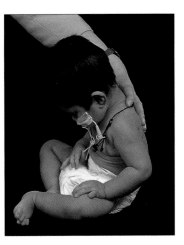

bolic disorders (such as phenylketonuria) are other preventive measures already operating. Similarly, early detection of amino acid disorders, hypothyroidism and galactosaemia in the neonate prevent such infants accumulating neurological damage.

Presentation

Feeding difficulties

Feeding difficulties are commonly amongst the earliest problems in the baby with cerebral palsy and are often managed within the family with great difficulty for prolonged periods of time. The problems usually revolve around persisting strong primitive brain stem reflexes. The natural cradling cuddle at feed time provokes a tonic neck reflex with the infant's head, trunk and arms extending stiffly away from the breast or bottle. Many mothers feel very self-conscious about the postures they need to adopt to break this extensor pattern, and avoid feeding in public. Feeds take a very long time and more than five hours a day may be so occupied. The mothers often severely restrict their social life. Excessive tongue thrust, poor bolus formation and protection of the airway in poorly coordinated swallowing all contribute to the difficulties. As much feed may spill out as is swallowed, with regular bouts of coughing and choking at feed time.

The infants are frequently chesty from recurrent aspiration. If a feeding problem is elicited in the history it should be observed. Feeding mechanisms should be routinely assessed in the history as well as assessing the amount of feed taken and weight gained.

The floppy infant

Floppiness may be an early presentation of any form of cerebral palsy. The characteristic picture is of visible limb movement, with better limb than axial tone (central

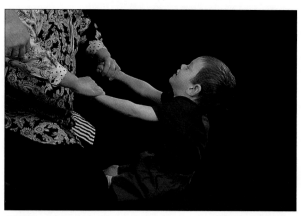
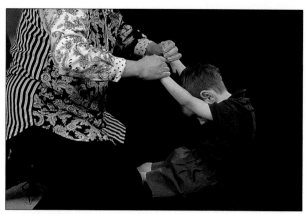

15.26 and 15.27 A 3-year-old with dyskinetic cerebral palsy showing central hypotonia.

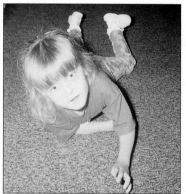

15.28 A hemiplegic pattern of crawling.

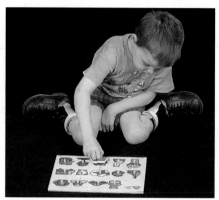

15.29 W-sitting in spastic diplegia.

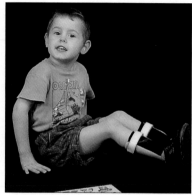

15.30 Straight-leg sitting cannot be achieved without hand propping to prevent a backward fall.

hypotonia) (**15.23–15.25**). Head lag is but one component of complete truncal lag and when the infant is held sitting, the back is rounded in forward flexion. Reflexes are preserved if not brisk, though they are frequently depressed in pure ataxic cerebral palsy. If this is the precursor of spastic cerebral palsy it is usually the tetraplegic form and is readily recognised by the infant's supine posture at five to six months of age. The arms are held asymmetrically abducted with adversion of the head in a persisting asymmetrical tonic neck reflex. This will give the impression of asymmetrical tone in the upper limbs, which disappears if the head is held in the midline. The hands are fisted and the primitive grasp and Moro reflexes persist. The infant's head cannot be held in the midline (normally achieved by three to four months of age). The legs are extended and adducted with plantar flexion of the feet.

Some of the most profound and persisting central hypotonias evolve later into athetoid (dyskinetic) cerebral palsy (**15.26 and 15.27**). Distinguishing them at an early stage from myopathic presentations can be difficult and some may have a muscle biopsy. The biopsy is often abnormal in its fibre size but not specific for a neuromuscular disorder. Hypotonia in infants with ataxic cerebral palsy may also be marked and reflexes

difficult to obtain. Contractures are not seen in the pure form of ataxic and athetoid cerebral palsy.

Patterns of movement

Non-ambulatory patterns of movement

The patterns of movement will reflect the nature of the underlying cerebral palsy. The child with a hemiplegia will crawl with the affected arm tucked under the trunk, or bottom shuffle, propelling with the sound arm (**15.28**). The faster the movement, the more obvious the flexed, adducted posture of the affected arm becomes. In a diplegia, the infant typically crawls commando-style with legs extended and progress almost entirely dependent on the pulling power in the arms. There is a notable lack of alternating flexion at the hips. Children with a diplegia may omit sitting before crawling and pulling to stand. Any attempt for them to straight-leg sit is made very difficult, as hamstring spasticity extends the hips, rocking them back on to the sacrum (**15.29 and 15.30**). When they do sit, it is usually in a W-pattern, with the buttocks on the floor between the heels, with hips

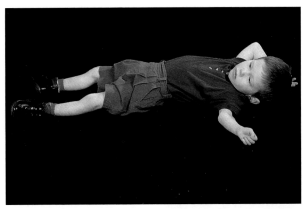

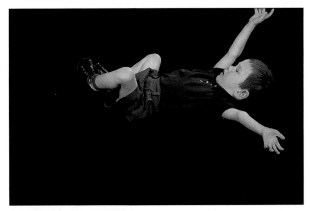

15.31 and 15.32 Persisting ATNR and Moro in a child with dyskinetic cerebral palsy (CP).

15.33 The child wants to walk but cannot achieve it.

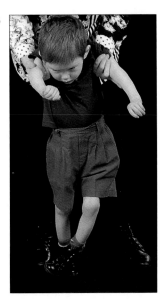

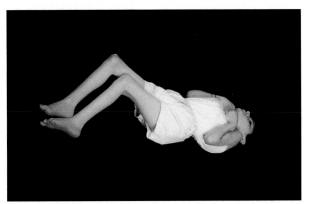

15.34 A 16-year-old with long-standing spastic four-limb CP and windswept posture.

markedly internally rotated. When they stand, they firmly rise up on to their toes. Many normal children go through a phase of toe-standing, but it is usually intermittent, even in habitual toe-walkers. Initially in the spastic child, a large component of toe-standing may be dynamic, but contractures eventually follow.

Infants with spastic tetraplegia or athetosis may be so hampered by primitive reflex patterns that no rolling or crawling can be achieved (**15.31–15.33**). Associated severe learning difficulties may deprive them of some motivation. One aspect of development should never be assessed independently of another. Children with a severe spastic tetraplegia may retain their early posturing: poor axial tone, extension of the legs with some degree of fixed flexion at the hips, knees and ankles, and arms held adducted with an asymmetrical tonic neck reflex persisting in a semi-obligatory way. Emotion or sudden changes in posture bring out reflex patterns of posturing and an increase in tone. In distress, the child's startle-like tonic abduction of upper limbs can look like a myoclonic seizure. As the child grows, the adversion of the head is accompanied by pelvic sweeping to the

same side (**15.34**). In this windswept posture the external hip is most at risk for dislocation and a scoliosis develops. A few well-motivated children can achieve crawling in a commando style with tightly fisted hands and limited upper limb movements.

In ataxic cerebral palsy, crawling is late developing and once achieved is prolonged. The crawling base is reasonably rectangular (compared with the widened crawling base of a child with the proximal weakness of a neuro-muscular disorder). Parents are often frustrated that the child pulls up on the furniture to stand but is afraid to let go, but four points are more secure and effective for movement than two.

The child with dyskinesia may have the most severe physical handicap with the most preserved intelligence. Irritability and fractiousness in the toddler age group may reflect the frustration this brings (*see* **15.33**). Initiating voluntary movements of any kind, including opening the mouth, releases a generalised pattern of dystonic movement. There is no articulation or respiratory control for the delivery of speech. Eye-pointing may be the earliest means of communication. Often the athetoid

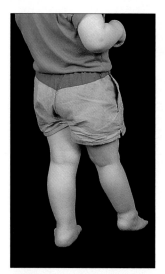

15.35 Hemiplegic toe strike. Note upper limb is adducted, flexed and pronated.

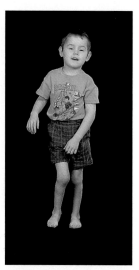

15.36 and 15.37 Diplegic gait with and without ankle–foot orthoses.

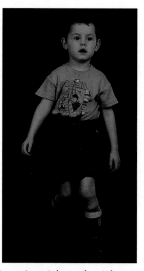

15.38 Asymmetric posturing during Fog's testing in aa adolescent with hemiplegia.

nature of the cerebral palsy becomes more easily recognised around the age of one year as the child begins to reach out. The effort leads to an obvious increase in tone with extension of neck and trunk and wide opening of the mouth. Though marked extension and inversion of the limbs accompanies this, there will be no contractures unless there is associated spasticity as the tone is dynamic. Applying splints is inappropriate as they only provoke dynamic posturing. Passive observation of the relaxed child will usually show a full range of joint movement and may be kinder than inducing dynamic posturing by grasping the floor. The child with athetoid cerebral palsy can show a remarkable fluctuation in tone only really evident during a wakeful state.

Milder patterns of dystonia may be transient in the first 18 months of life (Willemse, 1986). These may be postural, symmetrical or asymmetrical. Crawling on an internally rotated hand or persistent thumb adduction are examples. Other infants offer more concern: they may swim ineffectively, prone with arms and legs flailing in an alternating pattern of movement. Attempts to flex and extend the legs in a crawling fashion are clearly seen but the effect is so dislocated that no progress is made, except in circles, or the child finishes up rolling when the intention was to crawl. Confusion with spastic diplegia occasionally arises because of the marked dynamic increase in tone on handling. Again, passive observation can help to clarify that. These children may learn to walk late with developmental problems emerging in coordination and higher function.

Ambulatory patterns of movement

Most parents want the doctor to paint a picture of their child's future once a diagnosis of cerebral palsy is made. Shared markers can be helpful and learning to sit is one of the best. The majority of children who achieve reli-able independent sitting before the age of two years will learn to walk; half of those who do not sit until they are four years old will still go on to walk.

The gait of a child with marked diplegia or hemiplegia is characteristic (**15.35–15.37**), but mild abnormality is less obvious. Examination of associated movement on heel-walking, toe-walking or walking on the borders of the feet will reveal a reproducible marked asymmetry of upper limb posturing in a child with a hemiplegia (**15.38**). Exaggeration of posturing is seen on the affected side. Asking the child to run in a corridor will also bring out the hemiplegic posturing and in the diplegic child the running posture will be stiff (or impossible), lacking good extensor and flexor movements at the hips and knees.

Children with ataxic cerebral palsy walk immaturely, lacking a good heel-strike. Observation is best with the child barefoot, walking on a hard floor. A broad varying base is seen, sometimes with persistent abduction of the arms to assist balance. The lack of heel–strike is heard as a slapping sound on the floor. The child may not be able to attempt running, which, if achieved, is very awkward, like a fast walk with limited spring or elevation from the floor.

Manipulation

Early hand preference, certainly within the first year, points to a hemiplegia. This is often noted around five months of age when reaching out normally occurs. The affected hand is kept fisted with the thumb across the palm and the wrist held in flexion (**15.39**). Whole-hand grasp persists beyond nine months of age, the independent index finger approach failing to develop normally (**15.40**). In milder presentations, slow and awkward finger-thumb sequencing may be achieved. In ataxic cerebral palsy, delay in independent index-finger movement

15.39 A child reaching for a ball: the right hemiplegic arm remains relatively retracted and the fingers fail to extend.

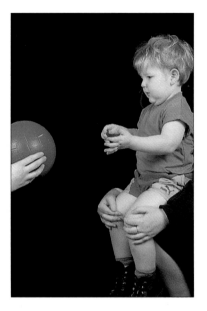

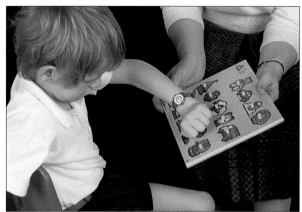

15.40 A 5-year-old boy with mixed spastic-athetoid CP showing whole-hand grasp.

is also found. In the toddler, tremor is best observed with form-board shapes or brick building. From three years onwards, the performance of threading beads, or placing pegs in slots is effective. There is notable awkwardness in handling objects and in removal of shoes and socks, when there is an overshoot as the item is finally removed, indicating a lack of refinement in the forces required (Eilassen *et al.*, 1991). The same is true of children with spasticity or mild athetosis, or those who are clumsy but who do not have cerebral palsy. Pencil control from three to four years onwards will also reveal an awkward grasp and shaky performance in children with cerebral palsy, particularly with ataxia.

The general examination

Clues to an underlying cerebral palsy may be revealed by comparing the growth on one side of the body with the other: hands, limbs and feet. A shortened leg demands examination and radiology of the hips. In hemiplegia, the shortening is commonly due to growth deficiency in the spastic side. It is important to note that such a growth differential will not be evident at birth. Obvious asymmetries at birth, notably in the lower limbs, demand a thorough search for an underlying spinal-cord lesion at an early stage.

Measurement of head circumference may reveal microcephaly or an enlarged head size. Dysmorphism or evidence of congenital infection should be sought. Mild dysmorphic features should be noted and may point to a genetic origin (Coorsen *et al.*, 1991). Skin stigmata or depigmentation may point to tuberous sclerosis, neurofibromatosis or one of the other neurocutaneous sydromes (*see* Chapter 11).

In continuing care, the general examination needs to take account of the problems which may be associated with cerebral palsy, especially the severe forms.

Recurrent chest infections may be related to aspiration of feeds or reflux. Vision and hearing assessments must be reviewed regularly. Constipation is a common problem related to immobility, poor voluntary muscle coordination and dietary factors. Recurrent urinary tract infections can occur due to bladder dysfunction. Associated urinary tract abnormality due to dysgenesis or a neurogenic bladder will need separate assessment and study. Specific complaints are unlikely to point to the cause for malaise in a severely handicapped child and much notice must be taken of parents or guardians who recognise the child to be unwell or out of sorts. The treatment of epilepsy is a common problem in this situation, when side effects of medication can be overlooked by those who do not know the child well.

Principles of management and preventable deformities

Once parents are given the news that their child has cerebral palsy, a system of social and professional support needs to be devised with due emphasis on how to manage everyday problems (**15.41**). Physio- and occupational therapists will advise on seating, posture, handling and feeding; speech therapists may also help parents to understand abnormal oral mechanisms as well as language development (*see* Chapter 3).

The hips and spine

The child who is not walking before three years of age, and an older immobile child with a scoliosis are both at high risk of hip subluxation (Cooke *et al.*, 1989). This can be painful, it restricts adequate seating and can hinder the development of walking skills. At risk children should be x-rayed at two and four years of age, or at any time clinical signs emerge. The risk of hip subluxation

211

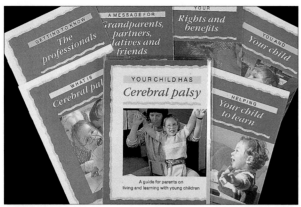

15.41 Information pack on cerebral palsy for parents, published by the Spastic Society.

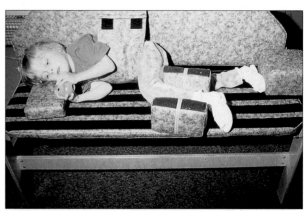

15.42 Side-lying board: an aid to improve posture in physiotherapy.

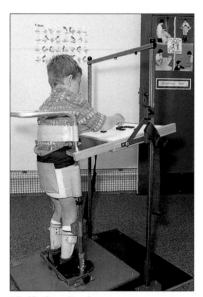

15.43 Standing frame.

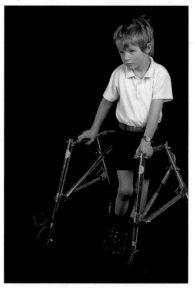

15.44. A boy with spastic athetoid cerebral palsy achieving an upright posture with a posterior Kaye–Walker.

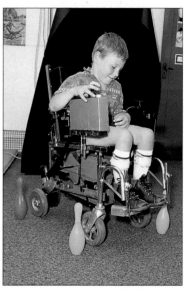

15.45 An electric wheelchair—well steered by a 6-year-old with four-limb spasticity.

may be minimised by maintaining an upright posture for periods of time (Scrutton, 1989). Standing frames enable this in the severely handicapped as long as contractures or profound hypotonia do not preclude this. Orthopaedic intervention may facilitate physiotherapy by the release of contractures, and in hypotonia prone-boards provide a degree of weight bearing through the hips and correct spinal deformities. In some children, an upright posture restores a degree of lumbar lordosis which is partially protective against progressive scoliosis.

In the very severely handicapped, side-lying boards may be all that the child can cope with to correct spinal posture for limited periods of the day (**15.42**).

Aids to posture and ambulation

The upright posture gives children added height and a fresh perspective on life (**15.43**). They adopt a more pos-

itive attitude as the new position brings more opportunity to participate and siblings and friends tend to include them more. The same advantage can be obtained from various technological advances such as mobile chairs with variable heights. There promises to be something of an explosion in such technology and, with advertising pressures added, there will be a need for well-resourced occupational therapists to guide families and doctors in their purchasing decisions. For children with adequate extensor tone, prone seating places the centre of gravity in front of the hip joints, instead of behind as in reclining seating, with postural and functional improvement for the child (Myhur *et al.*, 1992, p. 25). For those children who can walk with aids, posterior walkers may provide a better posture than foreward walkers (Logan *et al.*, 1991) (**15.44**). Electric chairs are usually viewed with enthusiasm by the child who toils with active physiotherapy (**15.45**). A degree of independence is achieved and children with athetosis can show great perceptual skills in steering their chairs in confined areas.

Antispasticity measures

Antispasticity agents such as baclofen may improve handling or function in spasticity. However, there may be side effects on general wellbeing and alertness which may be unacceptable to the parents, particularly of well-motivated children. Physiotherapy advice to parents and the child can help contain contractures. Night splints to ankles are an effective way of providing more than six hours each day of stretching the tendo-achilles (Tardieu *et al.*, 1988). Serial plastering over a few weeks may restore a range of movement. Knee contractures may be helped by soft splinting (Anderson *et al.*, 1988). Ankle-foot orthoses moulded in light plastic can be worn inside shoes and may be necessary to get more handicapped children into their standing frames. For valgus and varus deformities, footwear may be successfully adapted by wedging the soles to counteract the deformity, or in marked deformities, the attachment of below-knee calipers to footwear may be necessary.

Surgical measures

New techniques are being explored in a limited number of centres, to relieve spasticity by selective dorsal rhizotomy. Children likely to benefit are those with lower limb spasticity, high motivation and existing forward locomotion. Skilled pre-operative neurophysiological assessment is necessary but in well-selected cases spasticity will be reduced and gait improved (Neville, 1988, p. 257). Orthopaedic surgeons often face difficult decisions on the likely consequences of tendon release, tendon transfer or rotation osteotomies for the function of the child. Research coming from gait analysis laboratories promises to provide a more objective assessment (Patrick, 1991).

Communication

Computer systems open a new world of interaction and communication for those severely handicapped children who can operate a switch (**15.46**). No two handicapped children are identical in this regard. A painstaking search is required for solutions to the problems of adapting switches and programmes to the individual's needs. Cooperation must exist between computer scientists, the family, therapists, teachers and the child. Close ties are to be encouraged between therapists and University Departments with such skills. Finally, parents need to feel that their child's care is still in their hands. Advice must be shared at every level. Communication systems used at school should be learnt by parents as well. Advice on appropriate play and stimulating activities should make sure that home is a place of relaxed enjoyment, not an extension of school or a therapy session. The first reaction of parents, once they have begun to

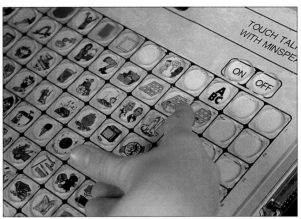

15.46 Dystonic posturing in this child still allows him to press the desired key for touch-talking.

cope with the shock and distress of knowing they have a handicapped child, is to want to know what they can do to help. Counselling sessions regarding diagnosis should be followed very soon by a therapy session in the Community. If there is one thing that the alternative therapies should have taught, it is that doctors often leave a vulnerable gap between delivering the diagnosis and constructing a positive approach.

Neuroradiology and the static encephalopathies

The development of neonatal ultrasound has allowed better definition and understanding of the contribution that haemorrhage and hypoxic-ischemic injury make to motor impairment; now magnetic resonance imaging (MRI) offers to improve our knowledge of the mechanisms involved in prenatal cerebral dysgenesis.

Ultrasound is the primary imaging modality in the neonate (see **Table 15.1,** overleaf). In certain clinical situations, CT provides a supplementary role as in the assessment of intracerebral mass lesions, certain congenital anomalies and in the demonstration of intracranial calcification. The use of MRI in this age group has also contributed to the further understanding of brain tumours, the pituitary gland, congenital anomalies and in the investigation of spinal congenital anomalies and mass lesions.

Normal anatomy

Role of imaging The demonstration of key signs including:

- The presence of blood
- Ventricular dilatation or asymmetry
- Periventricular white matter abnormalities
- Abnormal fluid collections
- Presence of intracerebral calcification
- Detection of abnormal intracerebral masses

TABLE 15.1 Grading of Periventricular/Intraventricular Haemorrhage

I	Subependymal haemorrhage
II	Intraventricular haemorrhage without ventricular dilatation
III	Intraventricular haemorrhage with ventricular dilatation
IV	Intraventricular haemorrhage with parenchymal haemorrhage

• Detection of abnormal intracerebral masses

These signs are present either individually or in combination in the following common groups of abnormalities encountered in this age group.

• Intracranial haemorrhage
• Intracranial infection
• Periventricular leukomalacia
• Cerebral neoplasms
• Congenital anomalies

Of these conditions, intracranial haemorrhage and periventricular leukomalacia will be considered further.

Intracranial haemorrhage

Germinal matrix haemorrhage is relatively easily diagnosed on ultrasound. Typically, it appears as an echogenic focus in the area of the caudate nucleus/caudothalamic notch. Germinal matrix haemorrhage may be unilateral but is frequently bilateral and symmetrical. Whilst such haemorrhages may remain confined to the subependymal germinal matrix, bleeding frequently breeches the overlying ependyma, extending into and expanding the entire ventricular system and subarachnoid space. Large intraventricular haemorrhages frequently lead to post-haemorrhagic hydrocephalus which in turn may cause further cerebral damage. Haemorrhages may involve almost the entire caudate nucleus and may obliterate the frontal horns by producing a mass effect upon the floor of the lateral ventricles. Although germinal matrix haemorrhages frequently completely involute over a period of weeks, a large germinal matrix haemorrhage often leaves behind a subependymal cyst. Small intraventricular haemorrhages may be somewhat difficult to diagnose with sonography but large intraventricular haemorrhages have typical appearances. Recent intraventricular haemorrhage is brightly echogenic. The internal echo characteristics of recent clots are homogeneous and isoechoic to the accompanying haemorrhage in the germinal matrix. In addition, haemorrhage is isoechoic with the normal choroid plexus. A small quantity of blood in the lateral ventricles presents a somewhat greater diagnostic challenge. Small isolated haematomas surrounded by CSF are most often found in the occipital horn or ventricular trigone. In addition, the formation of CSF-fluid levels is common in the dependent portions of the ventricles. Small intraventricular haemorrhages also commonly adhere to the rough surface of the choroid plexus.

On CT scanning, recent haemorrhage is readily identified by areas of increased attenuation. CT scanning accurately demonstrates the periventricular/intraventricular haematomas. The character and composition of blood clots change with time, becoming isodense and later hypodense over a period of 10 to 14 days.

Evaluation of post-haemorrhagic hydrocephalus (PHH) is usually accomplished by routine weekly cranial ultrasound examination. The size of the initial haemorrhage correlates reasonably well with the severity of the PHH. PHH is usually a self-limiting process. In patients with small haemorrhages, once stabilisation of the ventricular size has been established scans may be repeated less frequently than once a week. In patients with severe PHH, regular monitoring by means of ultrasound may be required. In severe cases of PHH, the sonographic appearances of hydrocephalus may be difficult to quantify because the effacement of the brain eliminates the normal anatomical landmarks. In cases of severe hydrocephalus, sonographic findings are frequently best interpreted in conjunction with the clinical measurements of head circumference.

Sequential ultrasound examinations reveal that the originally homogeneous clot undergoes central liquefaction, resulting in anechoic areas which gradually decrease in size, and eventually resolves. The absorption of the intraventricular blood clot may result in porencephaly developing weeks later. This is attributed to focal cerebral destruction. An area of porencephaly appears as a low lesion on CT and as an echoic area on ultrasound.

Periventricular leukomalacia

Periventricular leukomalacia (PVL) or infarction is the major non-haemorrhagic lesion found in pre-term infants dying in the neonatal period. Focal areas of necrosis are found particularly in the centrum semiovale, optic and acoustic radiations which are related to the frontal, occipital and temporal horns respectively. Ultrasonography demonstrates extensive bands of increased echogenicity around the lateral ventricles; sequential examinations showing the development of cystic areas in these sites. The areas of increased echogenicity are often bilateral and symmetrical. However, the sonographic diagnosis of PVL is complicated by the presence of areas of increased echogenicity that surround the lateral ventricles of normal neonates. Abnormal periventricular echogenicity is most likely the result of an acute infarctive process. As the initial infarction evolves, areas of liquefactive necrosis occur and small cysts begin to appear—cystic PVL. In more generalised cases, periventricular cysts may parallel both lateral ventricles. These cysts may be extremely small, measuring 2 to 3 mm. The identification of cystic degeneration about the lateral ventricles is diagnostic of PVL. Cystic degeneration, however, is not the end point of the infarctive process. Eventually, the cysts break down and form part of the lateral ventricles, resulting in 'pseudoventricle formation'.

On CT scanning, PVL is identified as areas of decreased attenuation. This appearance is very similar to undermyelination in a premature infant. Changes of cerebral atrophy in addition to the focal periventricular abnormalities indicate that the hypoxic insult may affect the entire brain.

CT is indicated for demonstrating blood in the subarachnoid spaces, in some cases of extensive intraventricular haemorrhage, and if the clinical findings are worse than suggested by the initial findings on ultrasound examination. Additional information from CT includes suspected haemorrhage within the posterior fossa, if a peripheral lesion appears most likely and if neurological signs are present.

MR is more sensitive than CT in the detection of subtle brain malformations and mild degrees of white matter damage. Babies born prematurely show periventricular white matter damage indicative of hypoxic-ischemic change though the timing of the insult is difficult. Truwit *et al.* (1992) showed half the babies born at term to have developmental anomalies, twice the rate reported with CT. Three major patterns of abnormality emerge:

• polymicrogyria consistent with mid-second trimester injury;
• isolated PVL reflecting late second or early third trimester injury;
• watershed cortical or deep grey nuclear damage consistent with late third trimester perinatal or post-natal injury.

Neuroradiology in the congenital infections

CT is more useful than sonography or MR in older children as many congenital infections produce calcification. The CT features are variable. Cerebral atrophy and calcification are the usual CT manifestations.

Neonatal herpes simplex encephalitis

CT shows the progressive development of patchy low attenuation in the deep white matter of both cerebral hemispheres. The cortex and central grey matter may become abnormally dense, due to multiple small haemorrhages initially, and calcification later. Atrophy becomes obvious within about three weeks. The early development of extensive calcification in gyri (especially along the grey-white matter junctions), basal ganglia and in the germinal matrix around the ventricles is a distinctive feature. Later, this becomes visible even on plain skull radiographs. Marked ventricular dilatation and heavy periventricular calcification is found especially when the disease was acquired *in utero*.

Cytomegalovirus   The commonest abnormalities are hydrocephalus and extensive periventricular calcification resulting from extensive subependymal necrosis.

Toxoplasmosis   Hydrocephalus and small multifocal intracerebral calcification, periventricular or cortical, may be seen. Occasionally, separation of the sutures may be present.

Chapter 16: Extrapyramidal Involuntary Movement Disorders

Pamela I. Tomlin, W. St. Clair Forbes

The extrapyramidal movement disorders encompass the most benign and the most progressive and distressing of neurological disorders. In the latter case, the search for amelioration with treatment has to be painstaking, as ready solutions are unlikely to be found. The extrapyramidal disorders manifest as distortions of posture which may be sustained or fleeting. Some forms are self-limiting, following reactions to drugs, intoxication or infection; others such as Wilson's disease, Segawa's syndrome and Gilles de la Tourette syndrome (TS) lend themselves more readily to treatment, whilst the neurodegenerative group is very difficult to modify.

The extrapyramidal system influences the motor system through polysynaptic connections via the basal ganglia and related subcortical nuclei (**16.1**). The caudate nucleus lies in the floor of the lateral ventricle, separated from the lenticular nucleus (composed of the putamen and globus pallidus) by fibres of the internal capsule. The subthalamic nucleus and the substantia nigra are functionally related to the basal ganglia (Clark, 1979).

The biochemical pathways which appear to predominate and around which treatments have evolved include dopaminergic, cholinergic and GABA fibres (**Table 16.1**, overleaf). The different syndromes may be thought of as those which have a poverty of movement; kinetic-rigid syndromes caused by dopaminergic underactivity and cholinergic overactivity; and dyskinesia with excessive involuntary movements caused by overactivity of dopaminergic pathways.

The quality of movement in the dyskinesias varies. It is best observed while the child tries to sustain a posture such as outstretching the limbs, or performing active movements such as in walking, taking a cup to drink, tying shoe laces or using a paper and pencil (**16.2 and 16.3**). Tremors are oscillatory. When the head is involved, this produces titubation, which may be noted on attempts to examine the fundi, when the examiner's hand supports the child's head. The movements of chorea are erratic and jerky, moving from one part of the body to another. Dystonia may be proximal, leading to

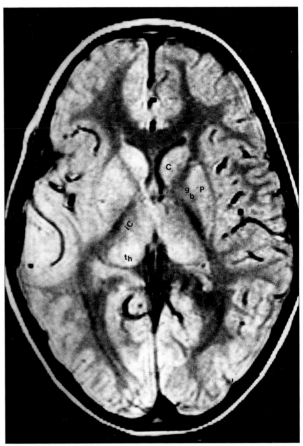

16.1 Basal ganglia on MR scan TI image: c = cordate nucleus; p = putamen; gb = globus pallidus; ic = internal capsule; th = thalamus.

rigid opisthotonic postures, or distal with the characteristic slow writhing movements of athetosis (**16.4 and 16.5**). Tics differ from chorea in that they are stereotyped, even if complex, for each individual. In all extrapyramidal disorders, the manifestations fluctuate in relation to emotional state, usually increasing with the patient's level of anxiety.

TABLE 16.1 The Rational Approach to Therapy in Extrapyramidal Movement Disorders

Rigid–akinetic states	Involuntary movements (tremor, chorea, torsion dystonia)
Dopamine agonists	*Dopamine antagonists*
L-Dopa (+ decarboxylase inhibitor)	Haloperidol ⎫
	Pimozide ⎬ Post-synaptic
Bromocriptine	Chlorpromazine ⎭
	Tetrabenazine Pre-synaptic
Anticholinergics ⎫	
Benzhexol ⎬	Tremor-responsive
Orphenadrine ⎮	Relatively high dose for dystonia
Benztropine ⎭	
	Cholinergics
	Choline chloride
	Lecithin

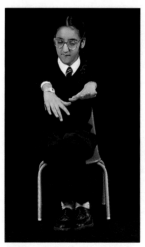

16.2 Familial recessive choreoathetosis: distal dystonic posturing.

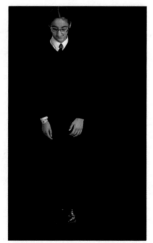

16.3 Familial recessive choreoathetosis: dystonic posturing of right leg held in adduction and flexion.

Benign forms

Tics

Tics are extremely common, and usually present in the juvenile years, particularly in relation to school entry. It is worth asking for some physical or mechanical origin to the repetitive movement. Persistent head jerking that began with a hairstyle that needed flicking from the eyes has been seen by the author. Contortions of the mouth and nose are common, as are eye-rolling movements. The child can demonstrate and control the movement at will. Prior to the movement, there is often a build up of tension and a compulsion is felt to perform the tic. The tic itself brings relief, acting as a source of comfort. The child often suffers too much attention by irritated observers, commonly parents or teachers. The movements are often most noticeable in moments of boredom or relaxation. Employing the child on a complex task will usually arrest the movements. Habits of eye rolling could be confused with absence attacks, but not if a careful description is obtained. The eye movements in tics span an elipse or part of an elipse rather than a direct vertical movement.

Myoclonic jerks are usually distinguished from tics by being simpler in form. Although they may not be accompanied by EEG changes, they are often only one form in a mixed epileptic disorder.

Another clue to the benign nature of tics is that one form is often given up for another over a period of time. Other nervous habits, like nail biting or lip licking leading to perioral soreness, may take their turn in this pro-

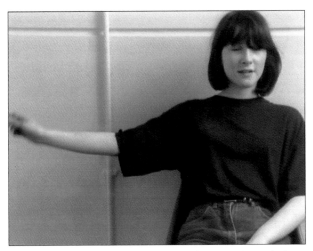
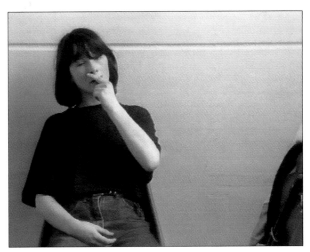

16.4 and 16.5 Video stills. (**16.4, left**) Distal writhing of athetosis. (**16.5, right**) Compromising accuracy of fine motor movement.

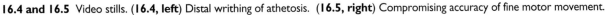

gression. It is worth looking for areas of predicament in the child's life. Children with learning difficulties may be under critical appraisal at home and at school. The capable child from whom much is expected may be under similar stress. Reassurance and advice on ignoring the tic is the most effective management.

Gilles de la Tourette syndrome

The similarities between TS and benign tics are the age of onset and the predominance of proximal and facial tics. Preliminary genetic studies suggest linkage withobsessive-compulsive disorder and Type II alcoholism. Shoulder shrugging movements are common and vocal tics, which are essential to the diagnosis, appear within a few years (Sweet *et al.*, 1973). These vary from barks, grunts, clicking and spitting to specific words or expletives which are often crude and embarrassing to the child. A sense of compulsion is experienced before the tic is exhibited. Although the tics canbe controlled for short periods, the affected person eventually must give way to the compulsion, with an associated feeling of relief. The compulsive experience of the child may be visible to the examiner as increasing restlessness and visible discomfort. Compulsive patterns of thought may be experienced. A family history of the disorder or of tics may be found. The presentation is juvenile or adolescent. A juvenile presentation in females carries a better prognosis with the chance of outgrowing the disorder in later years.

Clinical examination is essentially normal, although minorneurological asymmetries have been observed (Sweet *et al.*, 1973) with a predominance of left handedness. The EEG may show focal dysarrhythmias which do not coincide with the tic. Occasionally, cases may occur symptomatically as a result of infective or metabolic encephalopathy. The decision whether and how to treat is best in the hands of a practitioner with experience in the disorder. The necessary support and guidance on the social and psychological consequences often direct the children into the care of child psychiatry.

Haloperidol, benztropine, pimozide, clonidine and more recently fluoxitine have been used with success. Making the diagnosis does not make treatment obligatory. A decision to treat depends on the consequences of the disorder for the child's lifestyle.

Benign familial tremor

This is a tremor with an intentional element that makes it both embarrassing and disabling. It can present in childhood. Formal neurological examination of outstretched upper limbs and finger/nose testing reveal the signs, but they are better understood from the patient's point of view by observing activities. At the meal table, the child may prefer to have food cut up, using a fork in the dominant hand, reducing the reaching distance by lowering the head to the table and fixing the upper arm against the trunk. The embarrassed child may avoid taking drinks altogether at school or in company. Speed and legibilityof handwriting is compromised, making classwork and homework laborious. The skill of the occupational therapist is very valuable, both in monitoring treatment and in providing solutions such as lap-top computers at school. Extra time for examination should be considered in the 15–16 year olds. Drugs which maybe helpful include propanalol or primidone. Sometimes, patients find the intermittent use of propranolol helpful such as before weekend jobs such as serving at table.

Developmental dystonia

Transient dystonic patterns of movement have long been recognised in premature infants, whose extensor tone is predominant in the newborn period (Drillien, 1972). Follow-up shows that the majority of such signs disappear in the first year of life.

Other developmental dystonias have been reported, affecting upper and lower limbs, often on one side, when in turning of the leg and hyperpronation of the arm accompany movements (Willemse, 1986). The child may

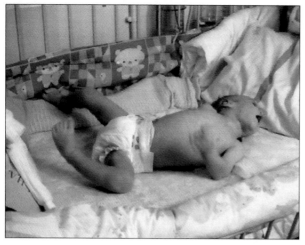

16.6 Severe choreoathetosis in early infancy: neck torsion, marked limb involvement.

crawl on the dorsal surface of one hand on the hyper-pronated side. Excessive bilateral adduction of the thumbs across the palm may also be seen. This can be an obvious nuisance to the well-motivated child reaching out at six months, but by 9–12 months the thumbs usually extend normally, allowing normal fine-finger performance to emerge.

Paroxysmal disorders

Paroxysmal dystonia on movement

These paroxysms may be of sustained dystonic posturing, often affecting only one side of the body, or choreic in form. They are shortlived, provoked by movement after a period of rest, with onset between six and 15 years of age. It is unusual, but helpful, for the clinician to have the opportunity to observe an episode, so a history is important. EEG monitoring during an episode may reveal a dysrhythmia, but standard recordings are usually normal. The condition usually responds to anticonvulsants. There may be a family history.

Paroxysmal dystonia of infancy

In this presentation, the predominant dystonia is truncal-with episodes of opisthotonus, limb extension and neck torsion (**16.6**). It can begin as early as three months (Andelini *et al.*, 1988) and the episodes can last from several minutes to two hours. They are not precipitated by movement, but can occur several times a day or only a few times per month. Awareness is maintained and because of reddening of the face and posturing, they may be mistaken for self-gratification episodes. There are no EEG abnormalities related and in Angelini's series all the children were normal developmentally and either outgrew their symptoms or experienced a dramatic reduction in frequency within two years. As this appears to be a benign disorder, which does not respond to anticonvulsants, treatment may not be required unless the symptoms cause distress, when clonazepam or haloperidol may help.

Drug reactions and intoxications

Acute extrapyramidal reactions to drugs are always dramatic with an almost uniformly good outcome. Dystonic reactions to drugs like metaclopramide have an onset within a short time of taking the dose, and are equally dramatically relieved by anticholinergic agents. It is less commonly realised that some regularly used anticonvulsants such as phenytoin, carbamazepine and diazepam, can rarely have the same effect. The problem subsides rapidly on cessation of medication and does not necessarily indicate that toxic doses are being taken, though that must be considered.

Tardive reactions, occurring after prolonged treatment with neuroleptic drugs, or after their withdrawal, are far less common in children. The outlook is good for children with the likelihood of recovery. Orofacial dyskinesia is a common presentation of the problem; choreiform reactions carry a better prognosis than dystonic reactions in the tardive form.

Carbon monoxide poisoning can lead to delayed extrapyramidal disorders. After a latent period of 7 – 10 days, the movements emerge. One such patient, known to the author, showed gross choreo-athetoid posturing especially in the supine position, and on attempting to do things for herself. Once on her feet she could walk correcting her balance, but needing an attendant. Retained alertness, with the variability and bizarre nature of the movements, together with the tendency to become worse under observation all conspire to raise the question of a functional disorder—a misjudgment to which all sufferers of dystonia are prone. In the case described, the choreo-athetoid phase subsided on clonazepam, only to be followed within a few weeks by an akinetic rigid Parkinsonian state. This responded to L-Dopa. The symptoms may take up to a year to subside.

Post-infectious disorders of movement

The choreic movements of Sydenham's chorea are very rarely seen now outside developing countries. As with many post-infectious neurological disorders, a viral illness is now likely to be implicated in causation and particularly since the decline in streptococcal virulence (**16.7 and 16.8**). The history of preceding infection is usually clear but specifying the agent may prove impossible. The symptoms are often predominantly unilateral.

When requested to outstretch the upper limbs, the patient does so with a poorly controlled shooting manoeuvre. 'Dinner-fork' posturing is seen, with an erratic dipping movement of the hand. On walking, there may be dystonic posturing of the leg with fidgety small movements to be looked for in the upper limbs. An associated dysarthria is common, with chewing and

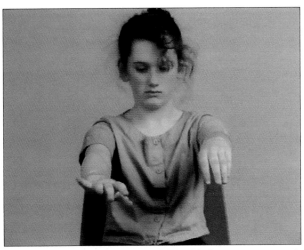 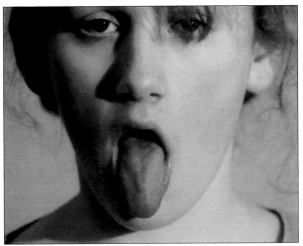

16.7 and 16.8 Video stills. (**16.7, left**) Post-streptococcal chorea: note asymmetry, distal athetosis. (**16.8, right**) Post strep-tococcal chorea: writhing of tongue.

swallowing difficulties. Formal examination of the palate is usually normal. The child can best describe for themselves the diffculties they have, with food lodging uncomfortably above the palate in the nasophary rnx. The child may complain of not always being able to draw breath normally, due to irregular involuntary movements affecting the trunk muscles. An explanation is warranted and reassurance. Some features may be subtle to the examiner who does not know the child well. Parents may comment that the child's facial expression is not normal for him, as well as noting the existence of facial grimacing. The quality of the voice may be altered, of which the parent and sometimes the patient will be aware.

A post-infectious diagnosis is one of exclusion. Important differential diagnoses include Wilson's disease (described in Chapter 14) and auto-immune disorders, especially systemic lupus erythematosis (*see* Chapter 9). Feelings of anxiety are not uncommon in those suffering from extrapyramidal disorder, but frankly psychiatric symptoms would alert to the possibility of Wilson's disease in the adolescent. The movement disorder in SLE may precede other arthritic or renal manifestations (King *et al.*, 1988). An associated arthralgia may support a post-infectious origin, or auto-immune basis, but it can also occur in Wilson's disease, as can a raised ESR. In Wilson's disease, the CT scan may show low attenuation in the basal ganglia and slit-lamp examination of the eyes should reveal evidence of Kayser–Fleischer rings. Copper studies should reveal low levels of serum copper and caeruloplasmin.

Other treatable or preventable extrapyramidal disorders

These are forms of dystonia which, though not benign or transient, are more readily controlled, or potentially preventable, than progressive neurodegenerative disorders.

A form of progressive dystonia which responds well to L-Dopa has been described by Segawa. The characteristic feature is the improvement after sleep and the progressive worsening of the symptoms as the day goes on (Deonna *et al.*, 1986). Wilson's disease untreated is progressive, but with dimethylcysteine therapy all the clinical symptoms can be reversed. Other correctable disorders with extrapyramidal consequences include hypocalcaemia, hypomagnesaemia, B_{12} deficiency and amino-acid and organic-acid disorders. In organic-acid disorders, such as proprionic acidaemia, early diagnosis may minimise cerebral damage; these children may have non-specific delayed development prior to the first acidotic episode. Dystonic and Parkinsonian presentations have been described in amino-acid disorders, such as homocystinuria (Kempster, 1988).

Head injury should be mentioned under the heading of a potentially preventable cause of dystonia. Sheering forces between the cortex and subcortical structures may be the mechanism of damage or deep contusions. The presentation is usually one of hemichoreoathetosis, delayed by a number of weeks after the injury (**16.9–16.12**). It may be very difficult to treat satisfactorily because of the unacceptability of side effects of treatment in an otherwise bright and normal child, and because of the limited benefit of drugs.

Herpes simplex encephalitis has been reported to relapse with extrapyramidal movements. CT-scan lesions remain confined to cortical areas (Shanks *et al.*, 1991) and the movement disorder disappears with time. Other viral infections or post-encephalitis illness may present with extrapyramidal features that gradually subside in time, so management should be supportive and reasonably optimistic.

Sandifer described abnormal truncal posturing associated with gastro-oesophageal reflux. Hyperextension or extreme lateral flexion of the trunk has been observed. This may occur during any activity including

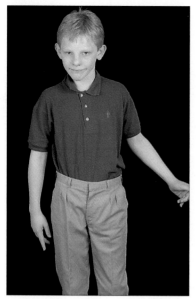

16.9 Post-traumatic chorea: ballis-
mic movement of left arm.

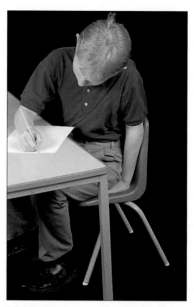

16.10 Post-traumatic chorea: same
boy as in **16.9**, sitting on arm to control movement to allow function.

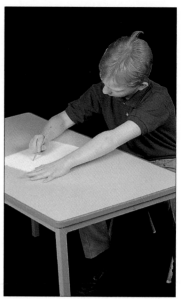

16.11 Post-traumatic chorea: the
arm freed, interfering with function.

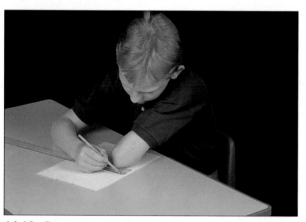

16.12 Post-traumatic chorea: control achieved with arm
flexed and adducted.

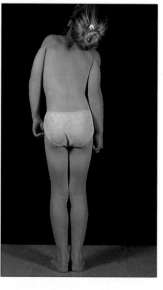

16.13 Bizarre posturing in
Sandifer's syndrome.

walking, giving rise to some bizarre forms of gait
(**16.13**). Confusion with torsion dystonia is possible, and
the diagnosis needs keeping in mind, as effective management of the hiatus hernia and reflux leads to complete resolution of the problem.

Neurodegenerative disorders

Dystonia musculorum deformans

This is one of the most distressing progressive disorders
presenting in childhood and idiopathic by definition. The
presentation may be focal, segmental or generalised.
Focal or segmental presentations under 10 years of age
are highly likely to become generalised, worsening over
five years on average, before plateauing (Marsden and
Quinn, 1990). Remissions are brief and drug management is difficult and disappointing, although a painstaking search for a response from L-Dopa, anticholinergic
agents, carbamazepine, baclofen or tetrabenazine is the
usual progression of treatment (Marsden, 1990).
Neurosurgical procedures are similarly undramatic in
their effect, but unilateral thalamotomy may benefit the
contralateral limbs.

The child is usually normal up to the mid-juvenile
years. The onset is insidious, with an altered gait first to
appear. An inverted dorsiflexed posturing of the feet is
accompanied by hyperextension of the knees and hips.
Posturing of the upper limbs in hyperextension and
hyperpronation may be seen alongside bizarre uncontrolled flexions of the upper limbs, which may end up
behind the child's back or behind the neck. In the gener-

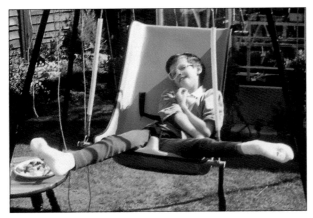

16.14 Hallervorden–Spatz disease: bizarre posturing in a progressive extrapyramidal disorder.

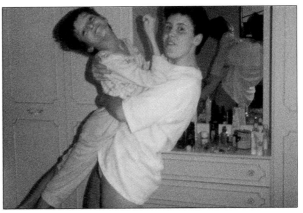

16.15 Hallervorden–Spatz disease: requiring tracheostomy.

alised form, the progression can involve the trunk and rob the child of mobility. Prolonged spasms can be exhausting to the child, accompanied by sweating and tachycardia. The quality of the voice changes, and occasionally, in the most severe cases, speech may be lost along with the ability to chew and swallow. Facial grimacing accompanies the spasms. With loss of control of the airway, feeding becomes an unpleasant experience accompanied by episodes of coughing and choking so that gastrostomy may be required. There is no intellectual deficit and a full multidisciplinary approach is needed to bring what comfort, interest and stimulation is possible to daily life.

Neurometabolic disorders

Children with progressive dystonia should be investigated for a neurometabolic diagnosis. White matter disorders such as metachromatic leukodystrophy and Pelizaeus–Merzbacher disease have extrapyramidal features. Globoid bodies are to be found in the basal ganglia in Hallervorden–Spatz disease, which is accompanied by cortical atrophy in time (**16.14 and 16.15**). These disorders lead to regression, with the emergence of pyramidal tract signs and intellectual deterioration in time.

Abnormalities of pyruvate metabolism, as in Leigh's encephalopathy, and mitochondrial cytopathies may also affect the extrapyramidal system (**16.16**). Estimation of plasma and CSF lactate can be helpful, although levels may only intermittently be raised. Mitochondrial disorders may be very difficult to diagnose in life when they affect the central nervous system, as they may be organ-specific, showing no mitochondrial abnormalities in accessible tissue such as muscle. Unfortunately, effective treatments do not yet exist and genetic understanding of mitochondrial disorders is still being researched (Harding, 1991). DNA deletions may be identified with a low recurrence risk.

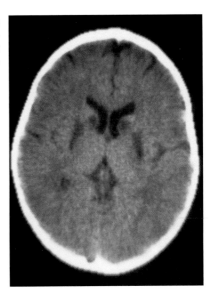

16.16 CT: Leigh's disease. Symmetrical low-density areas in basal ganglia.

Neuroradiology and the involuntary movement disorders

The CT and MR appearances of known metabolic and neurodegenerative disorders which lead to involuntary movements are discussed in Chapters 13 and 14. The most commonly encountered are probably the 'holes' (low attenuation areas seen on CT) in the basal ganglia seen in the mitochondrial cytopathies.

Basal ganglia calcification

Calcification of the basal ganglia is readily detected by CT; white has greater sensitivity than skull radiographs for the detection of calcium. Numerous disorders may have associated basal ganglia calcification. In many instances, there are distinguishing features, and the calcification will also be distributed throughout the cerebral parenchyma (*see* **Table 16.2**).

TABLE 16.2:   Basal Ganglia Calcification

Congenital	Idiopathic cerebrovascular ferrocalcinosis (Fahr's disease)
	Tuberous sclerosis
	Cockayne syndrome
	Kearns–Sayre syndrome
	Tay–Sach's disease
Infective	Cytomegalic inclusion disease
	Toxoplasmosis
	Post-viral encephalitis
	Congenital rubella
	Cysticercosis
Metabolic	Hypoparathyroidism
	Pseudo-hypoparathyroidism
	Pseudo-pseudo-hypoparathyroidism
	Secondary hyperparathyroidism
	Acquired immune deficiency syndrome
Vascular	Angioma
	Aneurysm
Neoplastic	Glioma
Toxins	Methrotrexate
	Carbon monoxide
	Lead
	Radiation

Fahr's disease

In this idiopathic group of conditions, there is an association of intracranial calcification with progressive mental deterioration, severe growth disorder and familial occurrence. CT reveals symmetrical calcification within the basal ganglia and cerebral cortex. Calcification may also be noted in the vermis, dentate nucleus and surrounding cerebellar white matter (**16.17**).

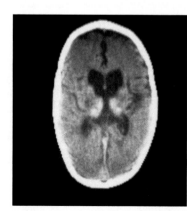

16.17 Fahr's disease. CT scan showing symmetrical basal ganglia calcification with ventricular enlargement and dilated whiter hemispheric fissure in cortical sulci.

Chapter 17: Diseases of the Spinal Cord

Michael J. Noronha

Symptomatology of spinal cord lesions

Clinical features which may follow a focal lesion of the spinal cord at a particular level include:

1. Radicular symptoms: An irritative lesion of one posterior spinal root causes pain referred to the corresponding dermatome; that is, the area of skin innervated by that root (*see* **Table 17.1**). Root pains are likely to be made worse by coughing and sneezing. The dermatome is likely to be hyperalgaesic and hyperaesthetic until the lesion interferes with conduction in the root, when appreciation of light touch and pin-prick is impaired over the dermatome.

A lesion of an anterior spinal root causes the features of a lower-motor-neurone lesion in the muscles innervated by the corresponding spinal segment.

2. Sensory impairment: A lesion of the posterior columns of the spinal cord leads to impairment of appreciation of posture, passive joint movement, and vibration below the level of the lesion on the same side. A lesion

TABLE 17.1 Neurological Pictures of Spinal Cord Injuries: Clinical Picture

A. Focal or transvere injuries	
C 1 - 4	Respiratory paralysis. Complete quadriparesis. Rapid death.
C 5 - 6	Flaccid quadriparesis in early stage – spastic later. Diaphragmatic movements spared. Sensory level at 2nd rib. Bilateral Horner's syndrome.
T 12 - L 1	Flaccid paralysis of lower limbs. Loss of sensation below inguinal ligament.
Conus medullaris	Urinary retention.
Cauda equina	Disturbance of rectal sphincter. Loss of sensation over lumbo-sacral dermatome. Flaccid paralysis of lower extremities.
B. Brown-Séquard	Unilateral muscle weakness. Contralateral disturbances of superficial sensation, especially pain or temperature.
C. Central cord lesion	Disproportionately more motor impairment of upper extremities (due to involvement of the more medial segments of lateral corticospinal tracts). LMN lesion of upper extremities. UMN lesion of lower extremities. Bladder dysfunction (usually urinary retention). Varying degrees of sensory loss, usually pain and temperature below level of lesion. Relatively good prognosis.

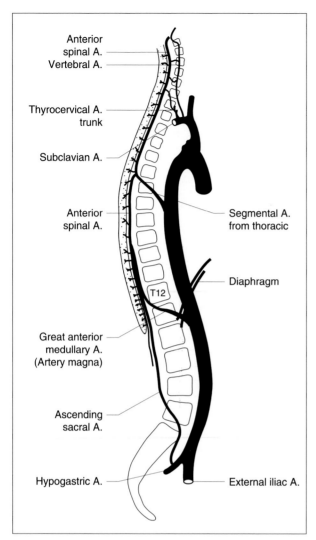

17.1 Blood supply of spinal cord: the anterior median spinal artery is joined at various levels by arteries which arise from the vertebral and subclavian arteries, the aorta, and the iliac arteries.

involving the spinothalamic tracts causes impairment of appreciation of pain, heat and cold on the opposite side of the body.

3. Corticospinal tract symptoms: damage to the corticospinal tract results in an upper-motor-neurone lesion, with weakness, spasticity, increased tendon reflexes, diminished abdominal reflexes, and an extensor plantar response below the level of the lesion on the same side.

4. Reflexes: A lesion of the spinal cord will impair or abolish a reflex whose arc passes through the segment involved. Reflexes mediated by segments below the level of the lesion willshow the changes characteristic of a corticospinal lesion.

5. Autonomic features: Sweating will be abolished over the area of skin which receives its sympathetic innervation from the segment of the spinal cord affected. Excessive sweating may occur over the area which

receives its sympathetic innervation from below the level of the lesion. The sympathetic outflow from the spinal cord is limited to the thoracic and first lumbar segments. The normal reflex activity of the urinary bladder and rectum is abolished in acute or rapidly developing severe lesions of the spinal cord, resulting in retention of urine and faeces. When reflex activity of the spinal cord is well established, reflex evacuation of the bladder and rectum occurs.

Spinal shock

This syndrome occurs in acute spinal cord lesions and represents a transient decrease of synaptic excitability in neurones distal to the injury. All deep tendon reflexes are lost, the plantar responses cannot be elicited or are downgoing, and there is flaccid paralysis below the level of the lesion. Sphincter tone is generally little affected and there is complete urinary retention. If the injury has not been too severe, reflexes return, voluntary control is re-established, and motor recovery begins within hours or days of injury. If cord injury is severe, recovery of reflexes is accompanied by reflex facilitation, which may occur within days or weeks and is unaccompanied by any evidence of improved sensation or voluntary motor activity below the level of the lesion.

Blood supply of the spinal cord

The arterial blood supply is derived from several sources. There are two posterior spinal arteries, each arising from the corresponding vertebral or posterior inferior cerebellar artery. The single anterior spinal artery is formed by the union of a branch from each vertebral artery, and the spinal arteries are reinforced by segmental arteries which enter the spinal canal through the intervertebral foramina (**17.1**). Three of these, which are of particular importance, are situated in the lower cervical, the lower dorsal (arteria magna) and the upper lumbar region. The spinal veins terminate in a plexus in the pia mater and pass upwards into the corresponding veins of the medulla oblongata. Additionally, segmental veins pass outwards along nerve roots from the internal vertebral plexus, in which blood also flows upwards to the intracranial venous sinuses.

Syringohydromyelia

Syringohydromyelia is characterised by the presence of a longitudinal, fluid-filled cavity within the spinal cord. Presentationis rare in childhood. Dissociated sensory loss is seen, with loss of pain and temperature, but retention of light touch in one or both arms, and wasting of the small muscles of the hand with pyramidal signs in the legs.

CT myelography will demonstrate a smoothly-enlarged cervical spinal cord, although in one third of cases the cord may be either normal or reduced in size due to atrophy. Delayed CT scanning (up to 24 hours) will in most cases demonstrate contrast medium within the cavity. The sagittal T1-weighted MR sequence usually provides the most useful information. T2-weighted images can be useful to demonstrate intra-cavitary fluid turbulence and movement (signal void). Multiplanar MR is the method of choice for demonstrating the presence of a syrinx and the presence of a an associated Chiari malformation (*see* Chapter 12).

Management involves decompression of the syrinx, accompanied by marsupialisation, shunting or decompressing the fourth ventricle outlet to minimise the risk of recurrence.

Tethered cord syndrome

The most common tethering lesions are a lipoma of the conus and filum, a thickened (tight) filum terminale, diastematomyeila and myelomeningocele. An associated defect in the overlying skin is seen in almost half the cases. The conus medullaris ascends the spinal column with foetal development, reaching its final position at three months of age. Subsequent differential growth of the spinal column and cord may lead to the appearance of, or deterioration in, existing neurological signs. These most commonly take the form of a distal segmental motor deficit in the leg and sphincter disturbance. Surgery should arrest the deterioration.

These abnormalities are demonstrated on either CT myelography or MRI scanning. The lipoma has a characteristic appearance on both CT and MRI scanning. On CT, the lipoma appears as a low attenuation (fat density) mass intimately related to the low tethered cord.

Diastematomyelia

This is the presence of a cleft within the spinal cord resulting in two hemicords, which usually extend over a limited number of segments. This usually lies between the ninth thoracic and first lumbar level. There may be associated neuronal and mesodermal hyopoplasia,with segmental neurological signs. Deterioration may result from mild trauma from traction at the level of the bony spur. Surgical intervention may arrest this progression.

Plain films are nearly always abnormal, but the bony spur may be difficult to detect. CT myelography and MRI will demonstrate the two hemicords, which are usually equal in size. The hemicords unite below the level of the defect to form one cord. The canal is invariably widened at the site of the split cord. The dura and arachnoid may be duplicated,with an osteocartilagenous or fibrous spur penetrating the lower part of the intradural cleft.

Spinal cord injury

Injury to the spine and spinal cord is an infrequent occurrence in the paediatric age group, and is often accompanied by a lack of radiological evidence of fracture or dislocation. Spinal cord injury is seen in accidents marked by sudden hyperflexion or hyperextension of the neck, or vertical compression of the spine by falls on the head or buttocks, as may occur from diving into shallow water or falling from a horse. In physically abused infants, spinal cord injuries may be induced by violent shaking of the head.

Spinal cord concussion

This may be seen occasionally in cases of blunt trauma to the spine, unassociated with flexion/rotation forces. In such cases, there may be temporary reversible loss of cord function. Signs of recovery usually appear within several hours, and the total loss of cord function beyond the first two or three hours is almost always associated with some degree of permanent neurological deficit. When the spinal cord is seriously compromised, the clinical picture is characterised by spinal shock affecting the distal segments, and the child experiences complete loss of motor and sensory function in the segments caudal to the injury. There is complete areflexia of variable duration, usually lasting two to six weeks. Depending on the severity of the spinal cord injury, the final picture may be one of purely reflex activity of the isolated cord. With less extensive injuries, muscular function and/or subjective sensation may return over the course of the next few months up to a year. The clinical picture of the most common spinal cord injuries is summarised in **Table 17.1**.

Disorders predisposing to spinal cord injury

Achondroplasia Neurological disorders may be produced by structural anomalies of the cranium (resulting in hydrocephalus) and spinal cord (producing spinal and radicular compression). The spinal canal has a decreased cross-sectional area and the intervertebral foramina are narrowed. Cervical-occipital compression is most frequent in childhood, and may occur in the first months of life.

Down's syndrome Abnormal anterio-posterior movement of the atlas on the axis, termed atlanto-axial subluxation, may be seen in children with Down's syndrome (**17.2**). A pathological degree of separation between the arch of the atlas and the odontoid peg is defined as greater than 3 mm on a lateral radiograph of the cervical spine in flexion. Myelopathy at this level may result from direct compression of the spinal cord and uncommonly as a result of vertebral artery compression.

Mucopolysaccharidoses Cervical myelopathy is a common complication of mucopolysaccharidosis Type IV (Morquio syndrome). Ligamentous laxity combined with a deformed, hypoplastic odontoid peg puts children thus affected at great risk of acute and/or chronic cervical cord disease.

Anterior atlanto-axial instability and the develop-

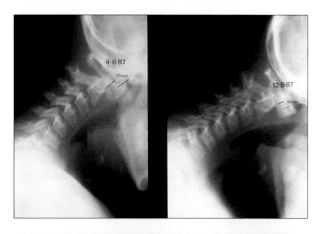

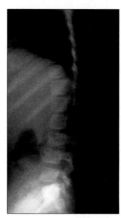

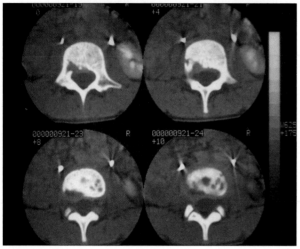

17.4 Discitis: CT scan of L3 vertebra showing destruction of body of vertebrae.

ment of anterior extradural soft-tissue thickening is the major cause of spinal cord compression at the craniocervical junction. This may be exacerbated by thickening of the posterior longitudinal ligament, invagination of the posterior arch of the atlas into the foramen magnum, or stenosis of the foramen magnum. The neurological insult may be acute and fatal, or more commonly, a chronic myelopathy develops over the early years of life.

Chronic myelopathy usually presents as reduced exercise tolerance, and progresses to frank pyramidal signs initially in the lower extremities, followed, if untreated, by weakness of the upper limbs. Eventual tetraparesis and respiratory paralysis lead to death in the twenties or thirties.

The clinical course can be modified by posterior occipito-cervical fusion,which stablises the upper cervical spine and prevents the progression of the myelopathy. In many cases at operation,the cervical cord is already seen to be damaged, and consideration should be given to performing the procedure early in life before the onset of cord damage.

Cervical myelopathy has been reported in other mucopolysaccharidoses (e.g. MPS I and II), but is much less common, and rarely requires active management.

Transverse myelitis

Transverse myelitis is an inflammation of the spinal cord, usually involving both grey and white matter in a considerable part of its transverse extent. It may be due to a variety of causes, some of which have not yet been identified. It may be caused by some form of demyelinating disorder, often complicating an infection, or may be due to the spread of bacterial infection, pyogenic (**17.3 and 17.4**) or tuberculous, to the cord. Pathologically, the spinal cord is generally softened, with the lower thoracic region most commonly involved. The lesion may be focally transverse or extend over several segments.

The onset of symptoms is acute or subacute, and there is usually some fever. Pain in the back at the level of the lesion is often prominent. There is usually rapidly progressive weakness of the lower extremities, accompanied by loss of sensation and sphincter control. In the ascending form of myelitis, there is a more or less rapid upward progression of the level of paralysis and sensory loss. Acute transverse myelitis must be distinguished from acute infectious polyneuritis, and from spinal cord compression caused by a space-occupying lesion. Cord compression is an acute neurosurgical emergency and must be excluded as soon as possible by metrizamide-myelography, which may be complemented by CT scanning if necesary. The prognosis of acute myelitis (non-bacterial) is usually good. About 60 % of patients have good return of function, and only 15 per cent fail to show any significant improvement. There is no evidence that corticosteroid therapy has any significant effect on the outcome of illness.

Spinal tumours

Tumours of the spinal canal are approximately 6–7 times less frequent than those in the intracranial compartment, and account for only 6–10 % of CNS tumours. A third of intraspinal tumours are intramedullary tumours, 24 % are intradural but extramedullary, and approximately 43 % are extradural.

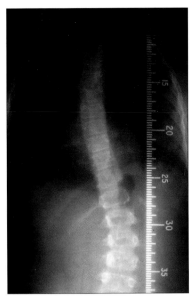

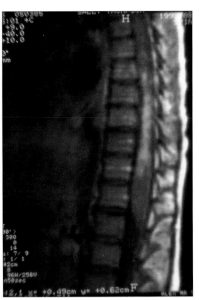

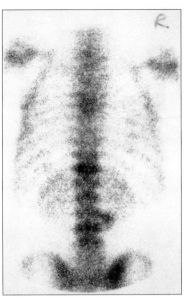

17.5 Spinal cord tumour: x-ray of dorso-lumbar spine illustrating scoliosis and narrowing of pedicles of D12–L1 vertebrae.

17.6 Spinal cord tumour: MRI scan—T2 imaging—illustrating widening of spinal cord at D11–L1 region with presence of hypodense areas suggesting an intramedullary tumour.

17.7 Gamma camera picture indicating increased uptake in mid-dorsal and lumbar vertebrae and right sacral region, suggesting multiple tumour deposits.

Clinical features

Presenting symptoms depend on whether the tumour arises within or outside the spinal cord. Intramedullary lesions usually produce symmetrical weakness and atrophy of the affected segments; extramedullary tumours tend to begin with unilateral pain in segmental distribution, often accompanied by paraesthesiae and numbness. Whether the tumour is situated within the cervical region or at the cranio-cervical junction, torticollis may result (**17.5**). In both types of tumour, impairment of gait, pain and stiffness in the back or legs commonly occur. Later, urinary incontinence and sensory deficits also appear. An expanding tumour may compromise the arterial or venous circulation to the cord, producing a sudden and irreversible paraplegia.

Imaging techniques

CT myelography (using water-soluble contrast media) and MRI are the two techniques for demonstrating intramedullary, extramedullary-intrathecal and extrathecal tumours. MRI has become the method of choice for investigating these tumours, in view of its multi-planar facility. MRI has a high sensitivity for detecting lesions within the spinal cord, and can show multiple lesions which may influence patient management. MRI will show a change in cord contour (best seen on T1-weighted images) and abnormal signal intensity that is often demonstrated on T2-weighted images (**17.6**). Similarly, cystic lesions are well demonstrated on MRI. MRI and CT will also evaluate any bone involvement. Bone metastases (**17.7**) exhibit a low signal on T1-weighted

images against a background of high signal marrow fat. Gadolinium DPTA allows the detection of small low-contrast lesions, and often reveals lesions which are not apparent on unenhanced MRI.

Role of imaging

1. Diagnosis.
2. Accurate location of abnormality.
3. Differentiation of cystic from solid lesion.
4. Detection of tumour recurrence.
5. Detection of post-irradiation or post-surgical changes.

Intrinsic cord tumours

These are either ependymomas or astrocytomas (**17.8**). Ependymomas are the commonest tumours of the lower cord, conus and filium terminale. Astrocytomas in children are found mostly in the cervical region. Cysts can occur within an intramedullary tumour which is surrounded by abnormal glial elements and containing haemorrhagic or xanthochromic fluid, which can be readily detected on MR scanning.

Myelography shows fusiform expansion of the spinal cord and, when followed by CT, the cord contour is clearly seen. The distinction between syringohydromyelia and cystic or even solid intramedullary tumours can be difficult on CT. MRI, however, can accurately differentiate between a solid and cystic lesion. Solid tumours may show heterogeneous enhancement following gadolinium DPTA. Sagittal-plane MRI will accurately demonstrate the superior and inferior extent of an infiltrating intramedullary tumour (**17.9 and 17.10**).

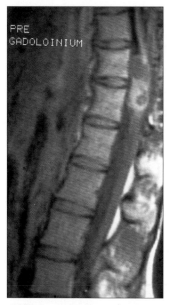

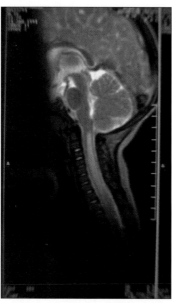

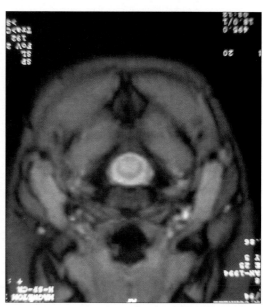

17.8 Intramedullary ependymoma (lower thoracic region)—MRI. Sagittal T1W pre-contrast. The cord is expanded and shows a well-defined mass.

17.9 Intramedullary tumour—MRI, sagittal. Diffusely expanded cord showing large area of increased signal extending from the foramen magnum to the first thoracic vertebra.

17.10 Lumbar meningocoele—MRI, axial T1W. Large lumbo-sacral spina bifida with meningocoele with dorsal tethering.

Intradural extramedullary metastases

Metastatic seeding from intracranial tumours such as medulloblastoma, ependymoma and pinealoma commonly occurs and influences both the management and prognosis. The diagnosis of drop metastases is usually made by CT myelography or MR. They appear as discrete spherical nodules attached to the nerve roots or spinal cord. Gadolinium-enhanced MRI matches the sensitivity of myelography supplemented with CT.

Arachnoid leukaemic infiltration is recognised on imaging as thickened roots of the cauda equina. However, the root thickening can also be a manifestation of neurofibromatosis.

Extradural tumours

Primary and secondary neuroblastoma (**17.11**) and sarcoma are the commonest extradural tumours. MRI is the preferred method to demonstrate the cord compression, the extradural soft-tissue mass. The bone destruction is best demonstrated on CT or plain films.

Other investigations

Where germ cell tumours are considered a possible diagnosis, blood serum levels of beta HCG (human chorion gonadatrophin) and alphafetoprotein are estimated prior to surgery. These markers, where raised, alter the management of such tumours from one of surgery to chemotherapy and radiotherapy. In such circumstances, even in the presence of raised serum markers, it may be considered advisable to carry out a stereotactic biopsy to confirm the histology.

Management of spinal cord disease

The acute stage

Emphasis at this stage is on establishing the diagnosis and ruling out a compressive lesion. If a compressing lesion is identified, urgent decompression by means of laminectomy should be secured. Ventilation should be supported where necessary and the bladder drained.

Long-term management

When recovery is not complete, children need help and long-term rehabilitation. There are a number of spinal cord injury centres in the UK where this process might begin. The largest hurdle is psychological readjustment to the level of disability.

Children with a newly acquired paraparesis usually go through a grief reaction; the process of readjustment can be facilitated with the expert help of the clinical psychology and child psychiatry service.

Periodic review of the non-physiological consequences of the spinal cord lesion is required:

Hypoventilation May require permanent ventilatory support or perhaps just night-time assistance by means of a cuirass or other device. Repeated chest infection may justify antibiotic prophylaxis.

Bladder disturbance Needs careful assessment with

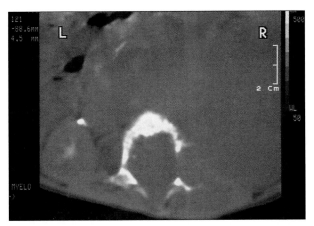

17.11 Neuroblastoma (spine). CT scan. Axial section through L1 showing a grossly expanded canal with a large, associated retroperitoneal soft-tissue mass extending into the right renal fossa.

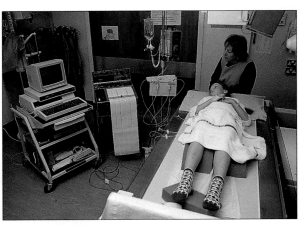

17.12 Cystometry in progress. Bladder pressure is measured as the urinary bladder is filled with contrast and video cystography performed.

radiological and urodynamic study (**17.12–17.14**). Only this will allow a rational decision to be made on the need for intermittent catheterisation, an indwelling catheter or even urinary diversion. The blood pressure needs checking regularly. Antibiotic prophylaxis may be needed.

Bowel disturbance   This requires attention to diet and laxatives. In general, a high lesion (above L1) is best treated with a low-residue diet, whereas a low lesion is best managed with a high-residue diet and regular laxatives or enemas.

Skeletal deformity   This may be avoided by due attention to seating, the control of spasticity with drugs, and regular physiotherapy.

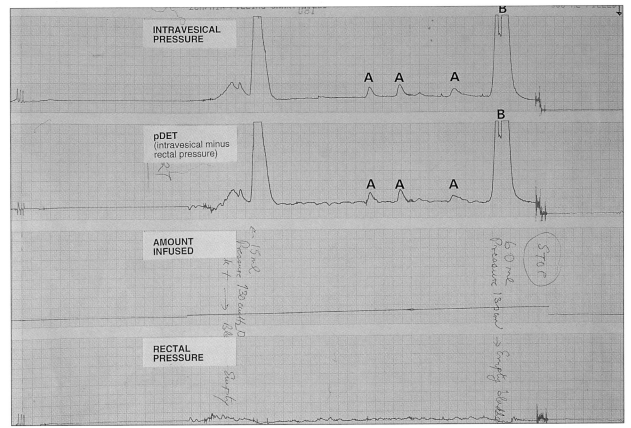

17.13 pDET is the detrussor pressure which is determined by subtracting intra-abdominal pressure measured with a rectal catheter from the intravesical pressure. The trace shows detrusor instability with uninhibited rises of bladder pressure (A) and then detrusor hyper-reflexia when the patient voids involuntarily (B).

Indications for cystometry

1. Spina Bifida cystica
2. Spinal dysraphism + neurological abnormality
3. Neurological disease + hydronephrosis
4. Severe urinary frequency
5. Incontinence of urine
6. A palpable bladder after voiding

17.14 Indications for cystometry.

Chapter 18: Genetics

Maurice Super

Genetics of childhood neurological disorders

This chapter will deal with recent advances in our understanding of some genetic disorders of the nervous system. Some are described in more detail, as examples of recent progress.

Disorders are recognised to have a chromosomal or genetic nature, because of either abnormal laboratory tests or the observation of inheritance patterns. Where the protein product of the gene is known, it is a fairly simple task to discover the chromosome localisation by somatic cell hybrid experiments with mouse and human chromosomes. Such hybrids shed human chromosomes selectively, allowing testing for the presence or absence of the gene product. Thus, the chromosome localisation of most enzyme defects is known.

For many diseases, the gene product is not known: it is the inheritance pattern which reveals the presence of a genetic disorder. The location and nature of many of these genes are now being elucidated, by studying families in which there is more than one affected individual. Normally occurring polymorphic markers are tested for in family members, searching for those which give the same patterns in affected individuals.

An example is seen in **some** families with Tuberous Sclerosis (TS), where there is linkage of the condition to the blood group locus on chromosome 9 (**18.1**) or 16.

Here, the TS gene appears to be segregating with blood group A. Obviously, the more people studied within a family, the higher the probability that the observation is correct. A log of the odds of this being correct or LOD score can be calculated. A LOD score of greater than three indicates odds of 1000 to one or greater that the disease and marker are linked, and that the chromosome on which the marker is known to be located is

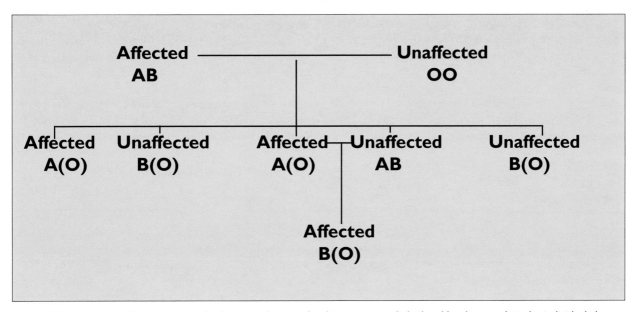

18.1 Linkage between blood group and tuberose sclerosis: the disease gene is linked to blood group A in the individual shown. A recombination in generation III leads to the diseased gene travelling with blood group O.

> **STAGES**
> - Recognition of genetic nature by pedigree analysis+/- laboratory test.
> - Finding a relevant linkage to allow chromosomal assignment.
> - Discovery of the actual gene and its defects, allowing pathogenesis to be better understood.
> - Application to diagnosis and family studies: DNA analyisis immunochemistry, *in situ* hybridisation.
> - Treatment.

18.2 Stages in gene localisation.

worthy of detailed study. Clinical usefulness of such marker studies in a family depends on the crossover rate, or distance between the marker and disease of interest. The distance is expressed in centiMorgans. Ten cM would indicate a 10 % error rate were such a marker to be applied to a family study. In the TS example above, if A(O)——AB from the second generation (*see* **18.1**) had an affected individual with blood group B, then this would indicate that a meiotic cross-over had occurred, with the TS gene now on the same chromosome as the O blood group. The estimated frequency with which this would occur gives the error rate in centiMorgans. It must be noted that linkage of TS with the ABO blood group locus can only be demonstrated in some families.

The number of polymorphic markers available for study has been greatly expanded artifically by the creation of restriction-fragment polymorphisms (RFLP's) with restriction enzymes which cut DNA at sites which they recognise by the occurrence of specific sequences of a few base pairs. Resulting differences in the lengths of the normally occurring fragments may allow the two chromosomes in an individual to be differentiated from one another in the region of the polymorphism, and this can be exploited in the family studies.

Once a gene has been localised to a particular portion of a chromosome, a series of experiments follow which may involve long- or short-range analysis close to the gene itself, with reducing error rates in using the linked markers so discovered (**18.2**). Eventually, the normal gene itself is isolated, recognised by promotional signals such as: the so-called TATA box, regions rich in the base pairs G and C; in open reading frames; in the occurrence of the gene in lower species (indicating its importance); and, ideally, recognition of the RNA from the gene in specific tissues known to be involved in the disease process. The discovery of the genes for dystrophin and cystic fibrosis transmembrane regulator are paradigms of this type of work.

Once the gene has been discovered, it can be used in diagnosis confirmation, family studies, and as a basis of

rational therapy. A Human Genome Project is being actively supported in North America and Europe, with the aim of locating all human genes. Figure **18.2** summarises the stages in gene localisation.

Chromosome disorders

It is of interest that partial monosomy or trisomy of any of the autosomes results in mental handicap. Presumably, this is the effect of enzyme or protein imbalance on our most sophisticated functions. Sex chromosome alteration has a lesser effect on intellectual function. Females with Turner's syndrome have difficulty with abstract mathematics as an isolated learning difficulty. Men with 47XXY Klinefelter's syndrome have no learning difficulties, but are vulnerable for psychiatric illness. Those with 48XXXY or 49XXXXY have significant intellectual impairment. Males with 47XYY are invariably tall; there is an increased incidence of behaviour disturbance in childhood and aggressive criminal behaviour in adults.

Studies of people who have a trisomy for different parts of chromosome 21 have determined that the genetic material responsible for the phenotypic expression of Down's syndrome lies on the long arm between segments 21q22.1 and 22.3. This small portion accounts for perhaps only 50 to 100 genes in all, the function of only a few of which has been established to date (**18.3–18.5**).

Mosaic chromosome disorders

When a mosaic of a normal cell line and an aneuploidic line co-exist, different tissues may demonstrate different proportions of the two types. In blood lymphocyte culture, there is a tendency, usually age-related, for the abnormal cell line to die off. Thus lymphocyte analysis may give a spurious normal result or show far fewer abnormal cells than are present in other tissues. When this is suspected, skin biopsy may be needed and fibroblast culture analysed. A specific disorder where this-

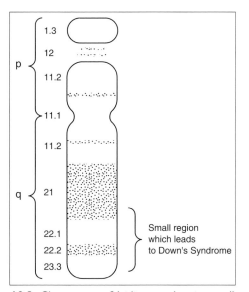

18.3 Chromosome 21 idiogram showing small region that, when trisomic, results in Down's syndrome.

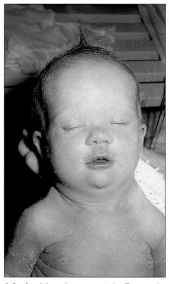

18.4 Newborn with Down's syndrome. Hypotonia, mongoloid slant to eyes, epicanthic folds.

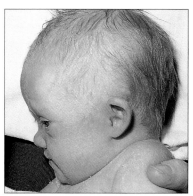

18.5 Newborn with Down's syndrome: flat occiput, small ears, hypoplastic nasal bridge.

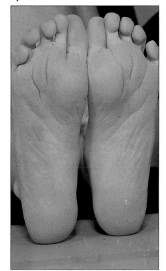

18.6 Trisomy 8 mosaic: longitudinal anterior plantar creases.

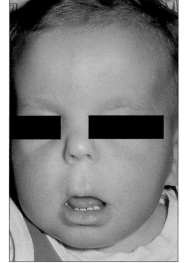

18.7 Tetrasomy 12p: anterior balding, thin upper lip, full lower lip, severe learning difficulties (diagnosis by skin biopsy).

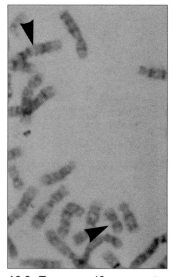

18.8 Tetrasomy 12p: composite extra chromosome, comprising 2 chromosomes, 12 short arms (arrowed) present in some cells.

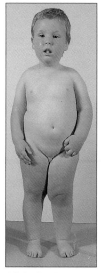

18.9 Prader–Willi syndrome: almond-shaped palpebral fissure, obesity, hypogenitalism.

might be necessary is Trisomy 8 mosaic, where characteristic 'cat's paw' creases of the anterior sole may point towards a hitherto unsuspected diagnosis (**18.6**).

In tetrasomy 12p or Pallister–Killian mosaic syndrome, there is such powerful selection against the abnormal cell line in blood that, even at birth, no abnormal cells are found on lymphocyte culture from blood and skin biopsy is needed to make the diagnosis. Clinically, it is suspected from a high birth weight, hypotonia, increased head circumference, sparse hair anteriorly, a long philtrum, thin upper lip and a full lower lip (**18.7 and 18.8** show the karyotype).

Microdeletion syndromes and imprinting

Increased sophistication of chromosome analysis, especially of longer, prometaphase spreads, has allowed a number of disorders with tiny chromosome deletions to be detected. Even more sophisticated analysis is possible by *in situ* hybridisation, using molecular probes representative of specific chromosome regions. (*See* **Table 18.1**, overleaf, for specific examples.)

Prader–Willi (PWS) and Angelman syndrome are examples of imprinting. In PWS, the deletion is paternal

TABLE 18.1 Microdeletion Syndromes Detectable on Chromosome Analyisis or *In Situ* Hybridisation

11p-	Aniridia, Wilm's genito-urinary abnormality mental handicap syndrome of contiguous genes
17p-	Miller Dieker or lissencephaly syndrome
15q-	Prader–Willi syndrome
15q-	Angelman syndrome

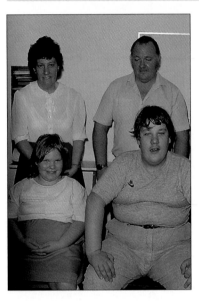

18.10 Brother and sister with clinical Fragile X syndrome. Mother is a transmitting female; father is unaffected.

in origin (**18.9**). In some cases where no deletion is found on chromosome analysis, it may be demonstrated by molecular methods, using probes from the relevant deleted segment. In yet others, the phenomenon of uniparental disomy has been demonstrated, with both chromosomes 15 of maternal origin and no paternal chromosome 15 present. This is **maternal imprinting.**

In Angelman syndrome, the opposite is the case—there is paternal imprinting: either a maternally derived deletion is present or paternal uniparental disomy. A family has been described with a translocation involving partial monosomy 15 in individuals with unbalanced products: both Angelman and Prader–Willi syndromes have occurred in the family, as could be predicted from the parent of origin.

In Fragile X syndrome (**18.10**), maternal imprinting may aggravate the severity of the clinical features. Molecular discoveries have allowed us to begin to understand the mechanisms which apply to certain autosomal disorders like myotonic dystrophy, too (*see* following section).

Autosomal dominant disorders

In myotonic dystrophy, we have a paradigm of a well-recognised clinical entity, with very well-understood clinical features including the inheritance of the congenital form invariably from the mother. At first, only the autosomal–dominant nature was known, then the unusual transmission of the congenital form was noted; linkage to secretor status was discovered, and then secretor and linked markers were located to chromosome 19q; closer and closer markers to the gene were found and eventually the gene itself discovered, when it was shown to demonstrate the same progressive alteration from generation to generation as had been demonstrated shortly before in Fragile X syndrome.

A third disorder which demonstrates the same feature is the rare disorder, progressive spino-bulbar muscular atrophy (SBMA) or Kennedy disease. In all three of these diseases a variable number of triplet base repeats, always including the bases C and G, occur within the gene, causing instability and severe alteration when the number of repeated sequences is above a certain critical threshold. The number of repeats may increase from generation to generation, markedly when the disorder passes through the female, thus the marked anticipatory effect and effect on severity of the phenotype, implicit in this type of imprinting. The three conditions, SBMA (Kennedy disease), Fragile X and myotonic dystrophy are examples of 'triplet repeat' diseases. The mechanism is likely to apply to other disorders too, including disorders lethal in foetal or early life.

In Neurofibromatosis 1, the gene has been located on chromosome 17q, and in some cases specific alterations of the gene have been shown. At present, there is no reliable link between the exact mutation and the clinical presentation. Furthermore, molecular methods are not widely available yet to identify those within families with the gene, but minimal or no clinical features, or to help in prenatal diagnosis. A familial tendency to malignancy has been observed in NF. The gene itself has recently been cloned. It codes for a protein termed Neurofibrin, itself a tumour supressor. Defects may result in a tendency to malignancy.

Neurofibromatosis II (bilateral acoustic neurofibromatosis) has been located to chromosome 22 and is much more regular in its clinical features than NFI. The gene itself has recently been identified.

The identification of the gene in Tuberous Sclerosis (TS) has proved to be extremely difficult. The condition is well recognised as autosomal-dominant with a high mutation incidence. The disorder shows a capacity to present in its most serious form with infantile spasms in infancy and severe mental handicap as a new mutation, often neither parent showing any sign even on detailed examination. Thus, an imprinting mechanism or progressive deterioration of a gene is unlikely, unless a premutation event can be demonstrated in TS too. At least four chromosomes have been implicated as possible sites of a TS gene, and yet there is no clinical evidence of heterogeneity according to the chromosome involved. Noonan syndrome is a variable dominant recently located to 12q.

Autosomal recessive disorders

The metabolic conditions are dealt with in Chapter 13. **Table 18.2** lists a few syndromes, at present still 'observational' with no diagnostic laboratory test. Parental consanguinity increases the chances of an autosomal-recessive disorder occurring.

TABLE 18.2 Autosomal-Recessive Syndromes

AR Microcephaly	—	'Large' face and ears relative to tiny cranium.
Smith–Lemli–Opitz	—	Microcephaly with bifrontal narrowing, syndactyly 2nd and 3rd toes, hypospadias, hypertrophied anterior palate; rare.
Seckel's syndrome	—	'Bird-headed', dwarfism, moderate mental handicap joint dislocations, abnormal cerebellar anatomy.
C-Trigonocephaly	—	Ridged metopic suture, especially in infancy, hypertrophied anterior palate common but features rather 'soft'; shares features with valproate embryopathy.
Bardet–Biedl syndrome	—	Obesity, polydactyly, mental handicap, retinitis pigmentosa, chronic renal failure.
Cockayne syndrome	—	Premature ageing DNA repair defect with UV light sensitivity.
Ataxia telangiectasia	—	Gene on chromosome 11 not yet cloned.
Friedreich's ataxia	—	Gene on chromosome 9 not yet cloned.
Wilson's disease	—	Gene on chromosome 13 not yet cloned.
Walker–Warburg or HARD+/-E	—	Hydrocephalus, agyria, retinal dysplasia +/- encephalocoele.
Coffin–Siris syndrome	—	Prominent nose; nail hypoplasia, especially 5th finger; posterior fossa defects.
Joubert syndrome	—	Cerebellar vermis hypoplasia with hypotonia, tongue thrusting and nystagmus, scalp wrinkling in infancy.

Disorders which may be recessive: cerebral palsy, especially ataxic; 'private syndromes', especially when affected children are born to consanguineous parents.

TABLE 18.3 Some X-linked Disorders Associated with Mental Handicap

Aqueduct stenosis-adducted thumb syndrome.

Duchenne muscular dystrophy.

Becker muscular dystrophy.

Coffin–Lowry syndrome — Full lips, fleshy hands, tapered large fingers, hypertelorism (X-linked dominant—female phenotype variable; male invariably serious [see 18.16]).

X-linked mental handicap, alpha-thalassaemia syndrome.

Fragile X syndrome.

X-linked recessive disorders

Learning difficulties form part of the picture of a great many recessive single-gene disorders of the X chromosome. In many of these, submicroscopic deletions or insertions of DNA material have occurred. In some of these disorders (see **Table 18.3**), the line between dominant and recessive is blurred; 'unlucky' lyonisation may result in females showing features of the disorder, termed manifesting heterozygotes as may occur for instance in Duchenne muscular dystrophy. Diagnostic precision is important. The wrong label of such a female as having 'limb-girdle' muscular dystrophy or spinal muscular atrophy would result in serious errors in genetic counselling.

Duchenne and Becker muscular dystrophy are alleles at Xp21. The disordered gene product is called dystrophin after the disease, and without the study of Duchenne and Becker, the nature and function of the gene and its products would remain unknown. The clinical variability resulting in a Duchenne or Becker phenotype can sometimes be ascribed to the type rather than the size of the mutation, and the effect this has on the dystrophin molecule. The template for dystrophin formation may be altered in a simple way with a deletion involving a direct multiple of three base pairs (giving a Becker phenotype). Another deletion may cause a frame shift after the mutation because the reading frame is entirely changed by the mutation. In many of these, dystrophin cannot be made and histochemical studies of muscle biopsy show no evidence of it—thus, Duchenne.

Mitochondrial inheritance

The ovum with its rich cytoplasm provides nearly all the mitochondria for the next generation. The sperm has almost no mitochondria, except for those needed to energise the tail.

The genetic material in mitochondria is laid out in a circle of DNA, unlike the double helix form of nuclear

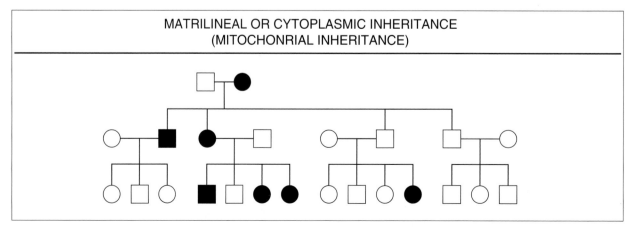

MATRILINEAL OR CYTOPLASMIC INHERITANCE
(MITOCHONRIAL INHERITANCE)

18.11 Mitochondrial disorders: matrilineal inheritance. Only females transmit the condition; more than half their offspring are affected (black shapes represent those clinically affected).

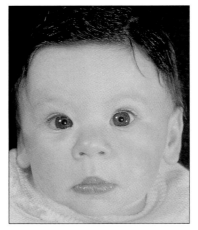

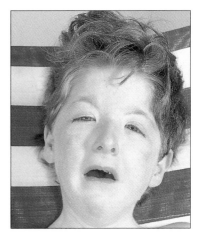

18.12 (left) Williams syndrome. Short palpebral fissures, epicanthic folds, long philtrum.

18.13 (right) Rubinstein–Taybi syndrome. Slanting palpebral fissures, hypoplastic maxilla.

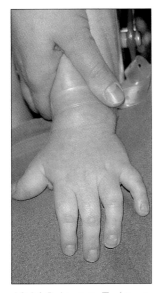

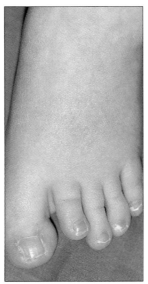

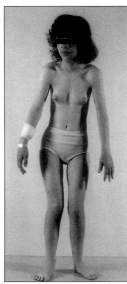

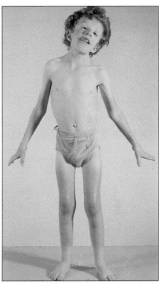

18.14 Rubinstein-Taybi syndrome. Broad thumbs.

18.15 Rubinstein–Taybi syndrome. Broad toes.

18.16 Coffin–Lowry syndrome. Learning difficulties, downslanting palpebral fissures, coarse facies, bulbous nose, tapering fingers, corticospinal degeneration, stooped posture.

18.17 Noonan's syndrome. Learning difficulties, neck webbing, lower pectus excavatum, pulmonary stenosis.

DNA. The genetic code of mitochondrial DNA differs somewhat to that of nuclear DNA, with mitochondrial triplet codons coding for amino acids which are different from those coded for on the equivalent nuclear triplet.

Most mitochondrial genes are under nuclear DNA control, but some are 'autonomous' mitochondrial genes, and inheritance of these is always matrilinial. One of the best-known examples, recently proved to be due to a point-mutation resulting in a defect in the detoxification of cyanide, is Leber's hereditary optic atrophy. More than half the offspring of affected women, male or female, develop the disorder, but affected men do not pass the condition on (*see* illustrative pedigree) (**18.11**).

There is further discussion on mitochondrial disease, under nuclear and non-nuclear control, in Chapter 13.

Recognisable syndromes with minimal recurrence risks

See **Table 18.4** (overleaf) and **18.12–18.17** for examples.

Prospects for treatment

To label a disorder genetic or even chromosomal may not necessarily imply that no definitive treatment is possible. Treatment possibilities based on knowledge of gene products or the insertion of genes into relevant tissues is now being documented. Insertion into nerve cells will prove difficult but hopefully not insurmountable.

Disorders in which genes on other chromosomes are 'switched off'

The X-linked mental handicap, alpha-thalassaemia syndrome, is a disorder of severe learning difficulties, dysmorphic features including mid-face hypoplasia, and H-body inclusions in red cells and haemotological features of alpha-thalassaemia. As the genetic abnormality is on the X chromosome, the alpha-globin gene does not function properly. The exact reason waits to be elucidated.

Noonan's syndrome (*see* **18.17**) is a well-known autosomal-dominant dysmorphic disorder. A number of clotting factors coded for on different chromosomes are poorly formed. Peripheral consumption of the clotting factors seems to be an unlikely explanation; it is more likely to be an effect on the coding genes. Resemblance of Noonan's syndrome to the Turner phenotype may be on this basis.

TABLE 18.4 Examples of Syndromes with Minimal-Recurrence Risks

Rubinstein–Taybi syndrome	—	'Punch' facial phenotype with broad thumbs and toes
Rett's syndrome	—	Autistic girls with normal very early milestones then marked slowing of brain growth, hyperapnoea and hand wringing
William's syndrome		

Chapter 19: Imaging

W. St. Clair Forbes

Introduction

The past two decades have seen the introduction of technological methods of imaging which have had a profound impact on paediatric neuroimaging. The introduction of computed tomography (CT), ultrasonography (US), and later magnetic resonance imaging (MRI) has lead to a re-appraisal of clinical investigative methods and applications. Nowhere is the contribution of non-invasive imaging more appreciated than when dealing with very young patients.

Imaging techniques

Neuroradiological techniques have traditionally been classified as either invasive or non-invasive. The important non-invasive imaging techniques are computed tomography, magnetic resonance imaging and ultrasonography (*see* Chapter 15), logically classified as those employing and those not employing ionising radiation (**Table 19.1**)

Ultrasound

This is the modality of choice in the neonate and infant prior to the closure of the anterior fontanelle.

Computed tomography

In CT scanning, a cross-sectional image is produced from the combination of x-ray transmission and computer technology (**19.1 and 19.2**).

Technical aspects

Modern computed tomography (CT) scanners employ collimated fan beams directed only at the layer under investigation. The transmitted radiation is detected by arrays of scintillation or ionisation detectors. The rotate/rotate principle is employed. In the third-generation scanner a rotating x-ray tube and rotating detector

TABLE 19.1 Non-invasive Imaging Techniques

A. No ionising radiation
- Ultrasound (US)
  - —High resolution
  - —Duplex
- Magnetic resonance imaging (MRI)

B. Ionising radiation
- Plain radiography
- Computed tomography
- Angiography
- Myelography
- Positron emission tomography (PET)

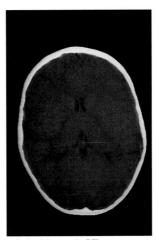

19.1 Normal CT scan, pre-contrast.

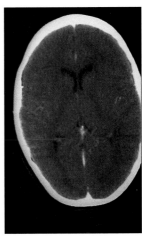

19.2 Normal CT scan, post-intravenous contrast medium.

241

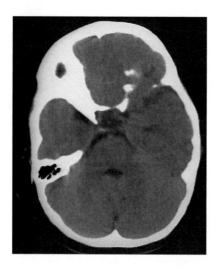
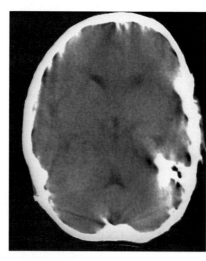

19.3 (left) Partial volume effect (PVE). CT scan. Note PVE of petrous ridge in the middle cranial fossa and interrupted orbital root on right, which might be mistaken for intracerebral calcification.

19.4 (right) Movement artefact seen as linear streaking.

array are used; the fourth-generation scanner uses a fixed ring of detectors with the x-ray source within the ring.

Advantages

The technical developments of modern CT scanners have resulted in shorter scan times, improved collimation leading to thin sections (1 mm or less), faster data acquisition, shorter reconstruction times per section, a high repetition rate of scanning due to improvements in X-ray tube technology, improved spatial resolution and an extended dynamic range (-1000 to +4000 Hounsfield Units (HU)). These developments have had a significant impact on patient handling and have resulted in improved diagnostic capability in craniospinal imaging. The advantages of third and fourth generation CT scanners are:

1. The scout projection radiographic facility ('scannogram') enables accurate anatomical registration and reproducibility of the sections with important implications for examination of the spine.

2. Easier patient positioning permits transaxial and direct coronal scanning.

3. The data obtained in the thin contiguous sections allow reconstruction in additional planes (coronal, sagittal, oblique), and with developments in software enables 3-dimensional reconstructions (3DCT) of bony structures.

4. Rapid sequence scanning of up to 30 sections in rapid sequence permits dynamic scanning and can provide information about the blood supply to normal or abnormal vascular structures.

5. The introduction of predetermined scanning protocols, with standardisation of technique, lessens the likelihood or operator error.

6. CT guided biopsy techniques can be introduced, including stereotaxy.

Assessment of detail has been improved by the spatial resolution of modern rotate/rotate scanners with picture element (pixel) size as low as 0.5 mm x 0.5 mm. Furthermore, density, discrimination of one part in 1000 may be obtained allowing high-resolution techniques. Use of limited field to view, bone filters and the extended dynamic range of modern scanners provides very detailed information which has resulted in improved diagnosis of craniospinal disorders.

Disadvantages

Tissue characterisation Despite its ability to discriminate amongst small differences in density, simple analysis of attenuation does not permit precise histological characterisation except when calcium (high density) or fat (low density) is present.

Partial volume effects The tissue contained within the small volume (voxel) examined, is unlikely to be homogeneous in composition. The measured Hounsfield unit (HU) is an average of the different components of the tissue within a voxel. This 'partial volume effect' (**19.3**) becomes especially important when normal and pathological processes interface within a section. The boundaries of the abnormality, therefore, may be difficult to define with accuracy.

Radiation dose All modern CT scanners allow the operator to ajust the dose level and image quality. Contiguous and overlapping sections result in higher doses than non-contiguous sections. High-resolution sections carry a higher dose penalty. Multiplanar reconstructions should be used in preference to direct scanning in planes other than the transaxial to reduce the radiation dose.

Movement Any movment will produce artefacts (**19.4**) which degrade the image quality even with the short scanning times of modern scanners.

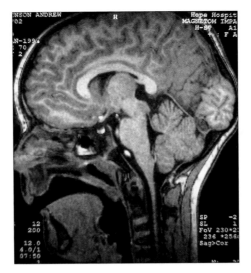
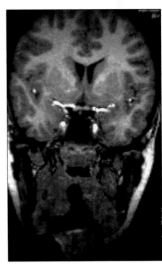

19.5 (left) Sagittal TIW. The IVth ventricular CSF shows low signal. Note the corpus callosum, brainstem, tentorium and cerebellum.

19.6 (right) Coronal TIW. Post i.v. Gadolinium. Note optic chiasm and enhancement of the carotid arteries.

Reproducibility Precise positioning and accurate reproducibility of thin sections present significant problems despite the scout-view facility. Careful external marking and a precise numbering code are helpful with follow-up examinations.

CT methods

General Thin sections in the transaxial plane as determined from the 'scannogram' are used for imaging a defined area where detailed information is required. Multi-planar reconstructions can be obtained allowing more accurate visualisation of the area being studied. Thick sections, usually 10 mm, with wider spacing, are used to sample a larger anatomical area, for example in the assessment of diffuse skeletal metastases or routine brain examinations.

Use of intravenous contrast media Administration of iodinated contrast media into the vascular system will raise the attenutation value of blood by 20–30 HU per mg/ml at 120 kVp. A rapid series of scans can be obtained using the dynamic scanning facility following a large bolus injection of contrast medium (Angio CT). The technique of dynamic sequential scanning requires a rapid series of scans at the same level. In dynamic incremental scanning, scans are performed at contiguous levels during a slower infusion.

Contrast enhancement occurs in those lesions whose vascularity is significantly different from that of the surrounding brain or in which the blood-brain barrier isdefective. Contrast medium is therefore administered in those cases where the plain scan shows evidence of a mass, in cases of suspected intracranial infection, for examination of thepituitary fossa and of the internal auditory canals, patients with focal epilepsy or where there is a focal EEG abnormality, in cases of vascular abnormality such as an aterio-venous malformation or giant aneurysm and where there are equivocal abnormalities requiring further evaluation.

Sedation and anaesthesia in CT Sedation or general anaesthesia (GA) may be required for some patients. Indications have become fewer with reductions in scanning times. The indications are:

1) Limited cooperation.
2) Critical illness.
3) Severe involuntary movements.
4) Behavioural disorders.

Sedation may be unnecessary in small infants, providing they are fed shortly before the study, kept warm and handled carefully. A number of sedation protocols have been proposed for larger children. Maintenance of the body temperature is particularly important when young children are being examined. The risks of combinations of sedatives given to young children should be recognised and appropriate resuscitation facilities must be available in the CT scanning room to cope with any emergency situation. Monitoring of seriously ill children should be carried out by skilled personnel during the CT scanning procedure.

Magnetic resonance imaging

MRI is established as the most advanced diagnostic imaging modality in paediatric neurology. Abnormalities of the brain and spinal cord are diagnosed non-invasively and without ionising radiation and with a greater degree of sensitivity. MRI has rapidly become the established primary modality in many clinical situations. The diagnostic usefulness of MR is further enhanced by its ability to image the brain and spine in multiple anatomical planes, sagittal, coronal, axial and oblique (**19.5 and 19.6**) (*see* **Table 19.2**, overleaf).

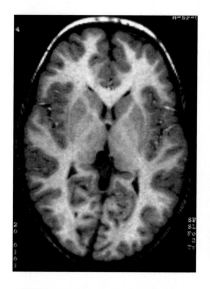 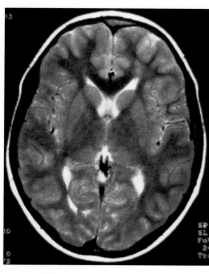

19.7 (left) Axial T1W. Note lateral ventricles and the grey and white matter structures. (Small co-incidental arachnoid cyst of the quadrigeminal plate cistern.)

19.8 (right) Axial T2W. The ventricular CSF shows increased signal. Note grey/white matter differentiation.

TABLE 19.2 Advantages

- High intrinsic soft-tissue contrast and discrimination
- Direct transverse, sagittal, coronal and oblique imaging
- Multisection imaging—axial, coronal, sagittal and oblique planes
- No bone or air artefacts
- Artefacts only from some metals
- No ionising radiation used
- Demonstration of normal development and function
- No known biological hazard

Image acquisition

Magnetic resonance is defined as the enhanced absorption of energy occurring when atomic nuclei with an odd number of protons or neutrons, e.g. H^+ within an external magnetic field, are exposed to radio frequency (rf) energy at specific frequency. This energy is recorded as an electrical signal, providing the data from which the digital images are constructed. This energy exchange following the removal of the rf pulse (the T1 and T2 relaxation times) is tissue-specific. T1-weighted (T1W) (**19.7**) images are best for evaluating normal or altered anatomical relationships (**Table 19.3**).

Pathological processes showing an increase in tissue fluid are best evaluated on T2W images (**19.8**) owing to the high signal on T2 due to proton density.

In outline, atomic nuclei with an odd number of protons and/or neutrons (e.g. proton (1H), sodium (23Na), phosphorus (31P) and carbon (13C)) possess an intrinsic spin, thus generating a magnetic moment. Nuclei of tissues placed within the main magnetic field tend to align along the direction of that field. Application of rf pulses can be used to induce resonance of particular sets of nuclei. The required frequency of the rf pulse is determined by the strength of the magnetic field and the particular nucleus under investigation. Resonance refers to a change in the alignment, and thus energy level, or the nuclei in the main field. The energy absorbed during this transition (higher energy state) is subsequently released to the environment when the rf pulse is turned off as the nuclei relax back to equilibrium (lower energy state).

The proton i.e. the hydrogen nucleus, is the one most suitable for conventional imaging. It is the most abundant in the human body and yields the strongest MR signal compared with the other spinning nuclei. The protons which give rise to the MR signal are mainly those in water lipids, with water protons in the majority. Protons which do not contribute significantly to the resultant MR signal include those in proteins, DNA and solid structures such as cortical bone.

The strength (amplitude) of the signal wall will depend not only on the number of measurable or mobile protons ('proton-' or 'spin-density') in the tissues, but also on a variety of other parameters such as relaxation times, blood flow, chemical shift or phase-contrast effects, magnetic susceptibility, diffusion, perfusion and rf absorption.

A variety of rf pulse sequences can be used to generate an image. The most commonly-used sequences are termed partial saturation recovery (PSR), inversion recovery (IR) and spin echo (SE). Different pulse sequences give different weighting in the received signal

TABLE 19.3 Signal Intensity of Anatomical Tissues on T1W and T2W Sequences

High signal on T1W and T2W images
Fat, marrow, haematoma/thrombus (varies with age). Slow-flowing blood.

Low signal on T1W and T2W images
Cortical bone, air/gas, ligaments/tendons, fibrocartilage, calcification, turbulent/fast-flowing blood.

Intermediate signal on T1W and T2W images
Muscle, nerves, spinal cord, hyaline (articular) cartilage, annulus fibrosis of disc, grey and white matter.

Low-intermediate signal on T1W and high signal on T2W images
Cerebrospinal fluid, urine, nucleus pulposus of disc, most tumours, infection, cysts, effusions.

to the various tissue parameters. A high signal intensity, using typical sequences, is observed from tissues with an increased proton density, short T1, or a prolonged T2. A low signal is produced by tissues with the opposite parameters. The MR signal related to flowing blood is a complex interplay of many factors, including blood velocity, direction of flow, flow profile (laminar or turbulent), pulse sequences employed and field gradients applied. Turbulent and fast-flowing (arterial) blood produces little or no signal, whereas static or slow-moving (venous) blood can give a higher signal. Thus arteries and veins can be detected.

Safety

No genetic or mutagenic effects have been demonstrated using presently available MRI instrumentation (**Table 19.4**, overleaf). There are three potential sources of hazard that exist relating to the different types of magnetic fields encountered in MRI:

1. Static main magnetic field   There is no evidence to suggest biological risk for those exposed to MRI from the static main field. Of practical concern is the attractive force on ferromagnetic objects which increases with field strength and inversely with distance from the magnet. Loose ferro-magnetic metal objects can thus become dangerous projectiles. Some vascular clips are, however, ferromagnetic and may be displaced by the static field. The degree of risk can be reduced or eliminated by

appropriate selection of alloys or implant manufacture such as high nickel-impregnated stainless steel alloys, tentallum and titanium.

2. Time-varying (gradient) magnetic field strengths Rapidly changing magnetic fields induce electric currents in tissue, since the body acts as a conductor. The magnitude of the effect is proportional to the rate of the change of field.

3) Radio-frequency magnetic field effects   Most of the rf pulse power used to excite nuclei is dissipated as heat in tissue. The recommendations on field limitations restrict exposure so as to avoid any significant rise in temperature of sensitive body tissues.

Monitoring of critically ill patients can be difficult within the tunnel of the magnet but intubated patients can be scanned successfully using non-ferromagnetic equipment.

Although no evidence exists to suggest that the embryo is sensitive to the magnetic and rf fields encountered in MRI, examinations in early pregnancy are restricted.

Single photon emission computerised tomography (SPECT)

Unlike PET scanning, SPECT is readily available in most Nuclear Medicine departments (**19.9 and 19.10**).

TABLE 19.4 Disadvantages of MRI Scanning

- Long scanning times

- Many protocol options

- Correct choice of rf pulse sequence parameters essential

- Poor bone calcium detail (including periosteal reaction)

- Motion artefacts with scanning thorax and abdomen

- Relative difficulty in monitoring/maintaining ill patients

- Patients with pacemakers restricted

- Claustrophobia (2 %–5 % cases studied)

- High capital and revenue costs

- Limited availability

- Long-term side effects (?)

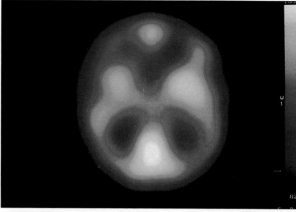

19.9 SPECT images of rCBF using Tc 99m–HMPAO. Blue areas denote low and red–white, high-blood flow.

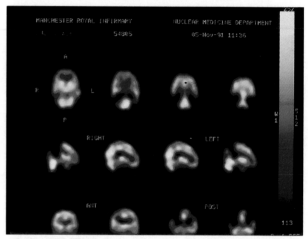

19.10 SPECT. Sagittal and coronal views allow accurate localisation of ictal change or structural abnormality.

Qualitative comparative estimates of blood can be made with 123I and technetium-99 misopropyliodo amphetamine using a rotating gamma camera.

The use of simple single-photon gamma emitters for cerebral tomography imposes a number of requirements. The radiopharmaceutical should be unaffected by its passage through the lungs, should be extracted rapidly in high concentrations by the brain tissues, and should be retained unaltered in the brain for a duration sufficient to allow the study to be performed.

After the initial very high first-pass extraction, the distribution is reasonably stable for about two hours, giving ample time for the investigation to be completed. After the initial high extraction there is a further slow uptake so that accurately-timed arterial blood concentrations must be measured if blood flow is to be assessed quantitively.

The expense and limited availability of cyclotron-produced isotopes such as 15 O and 123 I stimulated the development of a 99m Tc-labelled blood-flow radiopharmaceutical that was stable and crossed the normal blood-brain barrier very efficiently. The best known of the derivatives of the initial compound is 99m Tc-hexamethylpropylenamine oxine (HMPAO). It is a lipophilic compound with a high first-pass extraction fraction and its deposition is proportional to the blood flow. It crosses the blood-brain barrier. Following intravenous injection, the highest deposition is noted in the grey matter of the occipital and frontal poles and the basal ganglia. A steady state is attained within minutes and symmetrical stability maintained for about an hour. There is good visual correlation with tracers, such as those mentioned above, that show cerebral blood flow and glucose metabolism. Several useful applications have already been established for this compound.

HMPAO

This is taken up predominantly in grey matter, in rela-

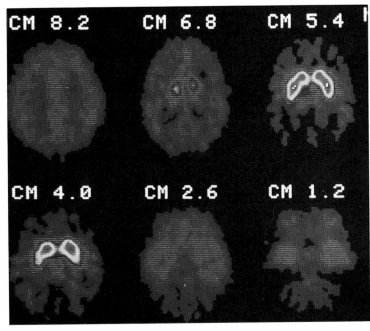

19.11 Positron emission tomography (PET) images of a normal subject injected with ¹⁸F-labelled N-methyl spiperone, demonstrating intense uptake of tracer in the basal ganglia. (Reprinted from Perkin, Hochberg, Miller, *Atlas of Clinial Neurology*, 2nd edition, Wolfe, 1993.)

tion to rCBF. In addition to demonstrating the cerebral cortex, the cerebellum, thalamus and basal ganglia are well shown. Difficulties in positioning the patient can be overcome by the use of oblique reconstruction, to obtain true transaxial slices. Although many studies are now performed using a single rotating conventional gamma camera, speed of aquisition can be increased using two opposing detector systems, or a custom-built multi-detector array.

HMPAO: in epilepsy Epileptogenic foci are seen in the interictal phase as areas of reduced perfusion. During the ictus, uptake is enhanced to well above normal levels. HMPAO has been used to localise a dysfunctional area prior to surgery, and to confirm its removal post-operatively. In some patients, HMPAO has been able to show the presence of several foci with a distribution which may render surgery impossible. HMPAO is superior to CT or MRI in this respect.

HMPAO: in cerebral tumours Some primary intracerebral tumours such as gliomas are seen as areas of increased uptake whereas metastases are frequently detected as hypoperfused areas due to local cerebral ischemia.

HMPAO: in head injuries Recent studies of the follow-up of closed head injury have indicated that HMPAO SPECT shows a greater number of abnormalities than either CT or MRI, with good correlation of clinical features. The impact of these findings on management or prognosis is not yet understood.

Positron emission tomography (PET)

PET, like conventional radionuclide imaging, requires the administration of a radiopharmaceutical to image physiology and function. The emitted radiation is then detected and reconstructed to form cross-sectional images of the isotope's distribution (**19.11**).

Positron-emitting isotopes of oxygen, nitrogen, carbon, fluorine, and rubidium are amongst those that have been developed for promoting research into the physiology of the brain.

With decay of the isotope, a positively charged positron is emitted which travels a few millimetres. This positron interacts with a normal electron, resulting in mutual annihilation, and the formation of paired gamma rays of equal energy (511 keV) which travel in precisely opposite directions. The patient is scanned between single or multiple pairs of opposed detectors, precisely aligned to detect, and by coincidence counting, matching pairs of gamma rays emitted by each annihilation reaction. The plane of disintegration can be localised by rotation of the detectors, and tomographic images constructed. This technique differs from SPECT in that two gamma ray photons are simultaneously registered, defining the axis along which the source is located.

The positron techique has two other advantages. First, since positron emitters possess short half-lives, the radiation dose to the patients is low and more radioactivity can be administered, to construct clearer images. Second, positron-emitting isotopes exist for carbon, oxygen, nitrogen and the halogen family. These atoms can be incorporated into biological molecules, and can be used to image aspects of cerebral physiology.

15 Oxygen is a positron-emitting nuclide which has a half-life of 122.5 seconds, equivalent to that of cerebral metabolic oxidation which it can be used to study. 15 O can also be used to measure cerebral blood flow (CBF), oxygen extraction and metabolism and blood volume. The most common positron emitters used for PET imaging are:

11 Carbon	half-life 20 mins
13 Nitrogen	half-life 10 mins
15 Oxygen	half-life 122.5 secs
18 Fluorine	half-life 110 mins

Unfortunately, the useful isotopes have short or very short half-lives, so that the PET equipment can only be sited close to a cyclotron, which limits its application.

Clinical applications

Regional cerebral blood volume (rCBV)   A small amount of carbon monoxide (CO) labelled with 15 0 is inhaled. The CO binds firmly to the haemoglobin and thus constitutes an intravascular marker. Tomographic images show differences in the blood-pool distribution, with the well-perfused grey matter seen in contrast against the white matter. Areas of vasodilation secondary to decreased perfusion can be seen.

Regional cerebral blood flow (rCBF)   15 O-labelled water (H_2 O15) can be used to study rCBF. H_2 15 O is a suitable pharmaceutical for this type of study, since it is easily produced, chemically stable, as well as being bio-

logically inert and a natural constituent of body tissue. It is infused by continuous intravenous administration or by inhalation of C 15 O, whereby the 15 O label is transferred to H_2 15 O, under the influence of carbonic anhydrase in the lungs. The method assumes that the tracer is freely diffusible across the blood-brain barrier, so that the observed uptake is purely dependent on rCBF.

Ammonia, labelled with 13N, has also been used to study rCBF. This agent is incorporated rapidly into glutamate, and its distribution is believed to reflect rCBF, although not in a direct linear fashion.

Cerebral oxygen metabolism   By using 15 O and PET, images of regional oxygen metabolism (rCMRO) and regional oxygen extraction fraction (rOEF) can be obtained.

Cerebral glucose metabolism   Glucose in the form of 2-deoxy-2-fluoro-D-glucose can be labelled with fluorine-18, a positron emitter, to form 18F-deoxyglucose (18F-DG), and PET studies can be performed to study cerebral glucose metabolism under different conditions.

Since glucose is not stored in the brain (although it provides 99 % of its energy requirements), the uptake of 18F-DG therefore reflects the cerebral glucose utilisation.

The relationship between sensory stimuli and regional cerebral metabolism can be studied in this way. Stimulation of one visual field causes increased metabolic activity in the contalateral visual cortex.

Other applications   Brain development, speech retardation, vision and movement can be studied using PET. In epilepsy, dysfunctional zones have been detected in areas of reduced perfusion and metabolism interictally, which, during the seizure, show dramatic increases in these parameters to well above normal levels.

References and Further Reading

Anderson, J. P., Sno, B., Dorey, F. J., Kabo, J. M. Efficacy of soft splints in reducing severe knee flexion contractures. *Developmental Medicine and Child Neurology*. 1988; 30: 502–508.

Angelini, L., Rumi, V., Lamperti, E., Nardocci, N. Transient paroxysmal dystonic in infancy. *Neuropaediatrics*. 1988; 19: 171–174.

Annegers, J. F., Hauser, W.A., Shirts, S. B., Kurland, L. T. Factors of unprovoked seizures after febrile convulsions. *New England Journal of Medicine*. 1987; 316: 493–498.

Aron, J. J., Marx, P., Black, M. F. *et al.* Ocular signs observed in the syndrome of Silverman. *Annals Occulistes*. 1970; 208: 533–546.

Begg, N. Reducing mortality from meningococcal disease. *British Medical Journal*. 1992; 305: 133–134.

Bille, B. Migraine in school children. *Acta Paediatrica Suppl.* 1962; 136, 51: 1–151.

Black, Eugene E., in: *Orthopaedic Management in Cerebral Palsy Clinics in Developmental Medicine.* MacKeith Press, 1990, Oxford.

Blau, J. N. Migraine; the theories of pathogenesis. *Lancet*. 1992; 339: 1202–1207.

Bloom, H. I. G., Wallace, E., Herk, J. M. The treatment and prognosis of medulloblastoma in children. A study of 82 verified cases. *American Journal Roentgenology*. 1969; 105: 43.

Clark, R. G. in: Clinical Neuroanatomy and Neurophysiology. Davis F. A., 1979, Philadelphia.

Cole, G. Acute encephalopathy of childhood. In: *Paediatric Neurology*. Brett E. M. Churchill Livingstone, 1991, London.

Cook, S. S. Children and dying: an explanation and selected biographies.Health Services Publishing Corporation, 1974, New York.

Cooke, P. H., Cole, W. G., Carey, R. R .P. L. Dislocation of the hip in cerebral palsy. *Journal of Bone and Joint Surgery*. 1989; 71-B: 441–446.

Coorsen, E., Msall, M., Duffy, L. Multiple minor malformations as a marker for prenatal aetiology of cerebral palsy. *Developmental Medicine and Child Neurology*. 1991; 33: 730–736.

Craft, Ann. Mental handicap and sexuality. Costello, 1989.

Cunningham, C. C., Sloper, S. Parents of Down's syndrome babies: their early needs. *Child Care Health and Development*. 1977; 3: 325–347.

Cunningham, C. C., Sloper, S. *Helping your handicapped baby.* Souvenir Press, 1978, London.

Cunningham, C. C. Early intervention in Down's syndrome. In: Hosking, G., Murphy, M. (eds) *Prevention of Mental Handicap: a World View.* Royal Society of Medicine, 1987, London, pp. 169–182.

Cushing, H. Intracranial Tumours of Preadolescence. *Am. J. Disease in Childhood*. 1927; 33: 551.

Cushing, H. Experience with cerebellar medulloblastoma. Critical review. *Acta Pathol. Microbiol. Immunol. Scand.* 1930; 7:1

Deonna, T., Fernandez, E., Gardner–Medwin, D. *et al.*

DOPA-sensitive progressive dystonic of childhood with fluctuations of symptoms—Segawa's syndrome and possible variants. *Neuropaediatrics.* 1986; 17; 81–85.

Dohnmann, G. J., Farwell, J. R: Intracranial neoplasms in children: a comparison of North America, Europe, Africa and Asia. *Diseases of the nervous system.* 1976; 37:696.

Drillien, C. N. M., Abnormal neurologic signs in the first year of life in low birth weight infants: Possible prognostic significance. *Developmental Medicine and Child Neurology.* 1972; 14: 575–584

Eilassen, A. C., Gordon, A. M., Forssberg, H. Basic coordination of manipulative forces of children with cerebral palsy. *Developmental Medicine and Child Neurology.* 1991; 33: 661–670.

Freeman, J. M., Nelson, K. B. Intrapartum asphyxia and cerebral palsy. *Pediatrics.* 1988; 82: 240–249.

Friedman, H. S., Schold, S. C. Rational approaches to the chemotherapy of medulloblastoma. *Neurological Clinics.* 1985; 3: 843.

Griffiths, M. and Russell, P. *Working together with handicapped children.* Souvenir Press, 1985.

Hanington, E., Jones, R. J., Amess, J. A. L., and Wachowicz, B. Migraine: a platelet disorder. *Lancet.* 1981; ii: 720–723.

Harding, A. Neurological disease and mitochondrial genes. *Trends in Neurological Science.* 1991; 14: 132–8.

Hobbs, C. J. Skull fracture in the diagnosis of abuse. *Archives of Disease in Childhood.* 1984; 59: 246–252.

Hockaday. Judith M. Migraine in childhood: and other on-epileptic disorders. Butterworth, 1988, London.

Hoffman, H. J., Hendrick, E. B., Humphreys, R. P. Metastasis from ventriculoperitoneal shunt in patients with medulloblastoma. *J. of Neurosurgery* 1970; 32: 83.

Jan, J. E. Head movements of visually impaired children. *Developmental Medicine and Child Neurology.* 1991; 33: 645–647.

Jan, J. E., Groenwel, H., Connolly, M. B. Head shaking by visually impaired children: a voluntary neurovisual adaptation which can be confused with spasmus nutans. *Developmental Medicine and Child Neurology.* 1990; 32: 1061–1066.

Kempster, P. A., Brenton, D. P., Gale, A. N., Stern, G. M. Dystonic in homocystinurian. *J. Neurol. Neurosurg. Psychiatry.* 1988; 51: 859–862.

King, J., Ankett, A., Smith, M. F. *et al.* Cerebral systemic lupus erythematosis. *Archives of Disease in Childhood.* 1988; 63: 968–70.

Ladybird Talkabout series: Willis & Hepworth Ltd. Loughborough.

Lance J. W., *et al.* Contribution of experiemental studies to understanding the pathophysiology of migraine. In *Migraine: A spectrum of ideas.* Eds. Sandler, M., Collins, G. M., 1990, OUP.

Lees, Janet and Urwin, Shelagh. *Children with language disorders.* 1991, Whurr, London.

Leggate, J. R. S., Lopez–Ramos, N., Genitori L., Lena G., Choux, M. Extradural Haematomas in Infants. *British Journal of Neurosurgery.* 1989; 3:533.

Logan, L., Byers–Hinckley, K., Ciccone, C. D. Anterior versus posterior walkers: a gait analysis study. *Developmental Medicine and Child Neurology* 1991; 32: 1044–8.

Louvois, J. de, Blackbourn, J., Hurley, R., Harvey, D. Infantile meningitis in England and Wales: a two year study. *Archives of Diseases in Childhood.* 1991; 66: 303–307.

Maclure reading type for children: Clement Clarke International Ltd, London.

Marsden, C. D., Quinn, N. P. The dystonias. *British Medical Journal.* 1990; 300: 139–144.

Myhur, U., Von Wendt, L. Improvement of functional sitting position for children with cerebral palsy. *Developmental Medicine and Child Neurology.* 1992; 33; 246–56.

Naeye, R. L., Peters, E. C., Bartholomew, M., Landis, J. R. Origins of cerebral palsy. *American Journal of Disease in Childhood.* 1989; 143: 1154–60.

Nelson, K. B., Ellenberg, J. H. Prognosis in children with febrile seizures. *Pediatrics*. 1978; 61: 720–727.

Neville, B. G. R. Selective dorsal rhizotomy for spastic cerebral palsy. *Developmental Medicine and Child Neurology*. 1988; 30, 3955–8.

Newton, R. W., Bergin, B., and Knowles, D. Parents interviewed after their child's death. *Archives of Disease in Childhood*. 1986; 61: 711–715.

Newton, R. W. Intracranial haemorrhage and non-accidental injury. *Archives of Disease in Childhood*. 1989; 64: 188–190.

O'Dwyer, N., Neilson, P. D., Nash, J. Mechanisms of muscle growth relative to muscle contracture in cerebral palsy. *Developmental Medicine and Child Neurology*. 1989; 31: 543–547.

O'Hare, A. E., Brown, J. K., Aitken, K. Dyscalculia in Children. *Developmental Medicine in Child and Neurology*. 1991, 33: 356–361.

Ozen, S., Besbas, N., Saatchi, U., and Bakkaloglu, A. diagnostic criteria for polyarteritis nodosa in childhood. *Journal of Pediatrics*. 1992; 120; 206–209.

Patrick, J. H. Use of movement analysis in understanding abnormalities of gait in cerebral palsy. *Archives of Disease in Childhood*. 1991; 66; 900–3.

Pembrey, M., Fennell, S. J., Van den Berghe, J. *et al*. The association of Angelman's syndrome with deletions within 15q 11–13. *Journal of Medical Genetics*. 1989; 26; 73–77.

Pharoah, P. O. D., Cooke T., Cooke, R. W. I., Rosenbloom, L. Birthweight specific trends in cerebral palsy. *Archives of Diseases in Childhood*. 1990; 65; 602–6.

Plum, F., Posner, J. B. *The diagnosis of stupors and coma*. Davis, 1980, Philadelphia.

Reilly, P. L., Simpson, D. A., Sprod, R., Thomas L. Assessing the conscious level in infants and young children: a pediatric version of the Glasgow Coma Scale. *Child's Nervous System*. 1988; 4: 30–33.

Robson, P. Shuffling, hitching, scooting or sliding. Some observations in 30 otherwise normal children. *Developmental Medicine and Child Neurology* 1970; 12: 608–617.

Sahlerr, O. J. *The child and death*. Mosby, 1978, St. Louis.

Scriver, C. R., Beaudet, A. L., Sly, W. S., Valle, D. *The metabolic basis of inherited disease*. McGraw–Hill, 1989, New York.

Scrutton, D. The early management of hips in cerebral palsy. *Developmental Medicine and Child Neurology*. 1989; 31; 108–16.

Sezen, F. Retinal haemorrhages in newborn infants. *British Journal of Ophthalmology*. 1970; 55: 248–253.

Shanks, R. D., Solomon, G. E., Wayne, H., *et al*. Neurological features of Gilles de la Tourette syndrome. *Journal of Neurology, Neurosurgery and Psychiatry*. 1973; 36: 1–9.

Sharief, N., Craze J., Summers, D., *et al*. Millier–Dieker syndrome with ring chromosome 17. *Archives of Disease in Childhood*. 1991; 66; 710–712.

Silverman, D. Agreeing not to intervene: doctors and parents of Down's syndrome children at a pediatric cardiology clinic. In: Lane, D., Stratford (eds.). *Current approaches to Down's syndrome*. Holt, Reinhart and Winston, Eastborne, pp. 363–385.

Sinha, S. K., D'Souza, S. W., Rivlin, E., Chiswick, M. L. Ischaemic brain lesions diagnosed at birth in pre-term infants. Clinical events and developmental outcome. *Archives of Disease in Childhood*. 1990; 65; 107–120.

Tardieu, C., Lespargot, A., Tarbay, C., Bret, M. D. For how long must the soleus muscle be stretched each day to prevent contractures? *Developmental Medicine and Child Neurology*. 1988; 30: 3–10.

Tasker, R. C., Matthew, D. J., Helms, P., Dinwiddie, R. Boyd, S. Monitoring in non-traumatic coma. Part I: invasive intracranial measurements. *Archives of Disease in Childhood*. 1988; 63: 888–894.

Tasker, R. C., Boyd, S., Harden, A., Matthews, D. G. Monitoring in non-traumatic coma. Part II: Electroencephalopathy. *Archives of Disease in Childhood*. 1988: 63: 888–894.

Torfs, C. P. P., Van den Berg, B. J., Oechsli, F. W.,

Cummins, S. Prenatal and perinatal factors in the etiology of cerebral palsy. *Journal of Pediatrics.* 1990; 116: 615–619.

Truwit, C. L., Barkovich, A. J., Koch, T. K., Ferriero, D. M. Cerebral palsy: MR findings in 40 patients. *American Journal of Neuroradiology.* 1992; 13: 67–78.

Wallace, G. B., Newton, R. W. Gower's sign revisited. *Archives of Disease in Childhood.* 1989; 64: 1317–1319.

Waters, W. E. *Headache* (Series in clinical epidemiology). Croom Helm, 1986, London.

Whitehouse, W. P., Newton, R. W., Evans, D. I. (1989). Platelet function in childhood migraine. In: *Headache in Children and Adolescents.* Eds: Lanzig, Balottin, U., and Cernibori, A. Elsevier.

Willemse, J. Benign idiopathic dystonie with onset in the first year of life. *Developmental Medicine and Child Neurology.* 1986; 28: 355–63.

Index